Aging in Liver and Gastrointestinal Tract

FALK SYMPOSIUM 49

Aging in Liver and Gastrointestinal Tract

EDITED BY

L. Bianchi
Institute for Pathology
University of Basel
Switzerland

P. Holt
Division of Gastroenterology
St Luke's-Roosevelt Hospital Center
New York
USA

O. F .W. James
Department of Medicine/Geriatrics
University of
Newcastle-upon-Tyne
UK

R. N. Butler
Department of Geriatrics
Mount Sinai School of Medicine
New York
USA

Proceedings of the 47th Falk Symposium held during Gastroenterology Week at Titisee, Federal Republic of Germany, June 10–12, 1987

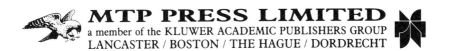

MTP PRESS LIMITED
a member of the KLUWER ACADEMIC PUBLISHERS GROUP
LANCASTER / BOSTON / THE HAGUE / DORDRECHT

Published in the UK and Europe by
MTP Press Limited
Falcon House
Lancaster, England

British Library Cataloguing in Publication Data

Falk Symposium (*47th: 1987: Titisee, Germany*)
Aging in liver and gastrointestinal tract.
1. Man. Gastrointestinal tract. Ageing
2. Man. Liver. Ageing
I. Title   II. Bianchi, L. (Leonardo), *1929–*
III. Series
612′.32

ISBN 0–7462–0066–8

Published in the USA by
Kluwer Academic Publishers
PO Box 358
Accord Station
Hingham, MA 02018–0358, USA

Library of Congress Cataloging-in-Publication Data

Falk Symposium (47th: 1987: Titisee, Germany)
Aging in liver and gastrointestinal tract.

Includes bibliographies and index.
1. Liver—Aging—Congress. 2. Gastrointestinal
system—Aging—Congresses. 3. Gastrointestinal system—
Disease—Age factors—Congresses. 4. Drugs—Metabolism—
Age factors—Congresses. I. Bianchi, Leonardo.
II. Gastroenterology Week (1987: Titisee, Germany)
III. Title. [DNLM: 1. Aging—congresses. 2. Gastro-
intestinal System—congresses. 3. Liver—congresses.
W3 FA17 47th 1987a / WI 700 F191 1987a]
OP185.F35 1987a   612′.32   88–12870

ISBN 0–7462–0066–8

Printed and bound in Great Britain by
Butler & Tanner Limited,
Frome and London

Contents

SECTION 3: LIVER MORPHOLOGY AND PHYSIOLOGY

SECTION 4: LIVER DRUG METABOLISM

CONTENTS

List of Contributors

I. B. ABRASS
Department of Medicine
University of Washington
Harborview Medical Center
325 – 9th Avenue, ZA-87
Seattle, WA 98104
USA

B. ANGELIN
Department of Medicine
Karolinska Institute
Huddinge University Hospital
S-14186 Huddinge
Sweden

H. J. ARMBRECHT
Geriatric Center (IIIG-JB)
St Louis VA Hospital
St Louis, MO 63125
USA

R. J. BARELDS
Department of Liver Cell Physiology
TNO Institute for Experimental
   Gerontology
PO Box 5815
NL-2280 HV Rijswijk
The Netherlands

J.-M. BEGUE
INSERM – U 49
Hôpital de Pontchaillou
35033 Rennes Cedex
France

L. BIANCHI
Institute for Pathology
University of Basel
Schönbeinstrasse 40
4003 Basel
Switzerland

W. S. BLANER
Department of Medicine
Columbia University of Physicians and
   Surgeons
630 West 168th Street
New York, NY 10032
USA

T. A. BRASITUS
Department of Medicine
University of Chicago
5841 South Maryland Avenue
Box 400
Chicago, IL 60637
USA

A. BROUWER
Department of Liver Cell Physiology
TNO Institute for Experimental
   Gerontology
PO Box 5815
NL-2280 HV Rijswijk
The Netherlands

S. J. BURWEN
Department of Cell Biology
Veterans Administration Medical
   Center and the University of
   California
San Francisco
4150 Clement Street
San Francisco, CA 94121
USA

J. A. BUTLER
Department of Chemistry
Illinois State University
Normal, IL 61761
USA

R. N. BUTLER
Gerald and May Ellen Ritter
  Department of Geriatrics and Adult
  Development
Mount Sinai Medical Center
One Gustave L. Levy Place
New York, NY 10029
USA

C. CHESNE
INSERM – U 49
Hôpital de Pontchaillou
35033 Rennes Cedex
France

M. T. CLANDININ
Nutrition and Metabolism Research
  Group
Division of Gastroenterology
University of Alberta
519 Robert Newton Research Building
Edmonton, Alberta T6G 2C2
Canada

B. CLEMENT
INSERM – U 49
Hôpital de Pontchaillou
35033 Rennes Cedex
France

C. K. DANIELS
Department of Anatomy and Cell
  Biology
Veterans Administration Medical
  Center and the University of
  California
San Francisco
4150 Clement Street
San Francisco, CA 94121
USA

H. DAVID
Institute of Pathology
Charité Clinic
Humboldt University Berlin GDR
Schumannstrasse 20/21
1040 Berlin
German Democratic Republic

A. M. de LEEUW
825 Lake Washington
Boulevarde South
Seattle, WA 98144
USA

F. DEINHARDT
Max v. Pettenkofer Institute
Pettenkoferstrasse 9a
D-8000 Munich 2
Federal Republic of Germany

K. EINARSSON
Department of Medicine
Karolinska Institute
Huddinge University Hospital
S-14186 Huddinge
Sweden

G. ESPOSITO
Institute of General Physiology and
  Biochemistry
School of Pharmacy
University of Milan
via Saldini 50
I-20133 Milan
Italy

A. FAELLI
Department of General Physiology and
  Biochemistry
University of Milan
via Celoria 26
I-20133 Milan
Italy

J. FEVERY
Department of Medicine
University Hospital Gasthuisberg
B-3000 Leuven
Belgium

B. FINCO
Ospedale Geriatrico
Piazza Mazzini
I-35100 Padovo
Italy

M. L. GARG
Nutrition and Metabolism Research
  Group
Division of Gastroenterology
University of Alberta
519 Robert Newton Research Building
Edmonton, Alberta T6G 2C2
Canada

D. GERSHON
Department of Biology
Technion-Israel Institute of Technology
Haifa 32000
Israel

R. A. GOODLAD
Royal Postgraduate Medical School
Hammersmith Hospital
Du Cane Road
London W12 0HS
UK

D. S. GOODMAN
Department of Medicine
Columbia University of Physicians and
    Surgeons
630 West 168th Street
New York, NY 10032
USA

C. GUGUEN-GUILLOUZO
INSERM – U 49
Hôpital de Pontchaillou
35033 Rennes Cedex
France

A. GUILLOUZO
INSERM – U 49
Hôpital de Pontchaillou
35033 Rennes Cedex
France

L. GULLO
Departments of Medicine and
    Gastroenterology
University of Bologna
Ospedale S. Orsola
I-40138 Bologna
Italy

H. F. J. HENDRIKS
Department of Liver Cell Physiology
TNO Institute for Experimental
    Gerontology
PO Box 5815
NL-2280 HV Rijswijk
The Netherlands

D. HOLLANDER
Division of Gastroenterology
University of California, Irvine
C340 Medical Science I
Irvine, CA 92717
USA

P. R. HOLT
Division of Gastroenterology
St Luke's-Roosevelt Hospital Center
114th Street and Amsterdam Avenue
New York, NY 10025
USA

G. J. M. HORBACH
Department of Organ and Cell
    Physiology
TNO Institute for Experimental
    Gerontology
PO Box 5815
NL-2280 HV Rijswijk
The Netherlands

A. M. HOYUMPA Jr
Division of Medicine/Gastroenterology
    and Nutrition
University of Texas Health Science
    Center
7703 Floyd Curl Drive
San Antonio, TX 78284–7878
USA

O. F. W. JAMES
Department of Medicine (Geriatrics)
University of Newcastle upon Tyne
Newcastle upon Tyne NE2 4HH
UK

W. JILG
Department of Virology
Max U. Pettenkofer Institute
Pettenkoferstrasse 9a
D-8000 Munich 2
Federal Republic of Germany

A. L. JONES
Departments Medicine, Anatomy and
    Cell Biology
Veterans Administration Medical
    Center and the University of
    California
San Francisco
4150 Clement Street
San Francisco, CA 94121
USA

M. KEELAN
Nutrition and Metabolism Research
    Group
Division of Gastroenterology
University of Alberta
519 Robert Newton Research Building
Edmonton, Alberta T6G 2C2
Canada

L. J. KING
Department of Biochemistry
University of Surrey
Guildford, Surrey, GU2 5XH
UK

Y. KISO
Pharmaceutical Institute
Tohoku University
Aoba-Yama
Sendai 980
Japan

K. KITANI
First Laboratory of Clinical Physiology
Tokyo Metropolitan Institute of
  Gerontology
35–2 Sakaecho
Itabashi-ku
Tokyo 173
Japan

D. L. KNOOK
TNO Institute for Experimental
  Gerontology
PO Box 5815
NL-2280 HV Rijswijk
The Netherlands

W. LENTON
Royal Postgraduate Medical School
Hammersmith Hospital
Du Cane Road
London W12 0HS
UK

C. LINDI
Department of General Physiology and
  Biochemistry
School of Pharmacy
University of Milan
via Saldini 50
I-20133 Milan
Italy

A. G. MALONEY
Cell Biology Aging Section (151E)
Veterans Administration Medical
  Center
4150 Clement Street
San Francisco, CA 94121
USA

E. MARCHIORI
Ospedale Geriatrico
Piazzo Mazzini
I-35100 Padovo
Italy

P. MARCIANI
Institute of General Physiology and
  Biochemistry
School of Pharmacy
University of Milan
via Saldini 50
I-20133 Milan
Italy

A. MARTIN
Cattedra di Malattie dell'Apparato
  Digerente
Istituto di Medicina Interna
Policlinico Universitario
via Giustiniani 2
I-35100 Padova
Italy

G. M. MARTIN
Department of Pathology SM-30
University of Washington
Seattle, WA 98195
USA

E. J. MASORO
Department of Physiology
The University of Texas Health Science
  Center at San Antonio
7703 Floyd Curl Drive
San Antonio, TX 78284–7756
USA

G. MONTICELLI
Department of General Physiology and
  Biochemistry
School of Pharmacy
University of Milan
via Saldini 50
I-20133 Milan
Italy

M. C. MONTINO
Cattedra di Malattie dell'Apparato
  Digerente
Istituto di Medicina Interna
Policlinico Universitario
via Giustiniani 2
I-35100 Padova
Italy

E. MUTCH
Department of Clinical Pharmacology
University of Newcastle upon Tyne
Newcastle upon Tyne NE1 7RU
UK

R. NACCARATO
Cattedra di Malattie dell'Apparato
  Digerente
Istituto di Medicina Interna
Policlinico Universitario
via Giustiniani 2
I-35100 Padova
Italy

M. N. ORSENIGO
Department of General Physiology and
  Biochemistry
School of Pharmacy
University of Milan
via Saldini 50
I-20133 Milan
Italy

D. V. PARKE
Department of Biochemistry
University of Surrey
Guildford, Surrey GU2 5XH
UK

W. PELEMANS
Department of Medicine – Division of
  Geriatrics
University Hospital Sint-Pieter
Brusselsestraat 69
B-3000 Leuven
Belgium

H. POPPER
The Stratton Laboratory for the Study of
  Liver Diseases
New York, NY 10029–6574
USA

N. E. PREECE
Department of Pharmacology
  (Toxicology Unit)
School of Pharmacy
University of Surrey
Guildford, Surrey GU2 5XH
UK

H. M. RABES
Institute of Pathology
University of Munich
Thalkirchner Str. 36
D-8000 Munich 2
Federal Republic of Germany

D. RATANASAVANH
INSERM – U 49
Hôpital de Pontchaillou
35033 Rennes Cedex
France

M. D. RAWLINS
Department of Clinical Pharmacology
University of Newcastle upon Tyne
Newcastle upon Tyne NE1 7RU
UK

N. W. READ
Sub-Department of Human
  Gastrointestinal Physiology and
  Nutrition
University of Sheffield
Floor K, Royal Hallamshire Hospital
Sheffield S10 2JF
UK

P. REINKE
Clinic of Internal Medicine
Humboldt University Berlin GDR
Schumannstrasse 20/21
1040 Berlin
Democratic Republic of Germany

A. RICHARDSON
Department of Chemistry
Illinois State University
Normal, IL 61761
USA

I. H. ROSENBERG
USDA-Human Nutrition Research
  Center on Aging at Tufts University
711 Washington Street
Boston, MA 02111
USA

R. M. RUSSELL
Departments of Medicine and Nutrition
USDA-Human Nutrition Research
  Center on Aging at Tufts University
711 Washington Street
Boston, MA 02111
USA

M. S. RUTHERFORD
Department of Chemistry
Illinois State University
Normal, IL 61761
USA

M. SANZARI
Ospedale Geriatrico
Piazza Mazzini
I-35100 Padovo
Italy

S. SCHENKER
Division of Medicine/Gastroenterology
  and Nutrition
University of Texas Health Science
  Center
7703 Floyd Curl Drive
San Antonio, TX 78284–7878
USA

D. L. SCHMUCKER
Departments of Anatomy and Cell
  Biology
Veterans Administration Medical
  Center and the University of
  California
San Francisco
4150 Clement Street
San Francisco, CA 94121
USA

E. L. SCHNEIDER
Andrus Gerontology Center
University of Southern California
Los Angeles, CA 90089–019
USA

I. SEMSEI
F. Berzar International Laboratory for
  Experimental Gerontology
University Medical Center
H-4012 Debrecen
Hungary

G. C. STURNIOLO
Cattedra di Malattie dell'Apparato
  Digerente
Istituto di Medicina Interna
Policlinico Universitario
via Giustiniani 2
I-35100 Padova
Italy

A. B. R. THOMSON
Nutrition and Metabolism Research
  Group
Division of Gastroenterology
University of Alberta
519 Robert Newton Research Building
Edmonton, Alberta T6G 2C2
Canada

M. TOSCO
Department of General Physiology and
  Biochemistry
School of Pharmacy
University of Milan
via Saldini 50
I-20133 Milan
Italy

C. F. A. van BEZOOIJEN
Department of Organ and Cell
  Physiology
TNO Institute for Experimental
  Gerontology
PO Box 5815
NL-2280 HV Rijswijk
The Netherlands

D. A. VESSEY
Liver Studies Unit
Veterans Administration Medical
  Center
4150 Clement Street
San Francisco, CA 94121
USA

R. K. WANG
Cell Biology Aging Section (151E)
Veterans Administration Medical
  Center
4150 Clement Street
San Francisco, CA 94121
USA

F. WILLIAMS
Department of Clinical Pharmacology
University of Newcastle upon Tyne
Newcastle upon Tyne NE1 7RU
UK

K. W. WOODHOUSE
Department of Medicine (Geriatrics)
University of Newcastle upon Tyne
Newcastle upon Tyne NE1 7RU
UK

N. A. WRIGHT
Royal Postgraduate Medical School
Hammersmith Hospital
Du Cane Road
London W12 0HS
UK

H. WYNNE
Department of Clinical Pharmacology
University of Newcastle upon Tyne
Newcastle upon Tyne NE1 7RU
UK

K.-Y. YEH
College of Physicians and Surgeons of
  Columbia University
St Luke's-Roosevelt Hospital Center
114th Street and Amsterdam Avenue
New York, NY 10025
USA

Section 1
Mechanisms of Aging

1
The aging process

R. N. BUTLER

First a personal note: Dr Hans Popper, a revered figure to so many, was working quietly, somewhat sequestered from the mainstream at Mount Sinai Medical Center, when I arrived in New York. I began visiting him and invited him to think about the liver and aging and to give a seminar on the topic in our Department. He did a fine job. I urged him to write reviews for the literature. One important practical application of his work has been the elevation of the donor age for liver transplants. Moreover, he has noted the potential role of the liver in pharmacological and dietary therapies that might intervene in aging (e.g. an anti-oxidant potential).

It is because of Dr Popper that we have this conference. We knew so little about the aging of the liver and the gastrointestinal (GI) tract. It is important that we systematically review aging from the molecular, cellular, tissue, organ and organismic level[1].

Why did nature give the liver so much redundancy? What does the liver have – what are its characteristics – so that it ages so little? What about the GI tract, so critical to alimentation? We will discuss some of these issues and more in this volume.

But first the framework. We in the industrialized world have gained an extraordinary, unprecedented, 25-year gain in life expectancy in this century, and it's not over yet. These 25 years nearly equal the gain that had been achieved during the preceding 5000 years of human history. Reductions in deaths from heart disease and stroke have complemented considerable reductions in maternal, infant, and childhood mortality rates, and 20% of the 25-year gain has come from base year 65.

This is not a function of biological evolution, of genetic expression. It is a social creation, a function of agriculture, industry, and in the broader sense, the industrial–technological revolution of which this demographic or 'longevity revolution' is a part. 'Baby boomers' were originally 76 million strong. In the years 2020 to 2030, when they will be 65 and over, they will constitute 20% of the population, or 1 out of every 5. The 85 + age group is now the most rapidly growing segment of the population.

Our continued longevity depends, of course, upon the outcome of efforts against the dreaded disease AIDS. Should it spread in the heterosexual population in Western societies, it would certainly curtail the new longevity dramatically.

In 1986, in collaboration with the National Institute on Aging and the American Museum of Natural History, we held a symposium at the Mount Sinai Medical Center that was supported by the Brookdale Foundation. We invited some of the world's finest scientists to examine modern biological theories of aging[2], and it was an excellent review.

There are multiple theories, and we see aging as multi-causal, complex, and variable. How to integrate them into a comprehensive whole is our challenge.

From the perspective of Medawar[3], we may question whether there is developmentally programmed aging. It is worth noting here that George Sacher in 1978 wrote of the 'biology of finitude of life in its three aspects of longevity, aging, and death', offering us a substitute for standard definitions of gerontology[4]. He adduced that some 100 genes are involved in longevity, and he conceptualized 'longevity assurance genes'. He noted that longevity has increased throughout the entire history of all mammalian species and has been especially rapid for human hominid ancestors.

Hayflick[5] also takes issue with the concept of developmentally programmed aging. He sees developmental longevity as up to 30 years of age and post-developmental from 30 to 85. His question is, 'why do we live as long as we do?', rather than, 'how do we age?'

Stochastic and random theories of aging appear to be more attractive to many. The value of Harman's free-radical damage theory[6] first proposed in 1954 is strengthened by the availability of outcome measures of thymine glycol, thymidine glycol, and 5-hydroxymethyluracil in the urine[7].

The heuristic and catalytic error catastrophe theory of Leslie Orgel has not been verified. Old cells appear to perform as well as young cells. On the other hand, the data of Dice and Goff[8] suggest that the cell disposal system alters with age.

Setlow[9] and Cerutti[10] discussed DNA damage repair at the Mount Sinai Medical Center symposium. Finch[11] led the discussion of neuroendocrine cascade and referred to Sapolsky's work. Certainly the new biology, including hybridoma technology and molecular biology, will assist in the further elucidation of these theories. The molecular biology of aging has been made a priority by the National Institute on Aging.

Cerami[12] of the Rockefeller University has described a mediator role for glucose in aging. He observed post-translational glycation of proteins and nucleic acids with cross-linking and loss of biological functioning. He is working towards an examination of the possible role of aminoguanidine as an effective intervention in this cross-linkage.

The Environmental Protection Agency and the National Institute of Environmental Health Sciences held a workshop in 1985 that recommended to the National Academy of Sciences that it form a Committee on Toxicity and Aging, co-chaired by Emil Pfitzer and myself, to develop a report on this topic (Committee on Chemical Toxicity and Aging, ref. 13). The challenge given to us was to:

4

- Define the current understanding of age-related changes in biochemical processes that affect the body's ability to metabolize/detoxify chemicals.

- Define the current understanding and the effects of chemicals on the aging processes and chronic disease states typical of the defined population(s) and on geriatric health.

- Define the current understanding of age-related changes in biochemical processes that affect the body's ability to metabolize/detoxify chemicals.

- Develop critical hypotheses for future needs in a well-founded research agenda concerning inter-relationships between human health, aging, drugs, and environmental pollutants.

This was one of the first organized efforts to bring together gerontologists and toxicologists. Our report proposed development of 'gerontotoxicology'. The proposal for gerontotoxicology indicated a need for model systems, for example, for outcomes of premature aging. It means a need for species of short life, predictable pathological changes with age, known genetics, economic feasibility. We noted the difficulty of distinguishing aging itself from toxic processes. We decided to call agents that accelerate particular aspects of aging 'gerontogens'.

A few words are now required about clinical aspects and what I call the 'new gerontology/geriatrics'.

NEW GERONTOLOGY/GERIATRICS

Revisionism

In the 1940s, in the beginnings of the fields of aging, there was very little money, and there were few researchers. The efforts of early researchers were to identify and measure changes. Nathan Shock[14] was a major leader. Most changes noted were decrements. But as time moved on, we came to realize that many of the decremental intellectual changes that were described occur later, are less serious than had been reported, and are more apt to be due to disease, e.g. Alzheimer's Disease and multi-infarct dementia.

Images of sexlessness have given way to the recognition that ability, desire, and satisfaction remain alive to the end of life if there is health and an interested and interesting partner.

Cerebral blood-flow measures, which we accomplished in the 1950s using the Kety–Schmidt technique, demonstrated that age *per se* did not lead to reductions in blood flow, oxygen consumption, and glucose utilization. More recently, positron emission tomography measurements are confirming this[15].

In the Baltimore Longitudinal Study on Aging population of Shock *et al.*[14], Lakatta has shown that cardiac output does not decline with age. Glomerular filtration rate is maintained or even increased in some one-third of the longitudinal subjects. Harman has shown that free and bound testosterone do not decline with age either, but rather in conjunction with chronic illness and alcoholism.

Mechanism

There has been movement from pure description and phenomenology to efforts to better understand the underlying mechanisms of aging. We have already briefly reviewed the modern theories of aging. However, this does not mean that we don't still need careful phenomenological studies since the field is still at an early stage of development.

Interventionism

The opportunity to control and moderate aging is now clear. The classic research intervention is McKay's food restriction study[16], which has been interpreted to increase lifespan. Socioeconomic contributions, such as Medicare and Social Security, have led to a healthier, more vigorous, longer-living population. There has been a reduction in death rates in old age since Medicare was passed in 1965.

Sociobehavioural interventions are effective in reducing morbidity and mortality. We see that women cope more effectively with bereavement, probably because of their support network, and Alvar Svanborg's work[17] shows the greater mortality and morbidity rates among men compared to women after the death of the spouse.

Biomedical interventions are possible too: calcium and exercise for osteoporosis, oestrogen for osteoporosis and for heart disease as well. Particularly exciting is the experimental basis for new possibilities of neuroplasticity.

Empowerment of older people

For older people, overcoming negative stereotypes, or ageism, is critical, along with increased self-regard and the mobilization of the continuing productivity of older persons – 'productive aging'[18]. We know from our NIMH studies[19] that the presence of a sense of purpose is associated with survival. Judith Rodin[20] has shown us the importance of control of one's situation to adaptation in old age. This is among the reasons why I oppose the term 'case management', arguing that if I were old and ill I would neither want to be a 'case' nor be 'managed'. I should prefer to work in collaboration with a physician and other health providers. This I call 'collaborative care', which gives one an important sense of control over one's own destiny.

The research imperative

There is a need to continue basic studies and better understand fundamental biological mechanisms of aging. It is also necessary to continue the conventional disease-mission approach, which certainly has helped us to understand the diseases that afflict older people. There are also the 'grey lands', the difficult area of separating aging from disease. Here Brody and Schneider[21] have helped us with the terms 'age-dependent' and 'age-related'.

We have seen the rise of geriatrics, first in the United Kingdom and then in Sweden, Japan, and, more recently, in the United States. We have established the first and only Department of Geriatrics at the Mount Sinai School of Medicine. In 1988, for the first time, the American Board of Internal Medicine and the American Academy of Family Practice will hold examinations for the Certificate of Competence in Geriatrics. The hope is, of course, to develop academic and consultative geriatrics, not a new practice specialty of geriatrics.

The three great antecedents of disease, intricately interconnected, are aging, genes, and the environment, broadly defined to include air, water, nutrition, diet, lifestyle – how we take care of ourselves. Some of the events of aging are nearly identical with environmental effects: UV light affecting cataract formation and photo-aging of the skin; noise pollution affecting hearing.

Social and individual responsibility are seen in the somewhat anaemic term 'health promotion/disease prevention'. We certainly know, for example, what a massive adverse effect tobacco has on health.

Lifespan extension research is always popular with the public. Some of the nonsense involved is nicely reviewed by Schneider and Reid[22]. I am hopeful that we will begin to have biomarkers of aging through the ten-year study of the National Institute on Aging and the National Center of Toxicology Research.

Let me end on a positive note with some language from the National Academy of Science's Committee on Chemical Toxicity and Aging report: 'Reduction of disease in old age is an obtainable objective that can be reached in part through modification of the environment'. That is quite a stunning statement. Perhaps the liver and the gastrointestinal tract might even have a role.

References

1. Popper, H. (1987). The liver in aging. In *Modern Biological Theories of Aging*. pp. 219–34 (New York: Raven Press)
2. Warner, H. R., Butler, R. N., Sprott, R. L. and Schneider, E. L. (eds.) (1987). *Modern Biological Theories of Aging*. (New York: Raven Press)
3. Medawar, P. (1957). *The Uniqueness of the Individual*. (London: Methuen)
4. Sacher, G. (1978). Longevity, aging, and death: an evolutionary perspective. *Gerontologist*, **18**, 112–19
5. Hayflick, L. (1987). Origins of longevity. In *Modern Biological Theories of Aging*. pp. 21–34. (New York: Raven Press)
6. Harman, D. (1987). The free-radical theory of aging. In *Modern Biological Theories of Aging*. pp. 81–8. (New York: Raven Press)
7. Saul, R. L., Gee, P. and Ames, B. N. (1987). Free radicals, DNA damage, and aging. In *Modern Biological Theories of Aging*. pp. 113–34. (New York: Raven Press)
8. Dice, J. F. and Goff, S. A. (1987). Error catastrophe and aging: Future directions of research. In *Modern Biological Theories of Aging*. pp. 155–76. (New York: Raven Press)
9. Setlow, R. B. (1987). Theory presentation and background summary. In *Modern Biological Theories of Aging*. pp. 177–82. (New York: Raven Press)
10. Cerutti, P. A. (1987). The role of DNA damage and its repair in aging: Evidence for and against. In *Modern Biological Theories of Aging*. pp. 199–218. (New York: Raven Press)
11. Finch, C. E. (1987). Neural and endocrine determinants of senescence: Investigation of

causality and reversibility by laboratory and clinical interventions. In *Modern Biological Theories of Aging*. (New York: Raven Press)

12. Cerami, A. (1985). Hypothesis, glucose as a mediator of aging. *J. Am. Geriatr. Soc.*, **33**, 624–34

13. Committee on Chemical Toxicity and Aging. (1987). *Aging in Today's Environment*. (Washington, DC: National Academy of Sciences)

14. Shock, N. W., Greulich, R. C., Andres, R., Arenberg, D., Costa, P. T. Jr, Lakatta, E. G. and Tobin, J. D. (1984). *Normal Human Aging: The Baltimore Longitudinal Study of Aging*. Publication No. 84–2450 (Washington DC: NIH)

15. Duara, R., Margolin, R. A., Robertson-Tchabo, E. A. *et al.* (1983). Cerebral glucose utilization, as measured with positron emission tomography in 21 resting healthy men between the ages of 21 and 83 years. *Brain*, **106**, 761–75

16. McKay, C. M., Crowell, L. A. and Maynard, J. (1935). The effect of retarded growth upon the length of lifespan and upon the ultimate body size. *J. Nutr.*, **10**, 53–79

17. Svanborg, A., Shibata, H., Hatano and Matsuzaki, T. (1985). Comparison of ecology, aging, and state of health in Japan and Sweden, the present and previous leaders in longevity. *Acta Med. Scand.*, **218**, 5–17

18. Butler, R. N. and Gleason, H. (1985). *Productive Aging*. (New York: Springer)

19. Butler, R. N. (1967). Aspects of survival and adaptation in human aging. Psychiatric report of five-year follow-up of NIMH study of healthy community-resident aged men. *Am. J. Psychiatry*, **123**, 1233–43

20. Rodin, J. (1986). Aging and Health: Effects of the sense of control. *Science*, **233**, 1271–6

21. Brody, J. and Schneider, E. L. (1986). Diseases and the disorders of aging, a hypothesis. *J. Chron. Dis.*, **39**, 871–6

22. Schneider, E. S. and Reed, J. D. (1985). Life extension. *N. Engl. J. Med.*, **312**, 1159–68

2
Genetics in aging

G. M. MARTIN

INTRODUCTION: RATIONALE FOR THE ROLE OF GENES

All phenotypes, including those associated with aging, result from interactions between nature (i.e. one's hereditary environment) and nurture (i.e. one's environmental experiences). One can cite at least three major lines of evidence, however, to illustrate the crucial role that genetics must have in the determination of the maximum life-span potential (MLSP) of an organism and of its pattern of aging. Most striking are the observations indicating that the MLSP is a constitutional feature of speciation. When a new species evolves, its newly modified genome, in ways that are still poorly understood, appears to set some general limits on the times of onset and rates of progression of age-oriented alterations in structure and function of molecules, cells and tissues and, thus, of the life span. For the case of eutherian mammals (i.e. those with highly-developed placentas), the range of MLSPs may be of the order of 30-fold, although much more reliable data are still required to more accurately establish that figure[1]. A somewhat more reliable parameter may be the doubling time of the mortality rate (T_d), i.e. the time required for the death rate to increase by a factor of two[2]. Reasonably reliable data are available for five eutherian mammalian species; these are listed in Table 2.1 and give about a 15-fold range.

Table 2.1 Doubling time of mortality rate (T_d) for five eutherian mammalian species for which reasonably reliable data exist (after Sacher[2])

Species	T_d (days)
Mus musculus domesticus (house mouse)	220
Peromyscus leucopus (white-footed deer mouse)	447
Canis familiaris (beagle dog)	812
Equus caballus (thoroughbred horse)	1332
Homo sapiens (U.S. white female, 1969 census)	3100

If we turn our attention to marsupial mammals, we discover a second line of evidence that underscores a major role for the genome. Like the life histories of flowering plants and migrating salmon, some species of marsupial mice undergo a single massive episode of reproduction (semelparity), following which there ensues more or less synchronous and precipitous pathologic alterations, most conspicuously involving the neuroendocrine, immune and reproductive systems, death ensuing in a few weeks. Such behaviour can be interpreted as support for a genetically programmed, neuroendocrine-mediated mechanism of aging. While most mammals are iteroparous, i.e. exhibit multiple rounds of reproduction, it would be surprising if elements of such deterministic aging were not of some importance in how we human beings age.

A third line of evidence derives from the work of medical geneticists, who have described a number of single gene mutations and conditions resulting from alterations in gene dosage that appear to bring forward in time and/or accelerate the rates of progress of particular aspects of senescence in man. Such mutations have been referred to as 'abiotropic', in that they ordinarily are not manifested until some time after birth and are characterized by degenerative and/or proliferative aberrations.

AGING IS UNDER HIGHLY POLYGENIC CONTROLS

In a previous study, Martin[3] systematically evaluated such abiotropic mutations in an effort to assess the proportion of the human genome that could potentially be involved in the modulation of various aspects of aging in human subjects. While one could criticize the particular set of criteria used to search for such genetic variations, the exercise was useful, I believe, in highlighting the large number of genetic loci which might have the potential, in different individuals, of altering the way we age. It was concluded that, at a maximum, close to 7% of human genes might act in this fashion. If we accept some estimates that there are between 30 000–100 000 different informational genes in man, this would give up to about 2000–7000 different genetic loci of potential significance to the pathobiology of aging. It might well be the case, however, that only a small proportion of these are of regular importance and of major importance for how most of us age. Certainly, there are some genetic loci that appear to be of major significance, the best example of which is that involved in the Werner syndrome. In that autosomal recessive condition, it is a reasonable hypothesis that a single enzyme deficiency leads to the acceleration of greying of hair, loss of hair, ocular cataracts, wrinkling and ulceration of skin, osteoporosis, diabetes mellitus, various forms of arterioscleroses (atherosclerosis, arteriosclerosis, medical calcinosis), and a large variety of neoplasms[4].

Using an entirely different approach, Sacher[5] and Cutler[6] have independently come to the conclusion that some 200–300 genetic loci were involved in the evolution of the MLSP of man from his humanoid precursors. These estimates were based upon unrealistically low mutation rates, however[7]. Moreover, they ignore the possibility that a simple chromosomal re-arrangement might lead, via both *cis* and *trans* effects, to changes in the expression of a large number of genes.

In any event, if we conclude that perhaps a few hundred genes are of major importance to aging, any geneticist would characterize such a system as being subject to highly polygenic controls. If a few thousand genes were involved in more subtle aspects of the phenotype, we could easily conclude that no two human beings ever have, nor ever will, age in precisely the same ways.

These conclusions are at variance, however, with the observations of the effects of dietary restriction on the life span of cohorts of rodents[8-10]. The fact that such a simple manipulation can significantly enhance life span argues against a highly complex genetic substrate for aging. As we have seen, however, genes can alter rates of aging, in mammals, by at least 1500% (Table 2.1), whereas dietary restriction increases longevity by only about 60%.

DOMAINS OF GENE ACTION IN AGING

Most gerontologists would agree that early development is a major arena of gene action in setting the stage for patterns of aging that unfold post-maturationally. For example, let us consider the eventual impact of age-related loss of dopaminergic neurons of the substantia nigra. Aging adults gradually lose these neurons, but the signs and symptoms of Parkinson's disease do not become clinically apparent until some 70% of neurons have been lost, dopamine levels declining with age by about 13% per decade[11].

Genetic controls surely exist in determining the extent to which the stem-cell precursors of that nucleus clonally amplify, attenuate, differentiate and migrate. Alterations in such genetic controls might lead to varying numbers of mature, functioning neurons and, hence, varying susceptibilities to the development of the 'threshold effect' of Parkinson's disease, independent of intrinsic and extrinsic variables determining the rates of loss of such cell types.

Parenthetically, I should add that studies of twins in Parkinson's disease have failed to document an important role for genetic susceptibility factors[12]. I am skeptical of these results, however, as the cohorts that have been studied so far were all exposed to the great 1918 influenza pandemic. That genes can potentially play a role in the susceptibility to Parkinson's disease is demonstrated by the existence of pedigrees exhibiting X-linked and, perhaps, autosomal recessive and autosomal dominant patterns of inheritance[13].

To further illustrate the importance of gene action during development, let me briefly review what is so far known about the natural history of the hereditary form of generalized lipodystrophy (the Seip syndrome)[14]. This autosomal recessive disorder is characterized by an apparently precocious development of the musculo-skeletal system and genitalia, accompanied by an extreme paucity of fat and abnormalities of lipids and carbohydrates. An enhanced rate of growth continues for about ten years. A variety of degenerative pathologies then ensues, including diabetic vasculopathies and, possibly, degeneration of the central nervous system.

The major focus of gerontologic research, however, has been upon the maintenance of macromolecular integrity after normal growth and development. Most popular theories of aging are of this type. They invoke particular subsets of genes as having seminal importance in the determination of life span. For example, the free radical theory[15,16] would emphasize genes that influence the generation and the scavenging of chemical free radicals. The intrinsic mutagenesis theory is mainly concerned with varying fidelities of the several DNA-dependent DNA polymerases and with the efficiencies and fidelities of the numerous enzymes involved in DNA repair. The genes of special significance to the protein synthesis error catastrophy theory of Orgel[17,18], would include the DNA-dependent RNA polymerases and the various proteins and enzymes involved in the fidelity of translation, as well as the proteases that recognize abnormal proteins. Investigators concerned with post-translational modifications of proteins would also be interested in the machinery of protein turnover and in genes that determine a variety of metabolic fluxes – for example, the levels of glucose in the case of protein glycations[19].

A third arena of gene action of relevance to aging involves the biology of cell–cell interactions. It is conceivable that, even in the absence of macromolecular alterations referred to above, age-related alterations in the proportion of various regulatory cell types (for example, those of the immune system) could be responsible for important components of the senescent phenotype. As in the case of development, there could be important components in the genetic control of the intrinsic rates at which different populations of stem cells attenuate and differentiate, resulting in alterations in cell–cell regulatory activities. Very little is known about such phenomena, but I believe they may have special relevance for the striking variety of inappropriate hyperplasias that are seen so commonly in the tissues of aging mammals[20]. These are paradoxical, in that they often occur in the face of tissue atrophy. Their importance is that they may act as tumour promotors[20].

INVESTIGATIVE APPROACH TO THE STUDY OF GENETIC AGING

Until recently, the major approach has involved correlative studies among groups of related species, in an attempt to implicate a particular subset of genetic loci in the determination of life span. The classical example is that of Hart and Setlow[21] who provided evidence for the importance of genes that determine the efficiency of UV-induced excisional DNA repair.

A related approach has been described above, in which spontaneous mutation in man has been exploited. In addition to such syndromes as the Werner syndrome, which I refer to as 'segmental progeroid syndromes'[3] there are numerous examples of single-gene mutations which affect, predominantly, one major aspect of the senescent phenotype. Examples would include xeroderma pigmentosum (aging of sun-exposed skin), the Gardner syndrome (loss of proliferative homeostasis of colonic epithelium) and familial Alzheimer's disease. I refer to such disorders as 'unimodal progeroid syndromes'[22].

Progress in the study of familial Alzheimer's disease has been especially gratifying. A major susceptibility gene and the gene controlling the synthesis of the amyloid protein has been mapped to chromosome 21 (see refs. 23–27). The deposition of this class of amyloid appears to be a concomitant of normal aging in many mammalian species[28].

Advances in experimental genetics now provide major opportunities to investigate the role of specific genes upon specific aspects of aging. In mammals, the most promising methodology involves transgenic mice. In fact, the first transgenic mice synthesized, involving the ectopic synthesis of growth hormone[29], now promises to be useful for the investigation of aspects of aging[30]. Moreover, the recent demonstration of the practicality of using genetically-modified cultivated embryonal stem cells for the synthesis of transgenic mice greatly extends the power of this approach[31,32]. In our own laboratory, we are using such systems for the evaluation of somatic mutational theories of aging[33,34]. Thus, experimental genetic applications to gerontology, as foreseen ten years ago[35], now appear to be coming to fruition.

References

1. Altman, P. L. and Dittmer, D. S. (1962). Lifespans: mammalians. In *Growth. Biological Handbook*. p. 445. (Washington DC: Fed. Soc. Exp. Biol.)
2. Sacher, G. A. (1977). Life table modification and life prolongation. In Finch, C. E. and Hayflick, L. (eds.) *Handbook of the Biology of Aging*. pp. 582–638. (New York: Van Nostrand Reinhold)
3. Martin, G. M. (1978). Genetic syndromes in man with potential relevance to the pathobiology of aging. In Bergsma, D. and Harrison, D. E. (eds.) *Genetic Effects on Aging. Birth Defects*: Original Article Series, **14** (1). pp. 5–39. (New York: Alan R. Liss)
4. Salk, D., Fujiwara, Y. and Martin, G. M. (eds.) (1985). Werner's syndrome and human aging. *Adv. Exp. Med. Biol.*, **190**. (New York: Plenum Press)
5. Sacher, G. A. (1975). Maturation and longevity in relation to cranial capacity in hominid evolution. In Tuttle, R. (ed.) *Antecedents of Man and After. I. Primates: Functional Morphology and Evolution*. (The Hague: Moutin)
6. Cutler, R. G. (1975). Evolution of human longevity and the genetic complexity governing aging rate. *Proc. Natl. Acad. Sci. USA*, **72**, 4664–8
7. Kirkwood, T. B. L. (1985). Comparative and evolutionary aspects of longevity. In Finch, C. E. and Schneider, E. L. (eds.) *Handbook of the Biology of Aging*. pp. 27–44. (New York: Van Nostrand Reinhold)
8. Masoro, E. (1985). State of knowledge on action of food restriction and aging. In Woodhead, A. D., Blackett, A. D. and Hollaender, A. (eds.) *Molecular Biology of Aging*. pp. 105–16. (New York: Plenum Press)
9. Holehan, A. M. and Merry, B. J. (1986). The experimental manipulation of ageing by diet. *Biol. Res.*, **61**, 329–68
10. Weindruch, R., Walford, R. L., Fligiel, S. and Guthrie, D. (1986). The retardation of aging in mice by dietary restriction: Longevity, cancer, immunity and lifetime energy intake. *J. Nutr.*, **116**, 641–54
11. Bujatti, M. and Reiderer, P. (1976). Serotonin, noradrenaline, dopamine metabolites in transcendental meditation-technique. *J. Neural. Transm.*, **39**, 257–67
12. Ward, C. D., Duvoisin, R. C., Inu, S. E., Nutt, J. D., Eldridge, R. and Colne, D. B. (1983). Parkinson disease in 65 pairs of twins and in a set of quadruplets. *Neurology*, **33**, 815–24
13. McKusick, V. A. (1986). *Mendelian Inheritance in Man*. 7th edn. (Baltimore: Johns Hopkins University)
14. Seip, M. (1971). Generalized lipodiptrophy. In Frick, P., von Harnack, G. A., Muller, A. F., Prader, A., Schoen, R. and Wolff, H. P. (eds.) *Ergebnisse der inneren Medizin und Kinderheilkunde*, **31**, 59–95. (New York: Springer-Verlag)

15. Harman, D. (1981). The aging process. *Proc. Natl. Acad. Sci. USA*, **73**, 7124–8
16. Balin, A. K. (1982). Testing the free radical theory of aging. In Adelman, R. C. and Roth, G. S. (eds.) *Testing the Theories of Aging*. pp. 137–82. CRS Series in Aging. (Boca Raton, Florida: CRC Press)
17. Orgel, L. E. (1963). The maintenance of the accuracy of protein synthesis and its relevance to ageing. *Proc. Natl. Acad. Sci. USA*, **49**, 517–21
18. Orgel, L. E. (1970). The maintenance of the accuracy of protein synthesis and its relevance to ageing: A correction. *Proc. Natl. Acad. Sci. USA*, **67**, 1476
19. Cerami, A., Vlassara, H. and Brownlee, M. (1987). Glucose and aging. *Sci. Am.*, **256**, 90–6
20. Martin, G. M. (1979). Proliferative homeostasis and its age-related aberrations. *Mech. Ageing Devel.*, **9**, 385–91
21. Hart, R. W. and Setlow, R. B. (1974). Correlation between deoxyribonucleic acid excision repair and lifespan in a number of species. *Proc. Natl. Acad. Sci. USA*, **71**, 2169–73
22. Martin, G. M. (1982). Syndromes of accelerated aging. *Natl. Cancer Inst. Monogr.*, **60**, 241–7
23. Goldgaber, D., Lerman, M. I., McBride, O. W., Saffiotti, A. and Gajdusek, D. C. (1987). Characterization and chromosomal localization of a cDNA encoding brain amyloid of Alzheimer's disease. *Science*, **235**, 877–80
24. Kang, J., Lemaire, H.-G., Unterbeck, A., Salbaum, J. M., Masters, C. L., Grzeschik, K.-H., Multhaup, G., Beyreuther, K. and Müller-Hill, B. (1987). The precursor of Alzheimer's disease amyloid A4 protein resembles a cell surface receptor. *Nature*, **325**, 733–6
25. Robakis, N. K., Wisniewski, H. M., Jenkins, E. C., Devine-Gage, E. A., Houck, G. E., Yao, X.-L., Ramakrishna, N., Wolfe, G., Silverman, W. P. and Brown, W. T. (1987). Chromosome 21q21 sublocalisation of gene encoding beta-amyloid peptide in cerebral vessels and neuritic (senile) plaques of people with Alzheimer disease and Down syndrome. *Lancet*, **1**, 384–5
26. St. George-Hyslop, P. H., Tanzi, R. E., Polinsky, R. J., Haines, J. C., Nee, L., Watkins, P. C., Meyers, R. H., Feldman, R. G., Pollen, D., Drachman, D. *et al.* (1987). The genetic defect causing familial Alzheimer's disease maps on chromosome 21. *Science*, **235**, 885–90
27. Tanzi, R. E., Gusella, J. F., Watkins, P. C., Bruns, G. A. D., St. George-Hyslop, P., Van Keuren, M. L., Patterson, D., Pagan, S., Kurnit, D. M. and Neve, R. L. (1987). Amyloid beta protein gene: cDNA, mRNA distribution and genetic linkage near the Alzheimer locus. *Science*, **235**, 880–4
28. Selkoe, D. J., Bell, D. S., Podlisny, M. B., Price, D. L. and Cork, L. C. (1987). Conservation of brain amyloid proteins in aged mammals and humans with Alzheimer's disease. *Science*, **235**, 873–7
29. Palmiter, R. D., Brinster, R. L., Hammer, R. E., Trumbauer, M. E., Rosenfeld, M. G., Birnberg, N. C. and Evans, R. M. (1982). Dramatic growth of mice that develop from eggs microinjected with metallothionein–growth hormone fusion genes. *Nature*, **300**, 611–15
30. Palmiter, R. D. and Brinster, R. L. (1986). Germ-line transformation of mice. *Annu. Rev. Genet.*, **20**, 465–99
31. Hooper, M., Hardy, K., Handyside, A., Hunter, S. and Monk, M. (1987). HPRT-deficient (Lesch–Nyhan) mouse embryos derived from germline colonization by cultured cells. *Nature*, **326**, 292–5
32. Kuehn, M. R., Bradley, A., Robertson, E. J. and Evans, M. J. (1987). A potential animal model for Lesch–Nyhan syndrome through introduction of HPRT mutations into mice. *Nature*, **326**, 295–8
33. Aizawa, S., Loeb, L. A. and Martin, G. M. (1983). Mouse teratocarcinoma cells resistant to aphidicolin and arabinofuranosyl cytosine: Isolation and initial characterization. *J. Cell Physiol.*, **115**, 9–14
34. Aizawa, S., Ohashi, M., Loeb, L. A. and Martin, G. M. (1985). Multipotent mutator strain of mouse teratocarcinoma cells. *Somatic Cell Mol. Genet.*, **11**, 211–16
35. Martin, G. M. (1977). Cellular aging – postreplicative cells. A review (part II). *Am. J. Path.*, **89**, 513–30

3
Molecular aspects of aging: changes in protein synthesis and the expression of α_{2u}-globulin

J. A. BUTLER, M. S. RUTHERFORD, I. SEMSEI and A. RICHARDSON

INTRODUCTION

A general characteristic of senescent organisms is the impairment in the ability of an organism to respond to stimuli. Because the response to stimuli at the molecular level occurs largely through protein-catalysed reactions, changes in protein synthesis may play a role in the inability of senescent organisms to respond to stimuli. Proteins are the most abundant macromolecules in a cell and make up approximately 50% of a cell by dry weight. More importantly, proteins are the molecular component through which genetic information is expressed.

Because proteins play an important role in cellular structure and function, it is not surprising that a large number of studies have been conducted in a variety of organisms on the effect of aging on protein synthesis[1-4]. An age-related decline in protein synthesis has been observed in organisms ranging from fungi to humans. Consequently, Richardson[1] suggested that the decline in protein synthesis is a universal characteristic of the aging process.

PROTEIN SYNTHESIS BY LIVER

The effect of aging on protein synthesis has been studied most extensively in liver tissue from laboratory rodents. Most of the studies in which cell-free systems have been used to measure protein synthesis have shown a decline in liver protein synthesis with increasing age[1-4]. However, the rate of protein synthesis in cell-free systems is approximately one-tenth that observed *in vivo*[1]. During the past decade, suspensions of hepatocytes have been employed to measure protein synthesis because the rate of protein synthesis in suspensions of hepatocytes is similar to the liver *in vivo*[5]. In 1977 and 1979, van Bezooijen *et al.*[6] and Coniglio *et al.*[7] demonstrated that the rate of protein synthesis by isolated hepatocytes decreased approximately 50% between 3 and 24 months of age and increased thereafter. The increase in protein synthesis after 24 months of age appears to be due, at least partially, to an increase in the synthesis of albumin[1].

Although the effect of aging on the total protein synthetic activity of liver has been studied extensively, very little information is currently available on the effect of aging on the synthesis of specific proteins by liver. The only information in this area is for albumin. Van Bezooijen *et al.*[8] showed that the synthesis of albumin by isolated hepatocytes increased dramatically with age.

During the past two years, our laboratory has studied the effect of aging on the synthesis of a variety of proteins by liver from male Fischer F344 rats to determine if the changes in total protein synthesis are similar to changes

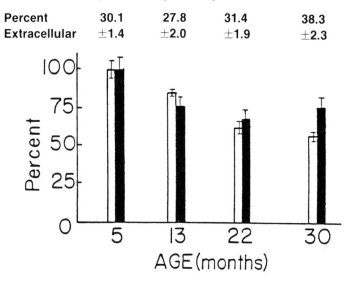

| Percent | 30.1 | 27.8 | 31.4 | 38.3 |
| Extracellular | ±1.4 | ±2.0 | ±1.9 | ±2.3 |

Figure 3.1   The effect of age on the synthesis of intracellular and extracellular proteins. The rate of [³H]-L-valine incorporation into intracellular (□) and extracellular (■) proteins in suspensions of hepatocytes isolated from male Fischer F344 rats was determined as described by Ricca *et al.*[5]. The data are expressed as a percentage of the 5-month-old animals. Values are expressed as the mean ± SEM of data obtained from 8 animals for each age. The synthesis of intracellular proteins declined significantly ($P<0.01$) between 5 and 22 months of age. The decline in extracellular protein synthesis was significant ($P<0.01$) between 5 and 13 months of age. The percentage extracellular protein synthesis given at the top of the graph represents the rate of incorporation of [³H]-L-valine into extracellular proteins divided by the rate of [³H]-L-valine incorporation into total protein. The percentage for 30-month-old rats was significantly higher ($P<0.05$) than the percentage for the other ages.

in the synthesis of individual proteins. Figure 3.1 compares the synthesis of intracellular and extracellular proteins by hepatocytes isolated from 5-, 13-, 22-, and 30-month-old rats. The incorporation of valine into intracellular proteins decreased continuously (by 30–35%) between 5 and 22 months of age. However, the incorporation of valine into intracellular proteins only decreased between 5 and 13 months of age and increased slightly between 22 and 30 months of age. Figure 3.1 also shows the percentage of the radioactivity incorporated into extracellular proteins. Between 5 and 22 months of age, approximately 30% of the radioactive valine was incorporated into extracellular proteins. However, in hepatocytes from 30-month-old rats, over 38% of the radioactive valine was incorporated into extracellular proteins. Thus, the synthesis of extracellular and intracellular proteins by liver change differently with increasing age. In the old animal, extracellular proteins make up a greater fraction of the proteins synthesized by the liver.

To compare the patterns of specific proteins synthesized by hepatocytes isolated from rats of various ages, we used two-dimensional gel elec-trophoresis and fluorography. Figure 3.2 shows fluorographs of samples taken from 5- and 30-month-old rats. It is evident that the relative synthesis of most (we estimate 95% or more) proteins was similar for young and old rats. In other words, we did not observe the appearance or disappearance of a large number of proteins with age. Thus, senescence is not a simple continuation of development in which a different spectrum of gene products are synthesized. We quantified the rate of synthesis of 36 proteins, which were randomly selected from the fluorograms. The synthesis of 35 of the 36 proteins decreased with age and the decrease was statistically significant for 58% of the proteins. Thus, it appears that the synthesis of most proteins declines with age in a manner very similar to the age-related decrease in total protein synthesis.

EXPRESSION OF α_{2u}-GLOBULIN BY LIVER

Although the relative synthesis of most proteins appears to remain constant with age (Figure 3.2), the synthesis of several proteins (approximately 5%) changes dramatically with age, i.e. there is either the appearance or dis-appearance of newly synthesized proteins. From Figure 3.2, it is apparent that the synthesis of a group of low molecular weight proteins is greatly reduced in the 30-month-old rats. These proteins correspond to α_{2u}-globulin. α_{2u}-globulin is a male-specific protein that is synthesized by hepatic paren-chymal cells. Roy's laboratory has shown previously that the levels and synthesis of α_{2u}-globulin decline dramatically with age in rats[9], and he pro-posed that α_{2u}-globulin was a 'senescence marker protein'[9,10]. Roy et al.[9] also showed that five major isoelectric variants of α_{2u}-globulin could be detected by two-dimensional gel electrophoresis. Figure 3.3 shows fluorographs of two-dimensional gels, which compare the synthesis of the five isoelectric variants of α_{2u}-globulin in 5- and 30-month-old rats. The synthesis of all five isoelectric variants of α_{2u}-globulin decreased dramatically with increasing age.

In young animals, α_{2u}-globulin is the major protein in the urine of male rats (Figure 3.4). The decrease in α_{2u}-globulin synthesis is paralleled by a decrease in the levels in α_{2u}-globulin in the urine. Figure 3.4 shows that the level of α_{2u}-globulin in the urine of 24-month-old rats is much lower than the level in the urine of 5-month-old rats. This decrease in α_{2u}-globulin occurs even though the total amount of protein excreted in the urine was greater for old rats. The age-related increase in proteinuria is well documented and

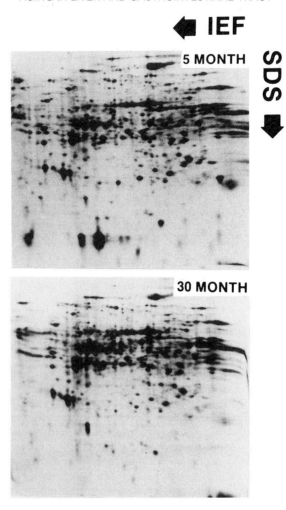

Figure 3.2 Two-dimensional gel electrophoresis of proteins synthesized by hepatocytes isolated from young and old rats. Hepatocytes isolated from 5- or 30-month-old male Fischer F344 rats were incubated with [^{35}S]-L-methionine for 2 h and the cellular homogenates subjected to two-dimensional gel electrophoresis as described by O'Farrell[14]. The gels were pH 5 to 8 in the first dimension and 12% acrylamide in the second dimension. The fluorographs for samples were pooled from 4 animals for the two ages shown. Equal amounts of acid-insoluble radioactivity were placed on each gel; therefore, the gels compare relative levels of protein synthesis because the total incorporation of [^{35}S]-methionine into protein is lower for the 30-month-old rats.

characteristic of laboratory rodents and arises from a decline in renal function[11].

Because the synthesis of α_{2u}-globulin by hepatocytes decreased with age, we measured the levels of α_{2u}-globulin mRNA in liver RNA using a cDNA probe to α_{2u}-globulin. Figure 3.5 shows the Northern blot analysis of α_{2u}-globulin mRNA in RNA isolated from liver of rats and mice. The cDNA

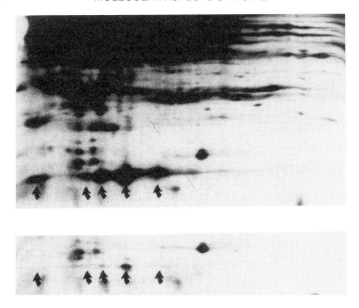

Figure 3.3 The effect of age on the synthesis of α_{2u}-globulin. Hepatocytes isolated from 5- and 30-month-old male Fischer F344 rats (top and bottom, respectively) were incubated with [35S]-L-methionine for 2 h. The culture supernatants from 4 animals for each age group were pooled, and equal amounts of radioactivity-labelled proteins from the supernatants were subjected to two-dimensional gel electrophoresis. The fluorographs of the gels are shown. The entire gel from the 5-month-old rats is shown, and the region of the gel containing the isoelectric variants of α_{2u}-globulin is shown for the 30-month-old rats. The fluorographs were over-exposed to enhance the detection of the isoelectric variants of α_{2u}-globulin. The isoelectric variants of α_{2u}-globulin, which are shown by the arrows, were identified according to the description given by Roy *et al.*[9].

probe hybridized to a 1.2 to 1.3 kb RNA species in RNA isolated from male Fischer F344 rats. It is apparent that the level of α_{2u}-globulin mRNA in RNA isolated from the liver of the rats decreased dramatically with increasing age. This decrease in mRNA levels of α_{2u}-globulin had been observed previously by Roy's laboratory[9,10]. We also used the cDNA probe to α_{2u}-globulin to measure the levels of the major urinary protein (MUP) mRNA in male C57Bl/6J mice. Male mice synthesize a urinary protein homologous to α_{2u}-globulin, which is known as MUP. This protein is encoded by a family of genes, which are approximately 90% homologous to the α_{2u}-globulin genes in rat[12]. Currently, there is no information about the effect of aging on the expression of MUP by mouse liver. The Northern blot in Figure 3.5 shows that the cDNA probe to α_{2u}-globulin hybridized to mouse RNA with a size of approximately 1.0 kb. The level of this mRNA species is much lower in RNA isolated from old mice compared to RNA isolated from young mice.

Figure 3.6 shows the expression of α_{2u}-globulin by liver of male Fischer F344 rats. There is an excellent correlation between the age-related decline in the synthesis, mRNA levels, and the transcription of α_{2u}-globulin. Thus,

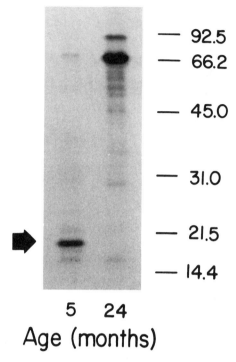

Figure 3.4 α_{2u}-globulin levels in the urine of young and old rats. Urine was collected from 5- and 24-month-old male Fischer F344 rats over a 24-h period as described by Ricketts et al.[11]. The urine was pooled from 4 rats for each age and was diluted to the same volume for the young and old rats. Equal volumes of the urine were subjected to SDS-polyacrylamide gel electrophoresis[15], and the gels were stained with Coomassie Blue. The migration of protein standards of known molecular weights is shown, and the arrow indicates the migration of α_{2u}-globulin.

Table 3.1 The expression of α_{2u}-globulin by liver of rats fed *ad libitum* and a restricted diet*

Expressed as:	Ad libitum	Restricted	Ratio†
Protein synthesis (dpm/10^3 cells)	7.5 ± 2.4	22.0 ± 4.6	2.9
mRNA levels (area/8 μg RNA)	0.37 ± 0.08	0.66 ± 0.12	1.8
Transcription (ppm)	554	1306	2.4

*These data were taken from Richardson et al.[17]. Male Fischer F344 rats were fed either *ad libitum* or 60% of *ad libitum* (restricted) beginning at 6 weeks of age. The expression of α_{2u}-globulin was measured at 18 months of age
† Ratio of restricted/*ad libitum*

the decrease in α_{2u}-globulin expression with increasing age is regulated primarily at the level of transcription.

Recently, we have measured the expression of α_{2u}-globulin in the liver of rats fed *ad libitum* and a restricted diet (40% of the diet consumed by the

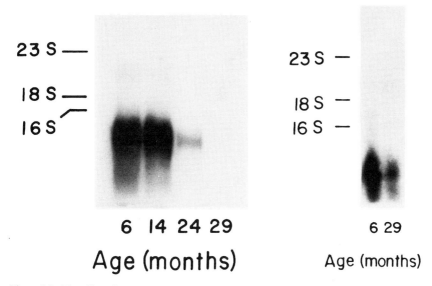

Figure 3.5 The effect of age on the levels of α_{2u}-globulin mRNA in rat and mouse liver. Northern blot analysis was performed as described by Rutherford *et al.*[16], and the autoradiographs of Northern blots are shown. The Northern blot on the left shows the hybridization of the α_{2u}-globulin cDNA probe to RNA isolated from male Fischer F344 rats of various ages. The Northern blot on the right shows the hybridization of the cDNA probe to RNA isolated from young and old male C57B1/6J mice. The RNA was pooled from 4 rats or mice for each age, and 8 μg of RNA was used for each age.

rats fed *ad libitum*). Dietary restriction, underfeeding not malnutrition, is the only experimental manipulation known to increase the longevity of mammals[13]. Because dietary restriction is believed to increase the longevity of rodents by retarding the aging process, we were interested in studying the effect of dietary restriction on the age-related decline in α_{2u}-globulin expression. Figure 3.7 shows the protein content of urine collected from 18-month-old rats fed either *ad libitum* or the restricted diet. There was a striking difference in the protein patterns observed in the two groups of rats. In all 10 rats fed the restricted diet, the level of protein in the urine was reduced and α_{2u}-globulin was detectable. Dietary restriction has been shown previously to reduce the age-related increase in proteinuria[11]. The urine from each of the 10 rats fed *ad libitum* contained high amounts of high molecular weight proteins and had no detectable α_{2u}-globulin. Table 3.1 shows the expression of α_{2u}-globulin by liver tissue from 18-month-old rats fed *ad libitum* or a restricted diet. At 18 months of age, the expression of α_{2u}-globulin has decreased 80–90% in rats fed *ad libitum* (Figure 3.6). The rats maintained on the restricted diet showed a higher expression of α_{2u}-globulin, e.g. the synthesis, mRNA levels, and transcription of α_{2u}-globulin was 1.8- to 3-fold higher for restricted rats than rats fed *ad libitum*. Thus, dietary restriction altered the age-related decline in α_{2u}-globulin expression, and this alteration

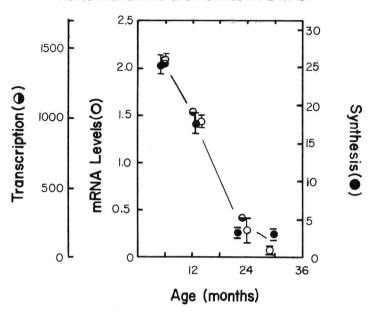

Figure 3.6 The effect of age on the expression of α_{2u}-globulin by the liver of male Fischer F344 rats. The data were taken from Richardson *et al.*[17]

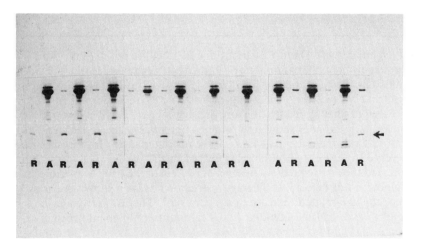

Figure 3.7 Effect of dietary restriction on the levels of α_{2u}-globulin in urine. The urine from 18-month-old male Fischer F344 rats fed *ad libitum* (A) or a calorie-restricted diet (R) was collected and analysed as described in Figure 3.4. The arrow shows the migration of α_{2u}-globulin.

occurred primarily at the level of transcription. This is the first evidence that dietary restriction has an effect at the level of gene expression.

SUMMARY

The effect of aging on the synthesis of specific proteins was measured in liver of male Fischer F344 rats. Although the rate of intracellular protein synthesis declined with increasing age, the synthesis of extracellular proteins increased significantly in old rats. Using two-dimensional gel electrophoresis, we found that the relative synthesis of most proteins remained constant with age. Less than 5% of the proteins visualized disappeared or appeared with increasing age. Therefore, we did not observe a dramatic change in the spectrum of genes expressed by liver with increasing age. In general, it appears that the synthesis of most proteins decreases with increasing age.

α_{2u}-globulin is a protein that disappears with increasing age. The decrease in the levels of α_{2u}-globulin in the urine of male Fischer F344 rats was correlated to a decrease in the synthesis of α_{2u}-globulin and a decrease in the mRNA levels and transcription of α_{2u}-globulin. Thus, the age-related decline in α_{2u}-globulin synthesis appears to arise from a decrease in the transcription of the α_{2u}-globulin genes. Dietary restriction, which increases the longevity of rodents, retards the age-related decline in α_{2u}-globulin expression. The regulation of α_{2u}-globulin expression by dietary restriction was again observed to occur primarily at the level of transcription.

Acknowledgements

This investigation was supported by grants AG 01548 and AG 04091 from the National Institutes of Health. The cDNA probe to α_{2u}-globulin was a gift from Dr Philip Feigelson.

References

1. Richardson, A. (1981). The relationship between aging and protein synthesis. In Florini, J. R. (ed.) *Handbook of Biochemistry in Aging*. pp. 79–101. (Boca Raton, Florida: CRC Press)
2. Richardson, A. and Birchenall-Sparks, M. C. (1983). Age-related changes in protein synthesis. In Rothstein, M. (ed.) *Review of Biological Research in Aging*. Vol. 1, pp. 255–73. (New York: Alan R. Liss)
3. Richardson, A., Roberts, M. S. and Rutherford, M. S. (1985). Aging and gene expression. In Rothstein, M. (ed.) *Review of Biological Research in Aging*. Vol. 2, pp. 395–419. (New York: Alan R. Liss)
4. Richardson, A. and Semsei, I. (1987). Effect of aging on translation and transcription. In Rothstein, M. (ed.) *Review of Biological Research in Aging*. Vol. 3. (New York: Alan R. Liss). (In press)
5. Ricca, G. A., Liu, D. S. H., Coniglio, J. J. and Richardson, A. (1978). Rates of protein synthesis by hepatocytes isolated from rats of various ages. *J. Cell. Physiol.*, **97**, 137–46
6. van Bezooijen, C. F. A., Grell, T. and Knook, D. L. (1977). The effect of age on protein synthesis by isolated liver parenchymal cells. *Mech. Age. Dev.*, **6**, 293–304

7. Coniglio, J. J., Liu, D. S. H. and Richardson, A. (1979). A comparison of protein synthesis by liver parenchymal cells isolated from Fischer F344 rats of various ages. *Mech. Age. Dev.*, **11**, 77–90

8. van Bezooijen, C. F. A., Grell, T. and Knook, D. L. (1976). Albumin synthesis by liver parenchymal cells isolated from young, adult, and old rats. *Biochem. Biophys. Res. Commun.*, **71**, 513–19

9. Roy, A. K., Nath, T. S., Motwani, N. M. and Chatterjee, B. (1983). Age-dependent regulation of the polymorphic forms of α_{2u}-globulin. *J. Biol. Chem.*, **258**, 10123–7

10. Chatterjee, B., Nath, T. S. and Roy, A. K. (1981). Differential regulation of the messenger RNA for three major senescence marker proteins in male rat liver. *J. Biol. Chem.*, **256**, 5939–41

11. Ricketts, W. G., Birchenall-Sparks, M. C., Hardwick, J. P. and Richardson, A. (1985). Effect of age and dietary restriction on protein synthesis by isolated kidney cells. *J. Cell. Physiol.*, **125**, 492–8

12. Dolan, K. P., Unterman, R., McLaughlin, M., Nakhasi, H. L., Lynch, K. R. and Fiegelson, P. (1982). The structure and expression of very closely related members of the α_{2u}-globulin gene family. *J. Biol. Chem.*, **257**, 13527–34

13. Richardson, A. (1985). The effect of age and nutrition on protein synthesis by cells and tissues from mammals. In Watson, R. R. (ed.) *Handbook of Nutrition in the Aged.* pp. 31–48. (Boca Raton, Florida: CRC Press)

14. O'Farrell, P. H. (1975). High resolution two-dimensional electrophoresis of proteins. *J. Biol. Chem.*, **250**, 4007–21

15. Laemmli, U. K. (1977). Cleavage of structural proteins during the assembly of the head of bacteriophage T4. *Nature*, **227**, 680–5

16. Rutherford, M. S., Baehler, C. S. and Richardson, A. (1986). Genetic expression of complement factors and α_1-acid glycoprotein by liver tissue during senescence. *Mech. Age. Dev.*, **35**, 245–54

17. Richardson, A., Butler, J. A., Rutherford, M. S., Semsei, I., Gu, M. Z., Fernandes, G. and Chiang, W. H. (1987). Effect of age and dietary restriction on the expression of α_{2u}-globulin. *J. Biol. Chem.*, **262**, 12821–5

4
Aging and disease

E. L. SCHNEIDER

INTRODUCTION

Today, record numbers of individuals are entering their seventh, eighth and ninth decades of life[1]. This trend will continue in all the developed nations on this planet. We have frequently heard about the growth of the number of individuals over the age 60 or 65. In the United States this group now comprises 12% of the population, up from 4% at the beginning of this century[1]. In Western Europe this number is even higher in certain countries. We are now beginning to witness a new development, the aging of the aged. The fastest growing age group in developed countries is the group aged 85 and above[1]. For physicians, this will have enormous consequences. Individuals in their sixties are largely a healthy population with only a small percentage, less than 5% requiring long-term care[1]. However, a considerably higher percentage, 35%, of individuals, in their eighties require substantial long-term care. A reflection of the disability of this age group is the finding that approximately 22% of this age group in the United States reside in nursing homes.

In this chapter, I will attempt to discuss the rationale for the separation of aging and disease with the full knowledge that this is not always possible. Since I have little background in gastroenterology and since our knowledge of the aging of the liver is small (it is expanded considerably in this volume), the examples that I will offer relate to other organ systems. However, I believe that the points to be made are quite valid for gastroenterology.

RATIONALE 1: THE NEED TO EXPLODE MYTHS RELATED TO AGING

Physicians and the general public have been exposed to decades of prejudice against aging[2]. This is reflected by the stereotype of the elderly individual as incompetent, incapable and incapacitated. Yet studies have shown that the vast majority of individuals over the age of 65 require little help in their activities of daily living[1]. The major causes of incompetency and incapacity are not aging processes but specific diseases that increase exponentially with aging, age-dependent diseases[3]. Examples of these conditions are Alzheimer's disease, Parkinson's disease and osteoarthritis.

Recognition that it is disease rather than aging that is the cause of disability is crucial to early diagnosis and the prevention of certain diseases. The best example is maculoretinal degeneration. This is the leading cause of blindness in individuals over the age of 65. The 'wet' form of this condition, in which neovascularization of the macular occurs, can be effectively treated by laser surgery[4]. If the diagnosis is made early in the course of this disease, blindness can frequently be prevented.

For many years, Alzheimer's disease was considered a rare disorder of relatively young individuals, those in their fifties and sixties. The common dementia seen in those individuals in their seventies and eighties was attributed to the aging process and was called 'senility'. Only in the last ten years have physicians realized that the most common cause of dementia in the last decades of life is Alzheimer's disease. Even more importantly, we have recognized that not all individuals develop dementia as they enter their eighties and nineties.

RATIONALE 2: ENCOURAGEMENT OF RESEARCH ON UNDER-INVESTIGATED CONDITIONS

Despite the enormous impact that age-dependent diseases have on an increasing proportion of our population, they have had relatively little research support until recently. The vast majority of disease-related research support was expended on the major killers: cardiovascular diseases and cancer. There was minimal support for the great disabling conditions such as Alzheimer's disease. The recognition that Alzheimer's disease rather than 'senility' is the cause of dementia in 2–3 million Americans has led to a 10-fold increase in support for this disease in the last 5 years in the United States[5]. However, we are still a long way from providing support proportional to the impact of this condition. In 1985, Alzheimer's disease resulted in direct costs[6] to Americans of $38 000 000 000. The research support for Alzheimer's disease that year was approximately $50 000 000 or about 0.1%[5]. It is projected that in the next century, the number of Alzheimer victims[7] will approach 10 000 000. If the costs for this condition increase proportionately, it will cost the United States about $200 000 000 000 which is the size of our biggest national budget deficit.

There are many other diseases and disorders which are still attributed to aging and have not received the research attention they deserve. An example is osteoarthritis, the most common cause of arthritis in those over the age of 65. This disease is the most common cause of disability in those over age 65, as measured by assessments of limitations in the activities of daily living[8]. Despite the importance of this condition, physicians often attribute the aches and pains from the joints of elderly patients to aging. However, osteoarthritis is no more a normal part of the aging process than Alzheimer's disease. Both are typical age-dependent diseases whose incidence and prevalence increase exponentially with aging and which merit research attention.

RATIONALE 3: PERMITS ADDITIONAL INSIGHT INTO THE NATURE OF AGING

Initial studies of the physiologic aspects of aging appeared to demonstrate that almost all physiological functions decline with aging[9]. However, many of these studies were flawed by two factors: the inclusion of many individuals with diseases in the older age groups and the inherent weakness of cross-sectional studies. Frequently these 'aging' studies compared young subjects, often laboratory workers and students, and older subjects, often clinic patients. Even excellently designed studies, like the Baltimore Longitudinal Study of Aging had the problem of including individuals with a number of diseases since increasing age is correlated with the accumulation of diseases. As an example, initial studies of cardiac output (represented by Cardiac Index in Figure 4.1A) suggested that this parameter declined with aging[9]. When this same population was screened for overt and latent coronary artery disease by stress electrocardiography and thallium scanning and only individuals free of disease were examined, no difference in cardiac output was found with aging[10] (Figure 4.1B).

Most studies of physiologic aging have been cross-sectional studies, that is, they involved examining individuals of all ages at a specific time. By contrast, longitudinal studies examine the same individual at different points in his/her lifespan. Cross-sectional studies can be confounded by cohort and secular trends. For example, a hypothetical cross-sectional study of computer skills might show differences with aging which are not due to the aging process but are due to the fact that the current cohort of young adults has had increased exposure to computers in their adolescence.

Cross-sectional studies of creatinine clearance in members of the Baltimore Longitudinal Study of Aging have shown an age-dependent decline in creatinine clearance[11]. However, longitudinal studies of these same individuals displayed three different patterns: individuals with an age-dependent decline that resembled that observed in cross-sectional studies, individuals that had a smaller decline in creatinine function than that observed in cross-sectional studies and individuals who exhibited no decline in creatinine clearance[12]. Therefore, this longitudinal study demonstrated that a decline in creatinine clearance is not an inevitable consequence of aging and raises the possibility that subtle age-dependent disease processes may affect this physiologic parameter.

RATIONALE 4: IMPROVES THE ATTITUDES OF PHYSICIANS CARING FOR OLDER PATIENTS

The medical profession has not been immune from bias against aging[2]. This has been manifested in the treatment of older patients as well as by the lack

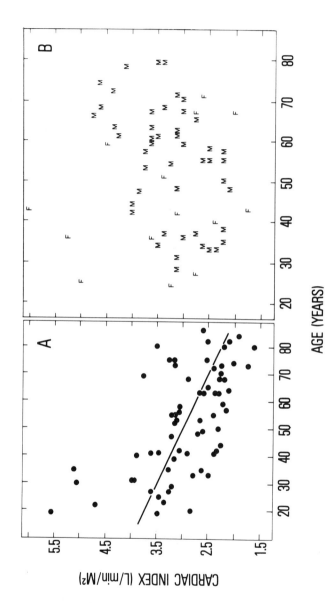

Figure 4.1 (A) The decline in various physiologic functions with aging. Note the apparent decline in cardiac index with aging. (From Brandfonbrener *et al.*[9]). (B) Cardiac output as a function of aging in individuals screened for coronary artery disease. Note no significant change in cardiac output with aging. M = male; F = female. (From Rodeheffer *et al.*[10])

of interest in the field of gerontology and geriatrics. There are many under-lying causes for this bias including the physician's own fear of growing old and the perception that care of the older patient is not as rewarding as the care of younger individuals in terms of personal satisfaction. Spokespersons for the field of geriatric medicine have tried to persuade physicians that older patients present a greater challenge; they have more diseases, take more prescription and non-prescription drugs and have more adverse drug responses[13]. However, the feeling still persists that it is more rewarding to deal with the younger patient with an acute disease than the older patient with multiple chronic conditions.

If physicians attribute the complaints of their older patients to aging, they will not only miss treatable and even curable conditions but they will also develop the attitude that aging is a series of inevitable unalterable losses of function. This attitude will certainly not promote a positive approach to their aged patients. By contrast, if vigorous attempts are made to discover the origin of a complaint and to restore function in disabled older individuals, a far more positive attitude will develop.

CAN WE ALWAYS SEPARATE AGING FROM DISEASE?

As I have indicated in this discussion, it is not always possible to make the separation of aging from disease. For example, with aging in humans, there is an accumulation in the cerebral cortex of senile plaques and neurofibrilla tangles, the hallmarks of Alzheimer's disease[14]. The age-dependent accumu-lation of these lesions can be so impressive that the cortex of a 'normal' 90-year-old individual can be difficult to discern from that of a 60-year-old with Alzheimer's disease. Are the plaques and tangles a normal part of the aging of the brain or does it represent a form of Alzheimer's disease?

This question can not be answered at this time. Perhaps further research can provide us with additional insight into the separation of disease from aging. However, for now, there are many age-dependent changes that occur with aging that are difficult to classify as being either caused by aging or by disease.

CONCLUDING COMMENTS

In this chapter, I have attempted to present a few rationales for the separation of disease from aging. It is clear that this cannot always be accomplished. Nevertheless, it provides an argument for the physician to vigorously search for a pathologic basis for the complaints of his/her older patients. If the physician recognizes that aging does not cause blindness, dementia or arthritis, he/she is prepared to find diseases which are treatable. If the phys-ician understands that the emphasis with many older patients needs to be on restoring function, there is an adequate challenge for his/her finest skills.

References

1. Guralnik, J. and Schneider, E. L. (1987). Prospects and implications of extending life expectancy. In Espenshade, T. J. and Stolnitz, G. J. (eds.). *Technological Prospects and Population Trends.* pp. 125–46 (Boulder, Colorado: Westview Press, Inc.)
2. Butler, R. N. (1975). *Why Survive? Being Old in America.* (New York: Harper & Row)
3. Brody, J. A. and Schneider, E. L. (1986). Diseases and disorders of aging: an hypothesis. *J. Chron. Dis.,* 39 (11), 871–6
4. Macular Photocoagulation Study Group (1982). Argon laser photocoagulation for senile macular degeneration. *Arch. Ophthalmol.,* **100,** 912–18
5. National Institute on Aging Annual Report 1986. (Bethesda, MD: United States Department of Health and Human Services)
6. Huang, L. F., Cartwright, W. and Hu, T. W. The Economic Cost of Senile Dementia in the United States, 1985. Public Health Reports. (In press)
7. Brody, J. A. (1985). Prospects for an aging population. *Nature,* **315,** 463–6
8. Manton, K. G. (1986). Past and future life expectancy increases at later ages: Their implications for the linkage of chronic morbidity, disability and mortality. *J. Geront.,* **41,** 672–81
9. Brandfonbrener, M., Landowne, M. and Shock, N. W. (1955). Changes in cardiac output with age. *Circulation,* **12,** 557
10. Rodeheffer, R. J., Gerstenblith, G., Becker, L. C. *et al.* (1984). Exercise cardiac output is maintained with advancing age in healthy human subjects: cardiac dilatation and increased stroke volume compensate for a diminished heart rate. *Circulation,* **69,** 203–13
11. Rowe, J. W., Tobin, J. D., Andres, R. A., Norris, A. and Shock, N. W. (1976). The effect of age on creatinine clearance. *J. Gerontol.,* **31,** 155–63
12. Lindeman, R. D., Tobin, J. D. and Shock, N. W. (1985). Longitudinal study on a rate of decline in renal function with age. *J. Am. Geriatr. Soc.,* **33,** 278–85
13. Schneider, E. L.. and Williams, T. F. (1985). Geriatrics and gerontology: Imperatives in education and training. *Ann. Intern. Med.,* **104,** 432–4
14. Tomlinson, B. E. (1972). Morphological brain changes in non-demented old people. In van Praag, H. M. and Kalverboer, A. F. (eds.) *Aging of the Central Nervous System: Biological and Psychological Aspects.* pp. 38–57. (Haarlem, The Netherlands: De Ervin F. Bohn NV)

5
Age-related alterations of proteins

D. GERSHON AND Y. KISO

Faulty enzyme molecules accumulate with age in cells *in vivo*. This phenomenon has been characterized by a 30–70% reduction in specific enzyme activity per unit of enzyme antigen as determined by immunotitration studies using

Table 5.1 Enzymes investigated for specific catalytic activity per unit antigen as a function of age

Enzyme	Source	Reference
A. Enzymes exhibiting reduced activity		
Aldolase A	Mouse striated muscle	18
Aldolase B	Mouse liver	19
Aldolase A	Rabbit erythrocyte, lens	20
Aldolase C	Rat lens	21
Isocitrate lyase	*Turbatrix aceti* (nematodes)	22
Enolase	*Turbatrix aceti* (nematodes)	23
Phosphoglycerate kinase	*Turbatrix aceti* (nematodes)	24
Aldolase	*Turbatrix aceti* (nematodes)	25
SOD	Rat liver, heart, brain, erythrocytes, lens	13, 26, 27
Lactic dehydrogenase	Rat liver	28
G6PD	Human erythrocytes	29
	Rat lens	2
Tyrosine aminotransferase	Mouse liver	30
3-Phosphoglycerate kinase (PGK)	Rat liver, brain, muscle	31
Glyceraldehyde-3-phosphate dehydrogenase	Rat striated muscle, lens	32, 33
B. Enzymes showing no reduced activity		
Tyrosine aminotransferase	Rat liver	34
Triose phosphate isomerase	*Turbatrix aceti*	35
Aldolase B	Mouse liver	36
Ornithine decarboxylase	Rat liver	37

antisera prepared against 'native' enzyme derived from young individuals. This has been described for a large number of enzymes in several organisms and tissue types. (Table 5.1) Other investigators have failed to find such an age-associated accumulation of faulty molecules (Table 5.1). It is our contention, however, that this accumulation with age is a universal phenomenon. These faulty molecules are not the result of errors introduced by the protein synthetic apparatus, i.e. misincorporation of amino acid residues, as was elegantly suggested by Orgel[1,2]. Random errors would lead to detectable alterations in properties of the enzyme molecules such as, K_m, K_i and total net charge, and would result in high levels of infidelity in DNA replication and transcription (see ref. 3 for an extensive discussion). However, such changes have not been detected in extensive studies conducted by our group[4] and that of Rothstein[5]. Also, no age-related infidelity of protein synthesis has ever been detected[6]. We thus conclude that the alterations in proteins which accumulate in cells of senescent organisms are of *post-translational* origin. We therefore, have been studying the nature of the alterations and the possible physiological consequences of the presence of these altered proteins in cells of aging organisms.

An early observation suggested a direction for our investigation of this phenomenon. In 1973, we found that in aging nematodes the half-lives of total soluble proteins and of aldolase were greatly extended[7]. Later studies confirmed these results for normal and amino acid analogue-bearing proteins in nematodes[8,9]. Similar observations were made in mouse liver for total proteins, for subcellular fractions and specifically for aldolase B[10,11] and other

Table 5.2 Half-life of protein as a function of age

Protein	Organism and tissue	Half-life (h)		Reference
		young	old	
A. Total proteins (cellular fraction)				
Nuclear	Mouse liver	38	75	10
Mitochondrial	Mouse liver	44	72	10
Lysosomal	Mouse liver	24	50	10
Microsomal	Mouse liver	30	38	10
Total soluble	Mouse liver	46	74	10
Total soluble	*Turbatrix aceti* (nematodes)	24–30	200–250	8
B. Individual proteins				
Isocitrate lyase	*Turbatrix aceti* (nematodes)	45–50	250–300	7
Aldolase	*Turbatrix aceti* (nematodes)	30–40	160–180	7
Enolase	*Turbatrix aceti* (nematodes)	10	>240	9
Orthinine decarboxylas	Mouse liver	0.16	0.33	30
Aldolase B	Mouse liver	25.6	37	10

enzymes (Table 5.2). The rate of degradation of puromycinyl peptides also was shown to be at least seven-fold slower in livers of old mice[11]. We have consequently suggested that faulty enzyme molecules that accumulate with age might be inactive molecules which are the normal intermediates of degradation. With age, the removal of these intermediates becomes very inefficient due to alterations in the degradation system itself[12]. In order to study this hypothesis we needed to devise means of identifying the altered molecules and distinguishing them from 'native' active forms. Following our hypothesis that altered molecules could perhaps have denatured domains which distinguish them from intact 'native' forms, an attempt was made to prepare specific antibodies which might preferentially interact with denatured, and thus presumably altered, regions of the molecules without interaction with those molecules with intact conformation. In order to avoid cross-reactivity between molecules with denatured domains and 'native' forms, purified enzyme was boiled in SDS and mercaptoethanol immediately before injection into rabbits in order to prevent the molecules from refolding into their 'native' conformation. Polyclonal antibodies were thus obtained against denatured molecules of purified rat and human cytosolic superoxide dismutases (SOD), glyceraldehyde-3-phosphate dehydrogenase (GAPD), glucose-6-phosphate dehydrogenase (G6PD), liver aldolase B and brain aldolase C. These antibodies have been compared in our recent studies to antibodies which had previously been prepared against the 'native' form of these enzymes.

Studies of SOD in liver and lens are examples of the approach we adopted. Immunotitration with anti-native SOD antibodies (ANA) showed that in liver homogenates of old rats and in old parts of rat lenses there was a considerable proportion of defective molecules (Figure 5.1). These results confirmed our original observations[13,14]. However, when homogenates of these organs first were subjected to incubation with anti-denatured SOD antibody (ADA), precipitated, and then titrated with ANA, the 'young' and 'old' preparations became essentially identical with regard to specific activity of SOD (Figure 5.1). It is important to note that ADA neither inactivated nor precipitated any SOD activity; full activity was completely retained in these preparations after the incubation with ADA and prior to the incubation with ANA. ADA thus removed cross-reactive material lacking catalytic activity without affecting 'native' forms of the enzyme. Results of similar studies using anti-denatured and anti-'native' antisera to aldolase B, aldolase C and GAPD have shown essentially similar results[15].

The use of ADA to aldolase B in Western blot analysis of proteins of liver and kidney showed that partially denatured, intact enzyme molecules existed in the liver. Very significantly, truncated peptides of aldolase B were also identified by this analysis in liver and kidney homogenates of young and old animals[16]. The peptide pattern was identical in all ages, however, 'old' homogenates contained much larger quantities of these truncated forms which we suggest are degradation intermediates. The quantitative differences are apparently due to reduced efficiency of the degradation system in cells of old organisms (see ref. 15 for detailed discussion).

Current studies are being conducted which aim to elucidate the nature of modifications which render a protein molecule more prone to denaturation intracellularly. We also are investigating the question of whether or not specific domains in protein molecules are initially denatured as a prerequisite for intracellular proteolysis. Furthermore, we are evaluating the possibility that the proteases involved in intracellular protein degradation can be identified. This will lead to an understanding of the causes of their age-related decline in activity which is responsible for the observed reduction in the rate

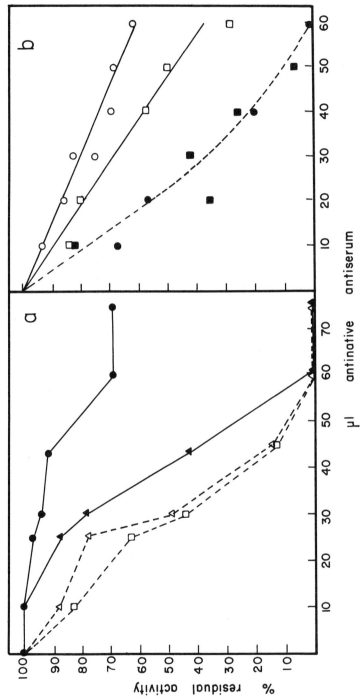

Figure 5.1 Immunoprecipitation of SOD with anti-native antiserum, with and without pre-incubation of tissue homogenates with anti-denatured SOD antiserum. (a) Liver homogenates of young (6 months) and old (27 months) rats: ▲——▲, ●——● Immunotitration with ANA of SOD from young and old rat livers, respectively; △--△, □--□ Immunotitration with ANA following pre-incubation with ADA of SOD from young and old rat, respectively. (b) Lens homogenates of young (4 months) and old (30 months) rats: ○——○, □——□ Immunotitration with ANA of SOD from young and old rat lenses, respectively; ○---○, ■---■ Immunotitration with ANA following pre-incubation with ADA of SOD from young and old rats, respectively

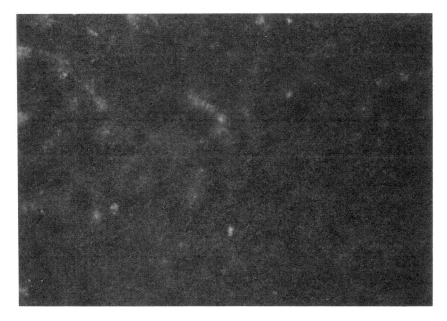

Figure 5.2 Immunostaining of young liver (5 months) with ADA against denatured aldolase B (× 120)

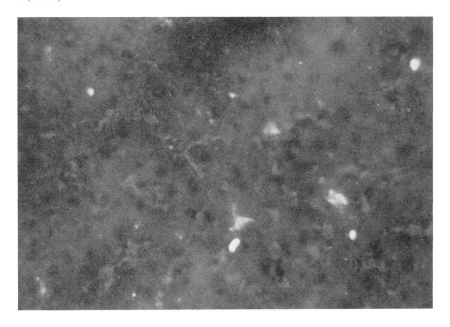

Figure 5.3 Immunostaining of old liver (34 months) with ADA against denatured aldolase B (× 120)

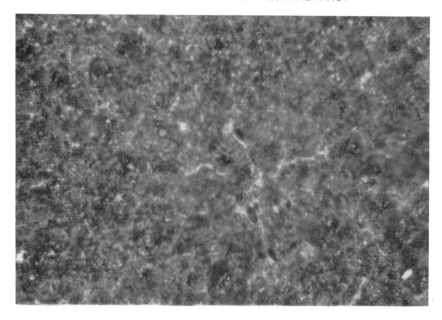

Figure 5.4 Immunostaining of young liver (5 months) with a Mab against denatured aldolase B (× 120)

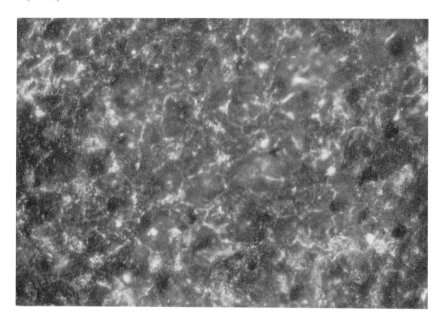

Figure 5.5 Immunostaining of old liver (34 months) with a Mab against denatured aldolase B (× 120)

of protein degradation. For all of these purposes it was decided to prepare monoclonal antibodies (Mabs) against denatured molecules of specific enzymes. If Mabs against various domains (sequences) in a denatured enzyme molecule are obtained it will be possible to identify those domains which denature intracellularly and the nature of the modifications which cause this denaturation. Also, the sub-cellular distribution of denatured enzyme molecules can be discerned by immune-histochemical studies.

Thirty-one Mab hybridomas have been produced against denatured aldolase B from rat liver and are being characterized. Some were shown to specifically interact with denatured aldolase B but not to inactivate nor precipitate active enzyme molecules and some identify peptides derived from aldolase by controlled proteolysis with *S. aureus* V8 protease. We anticipate that some of the 31 clones will be suitable for denatured domain analysis of aldolase molecules derived from liver.

ADA and several Mabs against denatured aldolase B have been used in immune-histochemical studies of sections from young and old frozen livers under conditions in which hepatic fine structure was well preserved. The sections were incubated with either ADA or Mab then with either FITC-conjugated goat anti-rabbit IgG antibody or FITC-conjugated goat anti-mouse IgG (H + L). Immunofluorescence with ADA was observed along the cytoplasmic membrane in both young and old livers (Figures 5.2 and 5.3); however, the intensity of fluorescence was much greater in the old. Sinusoidal cells and erythrocytes remained unstained (Figures 5.2 and 5.3).

Six Mabs already have been examined immunohistochemically in sections of young (5 month) and old (34 month) rat livers. Five have shown a pattern of interaction similar to that observed with ADA whereas the sixth Mab binds with a pattern following that of cytoskeletal proteins (Figures 5.4 and 5.5), noticeable only in old livers. This probably speaks against fortuitous cross-reactivity with unrelated proteins as was reported with anti-p60[src] Mab which cross-reacted with four unrelated cellular proteins, three of which were cytoskeletal[17]. Further studies are required to expand these data and to interpret their meaning. Generally, however, young cells do not store many denatured molecules while these accumulate in old cells.

Acknowledgements

The work presented here has been supported by U.S. PHS Grant AG 00459. D.G. is holder of the Skillman Foundation Chair in Biomedical Sciences. Y.K. is holder of a Lady Davis Post-doctoral Fellowship.

References

1. Orgel, L. E. (1963). The maintenance of the accuracy of protein synthesis and its relevance to aging. *Proc. Natl. Acad. Sci. USA*, **49**, 517–20
2. Dovrat, A., Scharf, Y., Eisenbach, L. and Gershon, D. (1986). G6PD molecules devoid of catalytic activity are present in the nucleus of the rat lens. *Exp. Eye Res.*, **42**, 489–96
3. Gershon, D. (1987). The 'error catastrophe' theory of ageing and its implications. In Warner, H. (ed.). *Modern Theories of Aging*. pp. 135–137. (New York: Raven Press)

4. Gershon, D. (1979). Current status of age-altered enzymes: alternative mechanisms. *Mech. Age. Dev.*, **9**, 189–96

5. Rothstein, M. (1983). Detection of altered proteins. In Adelman, R. C. and Roth, G. S. (eds.). *Altered Proteins in Aging*. pp. 1–9. (Boca Raton, Florida: CRC Press)

6. Hirsch, G. (1983). Measurement methods in aging research. In Adelman R. C. and Roth, G. S. (eds.) *Altered Proteins in Aging*. pp. 35–54. (Boca Raton, Florida: CRC Press)

7. Zeelon, P. E., Gershon, H. and Gershon, D. (1973). Defective aldolase in aging nematodes. Properties of the enzyme. *Biochemistry*, **12**, 1743–50

8. Reznick, A. Z. and Gershon, D. (1979). The effect of age on the protein degradation system in the nematode *T. aceti*. *Mech. Age. Dev.*, **11**, 403–15

9. Sharma, H. K., Prasanna, H. R., Lane, R. S. and Rothstein, M. (1979). The effect of age on enolase turnover in the free-living nematode, *T. aceti*. *Arch. Biochem. Biophys.*, **194**, 275–81

10. Reznick, A. Z., Lavie, L., Gershon, H. and Gershon, D. (1981). Age-associated accumulation of altered FDP aldolase B in mice. *FEBS Lett.*, **128**, 221–4

11. Lavie, L., Reznick, A. Z. and Gershon, D. (1982). Decreased protein and puromycinyl peptide degradation in livers of senescent mice. *Bioch. J.*, **202**, 47–51

12. Gershon, D., Reznick, A. Z. and Reiss, U. (1979). Characterization and possible effects of age-associated alterations in enzymes and proteins. In Cherkin, A. (ed.) *Physiology and Cell Biology of Ageing*. pp. 21–26. (New York: Raven Press)

13. Dovrat, A. and Gershon, D. (1981). Rat lens SOD and G6PD: studies on the catalytic activity and the fate of enzyme antigen as a function of age. *Exp. Eye Res.* **33**, 651–61

14. Reiss, U. and Gershon, D. (1976). Rat liver SOD: purification and age-related modifications. *Eur. J. Biochem.*, **63**, 617–23

15. Reznick, A. Z., Dovrat, A., Rosenfelder, L., Shpund, S. and Gershon, D. (1985). Defective enzyme molecules in cells of aging animals are partially denatured, totally inactive, normal degradation intermediates. In Adelman, R. C. (ed.) *Modification of Proteins during Aging*. pp. 69–81. (New York: Alan R. Liss, Inc.)

16. Reznick, A. Z., Rosenfelder, L., Shpund, S. and Gershon, D. (1985). Identification of intracellular degradation intermediates of aldolase B by antiserum to the denatured enzyme. *Proc. Natl. Acad. Sci. USA*, **82**, 6114–18

17. Nigg, E. A., Walter, G. and Singer, S. J. (1982). On the nature of crossreactions observed with antibodies directed to defined epitopes. *Proc. Natl. Acad. Sci. USA*, **79**, 5939–43

18. Gershon, H. and Gershon, D. (1973). Altered enzyme molecules in senescent organisms: mouse muscle aldolase. *Mech. Age. Dev.* **2**, 33–38

19. Gershon, H. and Gershon, D. (1973). Inactive enzyme molecules in ageing mice: liver aldolase. *Proc. Natl. Acad. Sci. USA*, **70**, 909–13

20. Mennecier, F. and Dreyfus, J. C. (1974). Molecular ageing of fructose biphosphate aldolase in tissues of rabbit and man. *Biochim. Biophys. Acta*, **364**, 320–8

21. Dovrat, A. and Gershon, D. (1983). Studies on the fate of aldolase molecules in the ageing rat lens. *Biochim. Biophys. Acta*, **757**, 164–7

22. Gershon, H. and Gershon, D. (1970). Detection of inactive enzyme molecules in ageing organisms. *Nature*, **227**, 1214–17

23. Sharma, H. K., Gupta, S. K. and Rothstein, M. (1976). Age-related alteration of enolase in the free-living nematode *Turbatrix aceti*. *Arch. Biochem. Biophys.*, **174**, 324–30

24. Gupta, S. K. and Rothstein, M. (1976) Phosphoglycerate kinase from young and old *Turbatrix aceti*. *Arch. Biochem. Biophys.*, **445**, 632–8

25. Reznick, A. Z. and Gershon, D. (1977). Age-related alterations in purified fructose-1-phosphate aldolase from the nematode *Turbatrix aceti*. *Mech. Age. Dev.*, **6**, 345–53

26. Reiss, U. and Gershon, D. (1976). Comparison of cytoplasmic superoxide dismutase in liver, heart and brain of aging rats and mice. *Biochem. Biophys. Res. Commun.*, **73**, 255–62

27. Glass, G. A. and Gershon, D. (1981). Enzymatic changes in rat erythrocytes with increasing cell and donor age: loss of SOD activity associated with increases in catalytically defective forms. *Biochem. Biophys. Res. Commun.*, **103**, 1245–53

28. Dreyfus, J. C., Kahn, A. and Schapira, F. (1983). Molecular mechanisms of alterations of some enzymes in aging. In Adelman, R. C. and Roth, G. S. (eds.) *Altered Proteins and Aging*. pp. 113–133. (Boca Raton, Florida: CRC Press)

29. Kahn, A. and Dreyfus, J. C. (1974). Purification of G6PD from red blood cells and from human leukocytes. *Biochim. Biophys. Acta*, **334**, 257–64

30. Jacobus, S. and Gershon, D. (1980). Age-related changes in inducible mouse liver enzymes: ornithine decarboxylase and tyrosine aminotransferase. *Mech. Age. Dev.*, **12**, 311–22
31. Sharma, H. K., Prasanna, H. R. and Rothstein, M. (1980). Altered phosphoglycerate kinase in aging rats. *J. Biol. Chem.*, **255**, 5043–8
32. Gafni, A. (1983). Molecular origin of the ageing effects in glyceraldehyde-3-phosphate dehydrogenase. *Biochim. Biophys. Acta*, **742**, 91–7
33. Dovrat, A., Scharf. A. and Gershon, D. (1984). Glyceraldehyde-3-phosphate dehydrogenase activity in rat and human lenses and the fate of enzyme molecules in the aging lens. *Mech. Age. Dev.*, **28**, 87–91
34. Weber, A., Guguen-Gullouze, C., Szajnert, M. F., Beck, G. and Schapira, F. (1980). Tyrosine aminotransferase in senescent rat liver. *Gerontology*, **126**, 9–16
35. Gupta, S. K. and Rothstein, M. (1976). Triose phosphate isomerase from young and old *T. aceti*. *Arch. Biochem. Biophys.*, **174**, 333–40
36. Weber, A., Gregori, C. and Schapira, F. (1976). Aldolase B in the liver of senescent rats. *Biochim. Biophys. Acta*, **444**, 810–17
37. Obenrader, M. F. and Prouty, W. F. (1977). Production of monospecific antibodies to rat liver ornithine carboxylase and their use in turnover studies. *J. Biol. Chem.*, **252**, 2866–72
38. Orgel, L. E. (1970). The maintenance of the accuracy of protein synthesis and its relevance to aging: a correction. *Proc. Natl. Acad. Sci. USA*, **67**, 1476

6
Adaptation in aging: lessons from receptor studies

I. B. ABRASS

INTRODUCTION

During senescence many hormonal responses decrease. Some do not change in old age but may be altered earlier in life, and there are a few in which responsiveness actually increases[1-3]. For the great majority, however, responsiveness declines either over the entire life span or during the post-maturational phase. Variations may be explained by the different rates at which individual cells, tissues and functions age.

A particular hormonally responsive system may be altered in aging at one or more levels. In complex tissues, which contain heterogeneous cell populations, changes could be due to a loss or gain of a particular cell type. Compared to simple fluctuations in cell numbers, altered molecular mechanisms could include biochemical processes within responsive cells. The *milieu interieur* of the organism could also influence hormonal responsiveness and result in either cellular or molecular changes, or both. The data for aging changes must therefore be considered in light of these mechanisms.

Molecular mechanisms of hormone actions in aging have received much attention. To consider these it is necessary to understand how hormones work. Steroid hormones with cytoplasmic receptors and hormones with cell-surface receptors have differing modes of action. Steroid hormones bind to specific cytoplasmic receptors after passively diffusing through the plasma membrane[4]. The receptor–hormone complexes are then translocated to the nucleus, where they attach to acceptor proteins or chromatin, inducing messenger RNA synthesis with subsequent synthesis of specific proteins. Cell surface-active hormones bind initially to specific cell membrane receptors[5]. Receptors for some of these hormones, e.g. catecholamines and glucagon, are linked to the enzyme adenylate cyclase. Binding of the hormone to its specific receptor activates this enzyme, which converts adenosine triphosphate (ATP) to cyclic adenosine monophosphate (cAMP). Cyclic AMP, in turn, activates protein kinase, which phosphorylates several proteins and leads to a number of biological effects. Other cell surface-active hormones, such as insulin, do not activate adenylate cyclase; although they may activate a tyrosine kinase, their other immediate biochemical events are largely unknown.

Many hormone actions and the subsequent biochemical events have been examined with regard to biological changes of aging. However, most studies on changes in the molecular mechanisms of hormone action during aging have been directed at hormone receptors[2,6]. This chapter will deal mainly with these studies, since receptor binding is the initial step in the mechanism of hormonal action and the biological response to hormones is largely dependent on the receptor–hormone complexes[4,5].

Receptors are protein molecules located either intracellularly or on plasma membrane. As opposed to binding proteins, receptors transduce information upon binding of the appropriate ligand (the molecule that forms a complex with a receptor). Such receptors are generally measured by incubating either whole cells or cytoplasmic, nuclear or membrane preparations with radioactive ligands, e.g. hormones, neurotransmitters or pharmacological agents, in the presence or absence of excess unlabelled hormone so that specific binding can be determined. Bound and unbound ligands are then separated by techniques such as charcoal absorption, gel filtration or membrane filtration. Finally, the samples are counted by scintillation spectrometry. Receptors must meet certain defined characteristics, such as time kinetics, saturability, specificity and, where appropriate, stereospecificity.

There have been many published investigations of hormone receptor changes during adulthood and senescence[2,6]. Most show that there are decreased concentrations of receptors during this stage of life. Many hormones have been analysed in human and animal cells and tissues, including corticosteroids, androgens, oestrogens, insulin, beta-adrenergic agonists, acetylcholine, gonadotropins, and dopamine and their respective target tissues. Four areas representative of the results, problems and controversies involved in hormone receptor changes in aging are glucose tolerance and insulin receptors, myocardial responsiveness and beta-adrenergic receptors, brain neurotransmitter receptors and adipocyte glucocorticoid receptors.

INSULIN RECEPTORS

It is generally agreed that glucose tolerance deteriorates with age[7]. Total insulin secretion and timing have been reported as similar in both old and young people, and therefore do not account for reduced glucose tolerance. However, the 'glucose clamp' technique, an indicator of peripheral sensitivity to insulin, demonstrates that the metabolic effect of insulin decreases with age[8]. This finding supports the hypothesis of a relative insulin resistance in the aged. Various mechanisms for this resistance have been proposed, including changes in insulin receptors.

The data on human insulin receptors with age are conflicting, although most investigators generally agree that changes in insulin receptors do not account for glucose intolerance. In a study of *in vivo* fibroblast aging, it was demonstrated that fibroblast insulin receptors actually increased with age[9]. In a presumably comparable study, an age-related loss of fibroblast insulin receptors was reported[10]. The latter investigation employed exponentially-growing cells, while the former used cells at confluency, when growth is inhibited by cell contact. In the study by Ito and coworkers[10], age differences were abolished if confluent cells were used. Whether confluent or growing cells are more appropriate for such studies is not clear, although a third study also has shown no age-associated differences in fibroblast insulin receptors[11]. In isolated lymphocytes[12] and circulating monocytes[13,14] insulin receptors also were reported to be unchanged with age.

When insulin receptors of fat cells from subcutaneous adipose tissue removed during elective laparotomy were studied, it was reported that these receptors were decreased in fat cells from older subjects[15]. The subjects were presumed to be metabolically healthy and of normal weight, but no data on their adiposity were reported. In studies of isolated adipocytes obtained on open biopsy of subcutaneous adipose tissue from healthy non-obese subjects, insulin binding was similar in the elderly and non-elderly groups[14].

These data do not preclude the possibility that insulin receptors are decreased in elderly individuals. However, they suggest that the reductions are more likely to be related to the *milieu* than to an intrinsic aging defect.

BETA-ADRENERGIC RECEPTORS

Myocardial responsiveness to stress and exercise is diminished in older humans and animals[16]. Both chronotropic (heart rate) and inotropic (force of contraction) responses to beta-adrenergic agonists are decreased with age[16-21]. Heart rate response to electrical stimulation and contractile response to calcium are, however, unaffected by age, which suggests that the intrinsic myocardial mechanism remains intact while the beta-adrenergic pathway is altered. Studies were therefore directed to the initial step of beta-adrenergic action, namely, the receptor. It was demonstrated that both beta-adrenergic receptor number and receptor antagonist affinity in hearts from senescent rats were unaltered[20,21]. However, agonist affinity does diminish with age in rat myocardium[22,23].

The next step in the proposed mechanism of beta-adrenergic action in myocardium is activation of adenylate cyclase with the formation of cAMP from ATP and the activation of cAMP-dependent protein kinase. Although unaltered stimulation of cAMP levels and protein kinase activation by beta-adrenergic agonists in aged-rat heart have been reported[21], we have found diminished myocardial adenylate cyclase activity in senescent rats, which may at least in part account for decreased myocardial beta-adrenergic responsiveness in aging[24].

The lymphocyte has been used as a marker for changes in the beta-adrenergic pathway, since myocardium is not easily accessible in man. As in the rat myocardium, we found human lymphocyte beta-adrenergic receptor numbers to be the same in old and young[25]. A study by others supports our results[26]. Although receptor number is unaltered, agonist affinity does diminish with age[27]. Since studies with human lymphocyte receptors or with rat myocardium showed no change in beta-adrenergic receptors, we investigated lymphocyte adenylate cyclase activity and found that it diminished with age. This suggests that diminished adenylate cyclase activity may account for altered catecholamine responsiveness also in this cell[28].

It appears, therefore, that receptor changes in rat myocardium and human lymphocyte do not alone account for the decreased beta-adrenergic responsiveness of aging, and that a post-receptor alteration needs to also be invoked.

BRAIN NEUROTRANSMITTER RECEPTORS

Dopamine receptors

The striatal dopaminergic system is progressively altered during aging with both degeneration and reduced responsiveness[29]. Such alterations in the basal ganglia are thought to be related to the increase of abnormal movements in the elderly[30]. The recent availability of radiolabelled dopamine antagonists, such as [³H]-spiroperidol, has made possible determinations of dopamine receptors in the aging brain. A marked loss of neostriatal dopamine receptors in aging animals has been reported[31-33] and investigations into the sensitivity of dopamine-stimulated adenylate cyclase in rat caudate nucleus and corpus striatum have revealed decreased enzyme activity over the maturational to postmaturational portion of the life span[34,35].

The difficulty of interpreting receptor changes in complex tissues composed of heterogeneous cell populations is evident. Since with age there is a significant decrement of neurons in the brain areas studied, the change in neurotransmitter responsiveness and the decrease in receptor number could be due to loss of a particular cell type, rather than to altered molecular mechanisms. Whether these changes in dopaminergic responsiveness are due to cellular loss or biochemical alterations does not detract from recent data demonstrating that they are preventable. Of the attempts to retard the aging process, only dietary restriction has extended life span in mammals[36]. (See also Chapter 7.) When the effects of dietary restriction on the normal age-related loss of dopamine receptors from rat corpus striatum were examined[37], it was found that as rats aged from 3 to 24 months, the progressive decrease in dopamine receptor concentration was substantially retarded in the brains of 24-month-old animals maintained on restricted diets after weaning.

Cholinergic receptors

Senile dementia of the Alzheimer type is associated with substantial atrophy of the cerebral cortex and hippocampus. Despite evidence for loss of central cholinergic neurons in Alzheimer's dementia[38,39], the cortical post-synaptic cholinergic receptors appear to be relatively intact in dementia[40,41].

Cholinergic input is decreased in senile dementia; post-synaptic cholinergic receptors are preserved. One therapeutic approach to this disease, therefore, has been to increase the acetylcholine delivered to the post-synaptic site by administering acetylcholine precursors, cholinergic agonists and/or acetylcholinesterase inhibitors. Some of the early experiments with dietary choline have not been as encouraging as anticipated, but solving the problems related to administration of cholinergic agonists and acetylcholinesterase inhibitors may bring more satisfactory results.

Beta-adrenergic receptors

As with dopaminergic receptors, decreased beta-adrenergic receptors have been reported in several parts of the aging rat brain, particularly the cerebellum and corpus striatum[42]. Again, these types of receptor studies are difficult to interpret, since they examine complex tissues which contain heterogeneous cell populations.

Following denervation, decreased neural input or treatment with antagonists, post-synaptic tissue becomes supersensitive to agonist stimulation. This supersensitivity is associated with an increase in post-synaptic receptor number. Denervation supersensitivity response appears to be blunted in the aging brain. Beta-adrenergic receptors are unaltered in the rat pineal gland with age[42]; catecholaminergic input to the pineal is regulated by light–dark cycles with concomitant regulation of beta-adrenergic receptors. This light–dark cycle regulation of pineal beta-adrenergic receptor number is lost in aging rats[42]. When cortical catecholamines are depleted by the administration of reserpine, young rats demonstrate beta-adrenergic receptor up-regulation. This regulatory response is blunted in aged rats[43]. If the inability of aged animals to up-regulate neurotransmitter receptors during receptor blockade is applicable to humans, it may explain, at least in part, the increased incidence of side effects from receptor antagonists in the elderly.

Other neurotransmitter receptor losses, such as serotonin receptors in the rabbit cortex, have been described[33]. However, interpretation of these data suffers from the same criticisms made earlier.

GLUCOCORTICOID RECEPTORS

The assessment of glucocorticoid action during adipocyte aging involves a cytoplasmic steroid hormone receptor in a tissue that has a relatively static cell number over most of the adult rat life span. The work in this area is essentially from a single laboratory and has been recently reviewed[44]. The studies have avoided some of the criticisms made earlier about heterogeneous cell populations, since collagenase digestion of rat epididymal fat pad yields a reasonably homogeneous population of cells. Differences with age cannot be due to shifts in cell populations or loss of a particular cell type.

Glucocorticoids are important regulators of adipocyte energy metabolism. When isolated rat epididymal fat-pad adipocytes are exposed to dexamethasone, glucose oxidation is inhibited. The extent of this inhibition is progressively reduced with increasing age[45]. Because receptor binding of glucocorticoids and responsiveness of inhibition of glucose oxidation in this tissue are closely linked, receptor concentrations were assessed in adipocytes obtained from rats of different ages. Glucocorticoid receptor levels were found to be progressively reduced with increasing age[45]. The data were the same when expressed as per cell or per milligram of protein.

The age-related loss of glucocorticoid receptors could be due to increased receptor degradation or decreased receptor synthesis. Glucocorticoid receptors were labelled by exposing isolated adipocytes to radioactive amino acids and isolating the receptors by affinity chromatography. The rate of synthesis of the putative glucocorticoid receptor in old cells was found to be less than half of that for mature adipocytes, whereas total protein synthesis was unaltered[46].

Thus these studies have demonstrated diminished adipocyte glucocorticoid responsiveness associated with reduced glucocorticoid receptors possibly due to a decrease in the biosynthesis rate of the specific hormone receptor.

References

1. Roth, G. S. (1975). Changes in hormone binding and responsiveness in target cells and tissues during aging. *Adv Exp. Med. Biol.,* **61**, 195–208
2. Roth, G. S. (1979). Hormone action during aging: alterations and mechanisms. *Mech. Age. Dev.,* **9**, 497–514
3. Finch, C. E. (1976). The regulation of physiological changes during mammalian aging. *Q. Rev. Biol.,* **51**, 59–83
4. King, R. J. B. and Mainwaring, W. I. P. (1974). *Steroid–Cell Interactions.* (Baltimore, MD: University Park Press)
5. Cuatrecasas, P. (1974). Membrane receptors. *Annu. Rev. Biochem.,* **43**, 169–214
6. Roth, G. S. (1979). Hormone receptor changes during adulthood and senescence: significance for aging research. *Fed. Proc.,* **38**, 1910–14
7. Davidson, M. G. (1979). The effect of aging on carbohydrate metabolism. A review of the English literature and a practical approach to the diagnosis of diabetes mellitus in the elderly. *Metabolism,* **28**, 688–705
8. DeFronzo, R. A. (1979). Glucose intolerance and aging. Evidence for tissue insensitivity to insulin. *Diabetes,* **28**, 1095–101
9. Rosenbloom, A. Goldstein, S. and Yip, C. C. (1976). Insulin binding to cultured human fibroblasts increases with normal and precocious aging. *Science,* **193**, 412–15
10. Ito, H., Orimo, H. and Shimada, H. (1976). Reduced insulin action *in vitro* and the binding of ^{125}I-insulin to the cultured human skin fibroblasts with aging. *Abstracts of 5th International Congress of Endocrinology (Hamburg),* p. 261
11. Hollenberg, M. D. and Schneider, E. L. (1979). Receptors for insulin and epidermal growth factor-urogastrone in adult human fibroblasts do not change with donor age. *Mech. Age. Dev.,* **11**, 37–43
12. Helderman, J. H. (1980). Constancy of pharmacokinetic properties of the lymphocyte insulin receptor during aging. *J. Gerontol.,* **35**, 329–34
13. Rowe, J. W., Minaker, K. L., Pollata, J. A. and Fleir, J. S. (1983). Characterization of the insulin resistance of aging. *J. Clin. Invest.,* **71**, 1581–7
14. Fink, R. I., Kolterman, O. G., Griffin, J. and Olefsky, J. M. (1983). Mechanisms of insulin resistance in aging. *J. Clin. Invest.,* **71**, 1523–35
15. Pagano, G., Cassander, M., Diana, A., Pisu, E., Bozzo, C., Ferrero, F. and Lenti, G. (1981). Insulin resistance in the aged: the role of the peripheral insulin receptors. *Metabolism,* **30**, 46–9
16. Lakatta, E. G. (1978). Perspectives on the aged myocardium. *Advances in Experimental Medicine and Biology, Philadelphia Symposium on Aging,* **97**, 147–69
17. Lakatta, E. G., Gerstenblith, G., Angell, C. S., Shock, N. W. and Weisfeldt, M. L. (1975).

Diminished inotropic response of aged myocardium to catecholamines. *Circ. Res.*, **36**, 262–9

18. Vestal, R. E., Wood, A. J. J. and Shand, D. G. (1979). Reduced beta-adrenoceptor sensitivity in the elderly. *Clin. Pharmacol. Ther.*, **26**, 181–6

19. Yin, F. C., Spurgeon, H. A., Greene, H. L., Lakatta, E. G. and Weisfeldt, M. L. (1979). Age-associated decrease in heart rate response to isoproterenol in dogs. *Mech. Age. Dev.*, **10**, 17–25

20. Abrass, J. B., Davis, J. L. and Scarpace, P. J. (1982). Isoproterenol responsiveness and myocardial beta-adrenergic receptors in young and old rats. *J. Gerontol.*, **37**, 156–60

21. Guarnieri, T., Filburn, C. R., Zitnik, G. Roth, G. and Lakatta, E. G. (1980). Contractile and biochemical correlates of beta-adrenergic stimulation of the aged heart. *Am. J. Physiol.*, **239**, H501–H508

22. Narayanan, N. and Derby, J. (1982). Alteration in the properties of beta-adrenergic receptors of myocardial membranes in aging: impairment in agonist–receptor interactions and guanine nucleotide regulation accompany diminished catecholamine responsiveness of adenylate cyclase. *Mech. Age. Dev.*, **19**, 127–39

23. Scarpace, P. J. and Abrass, I. B. (1986). Beta-adrenergic agonist-mediated desensitization in senescent rats. *Mech. Age. Dev.*, **35**, 255–64

24. O'Connor, S. W., Scarpace, P. J. and Abrass, I. B. (1981). Age-associated decrease of adenylate cyclase activity in rat myocardium. *Mech. Age. Dev.*, **16**, 91–5

25. Abrass, I. B. and Scarpace, P. J. (1981). Human lymphocyte beta-adrenergic receptors are unaltered with age. *J. Gerontol.*, **36**, 298–301

26. Landmann, R., Bittiger, H. and Buhler, F. R. (1981). High affinity beta-adrenergic receptors in mononuclear leukocytes: similar density in young and old normal subjects. *Life Sci.*, **29**, 1761–71

27. Feldman, R. D., Limbird, L. E., Nadeau, J., Robertson, D. and Wood, A. J. J. (1984). Alterations in leukocyte beta-receptor affinity with aging: a potential explanation for altered beta-adrenergic sensitivity in the elderly. *N. Engl. J. Med.*, **310**, 815–19

28. Abrass, I. B. and Scarpace, P. J. (1982). Catalytic unit of adenylate cyclase: reduced activity in aged human lymphocytes. *J. Clin. Endocrinol. Metab.*, **55**, 1026–8

29. McGeer, P. L., McGeer, E. G. and Suzuki, J. S. (1977). Aging and extrapyramidal function. *Arch. Neurol.*, **34**, 33–5

30. Potvin, A. R., Syndulko, K., Tourtellotte, W. W., Lemmon, J. A. and Potvin, J. H. (1980). Human neurological function and the normal aging process. *J. Am. Geriatr. Soc.*, **28**, 1–9

31. Govoni, S., Memo, M., Saiani, L., Spano, P. F. and Trabucchi, M. (1980). Impairment of brain neurotransmitter receptors in aged rats. *Mech. Age. Dev.*, **12**, 39–46

32. Severson, J. A. and Finch, C. E. (1980). Reduced dopaminergic binding during aging in the rodent striatum. *Brain Res.*, **192**, 147–62

33. Thal, L. J., Horowitz, S. G., Dvorkin, B. and Makman, M. H. (1980). Evidence for loss of brain [³H]-ADTN binding sites in rabbit brain with aging. *Brain Res.*, **192**, 185–94

34. Walker, J. B. and Walker, J. P. (1973). Properties of adenylate cyclase from senescent rat brain. *Brain Res.*, **54**, 391–6

35. Puri, S. K. and Volicer, L. (1977). Effect of aging on cyclic AMP levels and adenylate cyclase and phosphodiesterase activities in the rat corpus striatum. *Mech. Age. Dev.*, **6**, 53–8

36. Masoro, E. J., Yu, B. P., Bertrand, H. A. and Lynd, F. T. (1980). Nutritional probe of the aging process. *Fed. Proc.*, **39**, 3178–82

37. Levin, P., Janda, J. K., Joseph, J. A., Ingram, D. K. and Roth, G. S. (1981). Dietary restriction retards the age-associated loss of rat striatal dopaminergic receptors. *Science*, **214**, 561–2

38. Davies, P. and Maloney, A. J. F. (1976). Selective loss of central cholinergic neurons in Alzheimer's disease. *Lancet*, **2**, 1403 (Letter)

39. Perry, E. K., Perry, R. H., Blessed, G. and Tomlinson, B. E. (1977). Necropsy evidence of central cholinergic deficits in senile dementia. *Lancet*, **1**, 189 (Letter)

40. Davies, P. and Verth, A. H. (1978). Regional distribution of muscarinic acetylcholine receptor in normal and Alzheimer's-type dementia brains. *Brain Res.*, **138**, 385–92

41. Reisine, T. D., Yamamura, H. I., Bird, E. D., Spokes, E. and Enna, S. J. (1978). Pre- and postsynaptic neurochemical alterations in Alzheimer's disease. *Brain Res.*, **159**, 477–81

42. Greenberg, L. H. and Weiss, B. (1978). Beta-adrenergic receptors in aged rat brain: reduced number and capacity of pineal gland to develop supersensitivity. *Science*, **201**, 61–3

43. Greenberg, L. H. and Weiss, B. (1979). Ability of aged rats to alter beta-adrenergic receptors of brain in response to repeated administration of reserpine and desmethylimipramine. *J. Pharmacol. Exp. Ther.*, **211**, 309–16

44. Roth, G. S. (1980). Changes in hormone action during aging: glucocorticoid regulation of adipocyte glucose metabolism and catecholamine regulation of myocardial contractility. *Proc. Soc. Exp. Biol. Med.*, **165**, 188–92

45. Roth, G. S. and Livingston, J. N. (1976). Reductions in glucocorticoid inhibition of glucose oxidation and presumptive glucocorticoid receptor content in rat adipocytes during aging. *Endocrinology*, **99**, 831–9

46. Chang, W. C., Hoopes, M. T. and Roth, G. S. (1981). Biosynthetic rates of proteins having the characteristics of glucocorticoid receptors in adipocytes of mature and senescent rats. *J. Gerontol.*, **36**, 386–90

7
Extension of life span

E. J. MASORO

INTRODUCTION

Recently many articles and books have appeared which claim that life span can be extended and the aging processes slowed by appropriate modifications of life style and the environment[1]. Many of these publications propose nutritional manipulations or increased physical activity or both as the means of doing so.

In assessing the validity of these claims, the definition of terms has proven to be a key issue. Life span, as used by the gerontologist, refers to the maximum length of life that can be achieved by the members of a species (synonyms are maximum life span and life span potential). However, what is often referred to as an increase in life span by the books and articles on life span extension is, in fact, an increase in life expectancy. Life expectancy is defined by the gerontologist as the average length of life remaining for a population of a particular age; thus when projected from birth it is the mean length of life to be expected for a population born in a particular period of time (e.g. a given calendar year). In contrast to an increase in life span, an increase in life expectancy may not indicate a slowing of the aging processes. For example, in the United States life expectancy from birth has increased from 47 years in 1900 to 73 years in 1980[2]. This increase appears to be due primarily to the protection of the population from infectious diseases by technological and medical advances. The most reasonable interpretation is that this protection from infectious disease has permitted the population to age and that the extent to which this protection has influenced the aging processes is not defined by the life expectancy change.

In contrast, when an environmental manipulation increases the life span, it may well have done so by slowing the aging processes. The life span of Americans, unlike life expectancy, did not increase during this century but continued to be about 100 years. This fact indicates that the technological and medical advances of this century did not significantly influence the aging processes of Americans.

A similar issue in regard to effects on aging emerges in the report of

49

Paffenbarger et al.[3] showing that the life expectancy of Harvard University alumni who were physically active throughout life was greater than for those who were sedentary. Reductions in mortality due to cardiovascular and respiratory causes appear to be the major reasons for these mortality findings. Although these data are clearly of great importance, they do not provide evidence concerning the influence of physical activity on life span or the aging processes. It will take further research on this population involving many years of study to address these latter issues.

Why are gerontologists interested in life span extension? The major reason relates to the use of manipulations that extend life span as a basis for the exploration of the nature of aging. In spite of much thought and effort, the nature of the primary aging processes has yet to be identified. One general approach to the study of biological systems is the use of experimental manipulations that perturb the system. Are there ways to perturb the aging processes? Unfortunately, in general, it is very difficult to know if a manipulation has influenced the aging processes. However, as stated above, if a manipulation extends the life span of a species, it is likely that it does so by slowing the aging processes. It is the likelihood that the aging processes have been perturbed (i.e. slowed) which focuses the experimental gerontologists on the use of manipulations that extend life span as models for aging research.

The great interest of the general public in life span extension relates to the desire of the individual to have a long life of high quality for self and family. The goal of most people does not appear to be life span extension per se (i.e. the reaching of ages well in excess of 100 years) but what is desired is a good quality life into old age (and if this includes extension of the life span all the better). A question that must be addressed is whether the extension of the human life span is detrimental to, or of value to, society. The major problem posed by the elderly for society is the extent to which they utilize resources in excess of their contributions. Clearly, therefore, life span extension programs that do not increase the period of dependency should not adversely affect society other than being a contributor to possible overpopulation. The potential that extension of the human life span along with maintenance of the quality of life may have for benefitting society is rarely considered and yet there is strong possibility that it could do so. A most important route of human learning is by having experiences (the relating of experiences to others is much less effective). By providing a longer period of time to acquire experiences and a good quality of life, the extension of the life span may greatly increase the contributions a person can make to society. Indeed, humans are by far the longest lived mammals[4]. To what extent this long life has contributed to the accomplishments of humans is a question deserving attention.

CAN LIFE SPAN BE EXTENDED AND THE RATE OF AGING DECREASED?

On the basis of his actuarial analyses, Sacher concluded[5] that most of the chemical and physical treatments that have been found to increase longevity achieve this result by reducing vulnerability to disease and not by decreasing the rate of aging. Indeed, only two treatments were found to decrease the rate of actuarial aging. In the case of poikilotherms reducing body temperature and food restriction have been found to slow the rate of aging and increase life span. In mammals only food restriction has been shown to have such actions and this has been demonstrated only for rats, mice and hamsters[6]. However, they are the only mammals that have been rigorously studied in this regard and it is most important to learn if other mammals respond similarly to food restriction. Unfortunately, the resources required to do so are great. Also, to further explore the nature of aging and for the development of biomarkers of aging, additional manipulations that slow the aging processes and extend the life span would be invaluable. Indeed, having only one manipulation that has such an action in mammals hampers the development of experimental gerontology; therefore, research aimed at uncovering additional manipulations should be given high priority.

FOOD RESTRICTION OF RODENTS

Restricting the intake of food by a variety of means results in a marked extension of the life span of rodents. These many studies have been reviewed by Masoro[7] and Holehan and Merry[8]. A typical example is the study of Yu et al.[9] in which one group of rats was fed a standard semi-synthetic diet *ad libitum* and another provided 60% of the food intake of the *ad libitum* fed

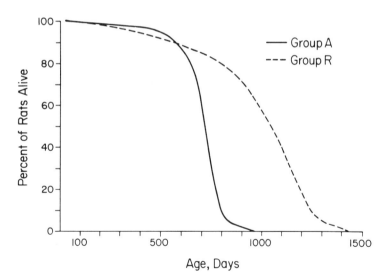

Figure 7.1 Survival curves for the *ad libitum* fed rats (Group A) and rats restricted to 60% of *ad libitum* intake (group R). (Reproduced from Yu *et al.*[9])

rats. The survival curves for the two groups of rats are shown in Figure 7.1. Note that food restriction not only increased the median length of life but also, to similar extent, the life span. Thus, these data, unlike those from the effects of technology and medicine on the survival curve of humans, indicate that food restriction has retarded the aging process. Moreover, analysis of these survival curves by the actuarial procedures of Sacher[5] also indicates that food restriction decreases the rate of aging.

Food restriction retards most of the age-related changes in the physiological processes ranging from slowing the aging of collagen to delaying the age changes in immune function to blunting age changes in the responses of target cells to hormones. These many actions have also been reviewed by Masoro[7] and by Holehan and Merry[8]. It should be noted that all age-related physiological changes are not slowed by food restriction, e.g. Yu *et al.*[10] reported that the age-related increase in systolic blood pressure in rats was not influenced by food restriction.

Food restriction retards or prevents most age-related diseases of mice and rats[7,11]. Most striking is its effects on chronic nephropathy. The lesions of this disease process are classified by the histopathologist as 0, 1, 2, 3, 4 and E based on increasing severity with 0 denoting no lesions and E denoting end-stage disease. The morphologic basis of this classification is presented in a report by Yu *et al.*[9]. The functional meaning of this classification in the case of the male Fischer 344 rats as indicated by serum urea and creatinine concentrations is presented[12] in Figure 7.2. Lesions of increasing severity through Grade 3 do not influence the serum urea and creatinine concentrations. Rats with Grade 4 lesions have a modest but significant elevation in serum levels of both. Rats with Grade E lesions have markedly elevated levels of serum creatinine and urea and most also exhibit parathyroid hyperplasia, osteodystrophy and metastatic calcification. Clearly, most rats with Grade E lesions are in renal failure. On the basis of rats sacrificed at 6, 12, 18, 24, 27 and 30 months of age (Figure 7.3), there is a clear age-related progression of the severity of these lesions in rats fed *ad libitum* and the rate of this progression is markedly reduced by food restriction. The extent of this protective action is even more clearly shown by the data on the pathologic analyses of the kidneys of rats that died spontaneously which are summarized in Table 7.1. More than 50% of the *ad libitum* fed rats had Grade E lesions and thus were probably suffering from renal failure. In contrast only 2% of the food restricted rats had Grade E lesions. Even more impressive is the fact that 72% of the *ad libitum* fed rats had either Grade 4 or Grade E lesions at death while only 2% of the food restricted rats had lesions of this severity.

In essence, food restriction prevents the clinical expression of a major age-associated disease process in rats. Although it influences almost all age-associated diseases it does not prevent the clinical expression of all. For example, although the occurrence of neoplastic diseases is delayed to older ages, the percentage of the food restricted rats with tumours at death is greater than for the *ad libitum* fed rats[12]. The latter undoubtedly is merely a reflection of the fact that food restricted rats die at older ages than *ad libitum* fed animals.

Clearly, the evidence which indicates that food restriction slows the aging processes is strong. Two questions arise: First, is this model of value for research on the nature of aging? And second, if so, what approaches should be taken to most effectively utilize this model? The answer to the first question

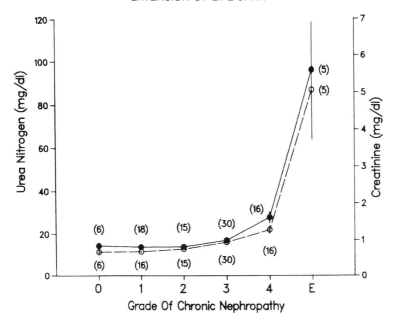

Figure 7.2 Serum creatinine and serum urea concentrations and the grade of chronic nephropathy (0 = no lesion; E = end-stage disease). The filled circles and solid line refer to serum urea concentration and the unfilled circles and broken line refer to serum creatinine concentration. Mean values plus or minus the standard error of the mean for the number of rats in parentheses. (Reproduced from Maeda *et al.*[12])

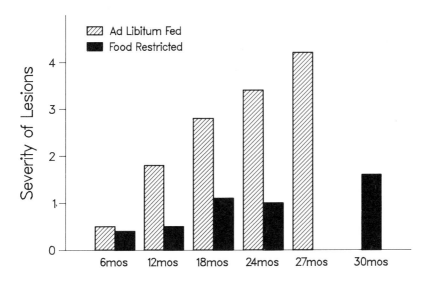

Figure 7.3 Age and the severity of chronic nephropathy in *ad libitum* fed and food restricted rats. At each of the ages noted and for each dietary group 10 rats were sacrificed. (Data for this figure are from Maeda *et al.*[12])

Table 7.1 Chronic nephropathy in male Fischer 344 rats that died spontaneously (data from Maeda et al.[12])

	Number of rats examined	% with lesions of grade:					
		0*	1	2	3	4	E†
Ad libitum fed	71	0	1	17	10	21	51
Food restricted	56	11	62	20	5	0	2

* No lesions
† End-stage disease

is 'yes', there are several important uses for this model. In regard to the second question in my opinion the most important and immediately compelling approach is research aimed at determining the mechanisms by which food restriction retards the aging processes. Understanding these mechanisms almost certainly will provide important insights on the basic nature of aging. Indeed, currently the research in our laboratory is almost totally focused on searching for these mechanisms.

Our initial work in this area was to experimentally explore the major hypotheses that have been proposed for the action of food restriction on the aging processes. McCay et al.[13] suggested in 1935 that food restriction delayed the aging processes by slowing growth and development. Our work with male Fischer 344 rats indicates that this is not the mechanism[10]. The design of our study and the longevity findings are summarized in Figure 7.4. Four dietary groups were utilized: Group 1 was fed ad libitum throughout life; Group 2 was food restricted from 6 weeks of age on; Group 3 was food restricted from 6 weeks to 6 months of age and ad libitum fed thereafter; Group 4 was fed ad libitum until 6 months of age and food restricted thereafter. The important finding is that food restriction started at 6 months of age (Group 4) was as effective as food restriction started at 6 weeks of age (Group 2) in regard to the age of tenth percentile survivors and the maximum length of life while food restriction from 6 weeks to 6 months of age was much less effective. Also, the Group 4 rats had the same retardation in age changes in the physiological systems and in the occurrence and progression of age-related diseases as the Group 2 rats while such was not the case with Group 3 rats. The data strongly indicate that food restriction acts post-maturationally in regard to its influence on the aging processes and that retarding growth and development has little to do with this action.

It was proposed by Berg and Simms[14] that food restriction increases longevity by reducing body fat content. Our work also does not support this view[15]. Using the Fischer 344 rat we found that, as would be expected, food restriction decreased body fat content. However, in the case of the ad libitum fed rats, there was no correlation between body fat content and the length of life and with the food restricted rats more body fat was associated with a longer life. Work by Harrison et al.[16] in mice is in accord with these findings. Thus, it may be concluded that reducing body fat content does not play a major role in life span extension by food restriction.

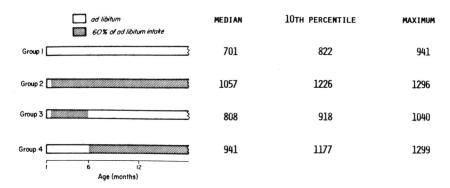

Figure 7.4 Design and longevity results of study testing hypothesis that food restriction retards the aging processes by slowing growth and delaying maturation. (Data are from and the design is that of Yu et al.[10])

Sacher[5] proposed that food restriction retards the aging processes by reducing the metabolic rate. This view has been widely embraced and is particularly attractive because it can easily be linked to the free radical theory of aging[17]. Direct testing of this hypothesis has been carried out in our laboratory and the data convincingly show that it is not valid. The data on the 6 month old rats has been published[18]; the metabolic rate per kilogram of lean body mass or kilogram of body mass to the power $\frac{2}{3}$ or kilogram of body mass to the power $\frac{3}{4}$ did not differ between *ad libitum* fed and food-restricted rats. Similar unpublished findings have been obtained for rats through most of the life span.

These results on metabolic rate challenge the classic view that food restriction influences the aging processes by reducing the intake of calories or other nutrients per unit of metabolic mass. Direct evidence in this regard comes from measuring food intake per unit of body mass; the findings[6] are summarized in Figure 7.5. The food-restricted rats consumed more food rather than less per unit body mass but if related to the lean body mass there was no difference in food intake between the two groups[9]. What clearly happens is the lean body mass is maintained so as the food intake per unit lean mass is the same for the *ad libitum* fed and food-restricted rats. As a consequence, the following conclusion may be drawn: reducing the nutrient input per animal rather than per unit of metabolic mass retards the aging process.

If the flux of calories or other nutrients per unit of metabolic mass is not the factor responsible for the action of food restriction on the aging processes, what other general mechanism can be envisioned? The most likely possibility in our view is that food restriction acts by modulating the neural and endocrine regulatory systems. Thus, the following is our working hypothesis: food restriction is coupled to the aging processes through its action on the endocrine and/or neural regulatory systems.

How can this general hypothesis be approached experimentally? There are

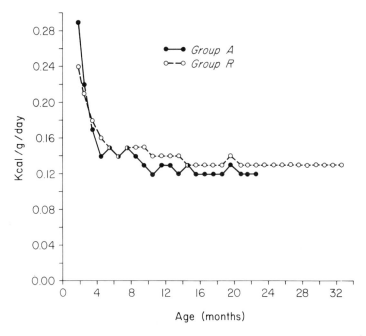

Figure 7.5 Food intake per unit body mass. The closed circles designate *ad libitum* fed rats (Group A) and the open circles rats fed 60% of the *ad libitum* intake (Group R) from 6 weeks of age on. (Reproduced from Masoro[6])

two guides. The first is the likelihood that a particular neural–endocrine regulatory process can be influenced by food restriction. And the second is the potential for the neural–endocrine regulatory process to be involved in the aging processes.

Several years age Everitt[20] proposed that food restriction decreases the secretion of an aging factor by the pituitary gland. The evidence that has emerged in support of this view has not been strong nor has the precise nature of the endocrine factor been defined. However, recently a possible definition has emerged in the form of the Glucocorticoid Cascade Hypothesis of Aging proposed by Sapolsky *et al.*[21]. The possible role of the hypothalamic–pituitary–adrenal cortical system in the action of food restriction warrants exploration.

It is also quite likely that food restriction could modulate the insulin–glucose homeostatic system. Cerami[22] has proposed that glucose by means of glycation reactions ultimately yielding advanced glycosylation end products can be a mediator of aging. Clearly, the glucose–insulin system as a potential coupler between food restriction and the aging processes deserves study.

Although it is not likely that food restriction acts directly on most tissues and organs, it must influence their functioning through the action of the neural and endocrine systems at these target sites. It is important to determine the nature of the effects at those target sites. In this regard, Cheung and Richardson[23] have discussed the importance of the rate of protein turnover in the maintenance of physiological responsiveness and pointed out that the rate of protein turnover decreases with increasing age. Cheung and Richardson[23] propose that food restriction delays age-related physiological deterioration by retarding the decline in protein turnover. This proposal clearly should be studied.

Although Harman's hypothesis[17] that food restriction influences aging by reducing free-radical generation due to a reduction in metabolic rate has been proven to be incorrect, food restriction still may act by reducing free-radical damage. This is clearly another area that should be explored. Further effort is needed both conceptually and experimentally aimed at understanding the actions of food restriction on cellular activities of target sites.

RELEVANCE OF FOOD RESTRICTION TO HUMANS

Does food restriction influence the aging processes of humans in a fashion similar to that in rodents? Of course, this question is always asked. The answer is that it has not been shown to be true in humans or for that matter in any mammalian species other than rodents. This does not mean that it does not have this action in all or most mammalian species but rather that it has not been carefully studied in a mammalian species longer lived than rodents. The reason for this is that the resources needed to execute such a study even in a species with the life span of dogs is enormous.

Nevertheless, Walford[24] proposes a life span extension diet for humans based to a great extent on the food restriction dietary regimens that have extended rodent life span. He states that there is not absolute proof that it will be effective in humans. However, he feels that different mammalian species age by essentially identical mechanisms and thus it is likely that their aging processes should be similarly influenced by food restriction.

This view of Walford[24] is reasonable and it would be appropriate to encourage those who desire life extension to follow his regimen except for two issues. First, do we know enough about the life long effects of nutrition to safely prescribe marked manipulations of usual dietary regimens? I do not believe we do and thus the element of uncharted risk emerges. The other issue is the possibility that a fraction of the human population has already chosen dietary lifestyles that permit the full human life span to be expressed. If so, it will not be possible to develop dietary programmes that will extend the human life span; but, of course, the use of such programmes may well enable more of the population to achieve the full human life span whatever it may be.

References

1. Schneider, E.-L. and Reed, J. D. (1985). Life extension. *N. Engl. J. Med.*, **312**, 1159–68
2. Fries, J. F. and Crapo, L. M. (1981). *Vitality and Aging*, (New York: W. H. Freeman & Co.)
3. Paffenbarger, R. S., Jr, Hyde, R. T., Wing, A. L. and Hsieh, C. (1986). Physical activity, all-cause mortality and longevity of college alumni. *N. Engl. J. Med.*, **314**, 605–13
4. Kirkwood, T. B. L. (1985). Comparative and evolutionary aspects for longevity. In Finch, C. E. and Schneider, E. L. (eds.) *Handbook of the Biology of Aging.* 2nd edn. pp. 27–44. (New York: Van Nostrand Reinhold Co.)
5. Sacher, G. A. (1977). Life table modification and life prolongation. In Finch, C. E. and Hayflick, L. (eds.) *Handbook of Biology of Aging.* pp. 582–638. (New York: Van Nostrand Reinhold Co.)
6. Masoro, E. J. (1985a). Metabolism. In Finch, C. E. and Schneider, E. L. (eds.) *Handbook of Biology of Aging.* pp. 540–63. (New York: Van Nostrand Reinhold Co.)
7. Masoro, E. J. (1985b). Nutrition and aging. A current assessment. *J. Nutr.*, **115**, 842–8
8. Holehan, A. M. and Merry, B. J. (1986). The experimental manipulation of ageing by diet. *Biol. Rev.*, **61**, 329–68
9. Yu, B. P., Masoro, E. J., Murata, I., Bertrand, H. A. and Lynd, F. T. (1982). Life span study of SPF Fischer 344 rats fed *ad libitum* or restricted diets: longevity, growth, lean body mass and disease. *J. Gerontol.*, **37**, 130–41
10. Yu, B. P., Masoro, E. J. and McMahan, C. A. (1985). Nutritional influences on aging of Fischer 344 rats. I. Physical, metabolic and longevity characteristics. *J. Gerontol.*, **40**, 657–70
11. Weindruch, R. (1985). Aging in rodents fed restricted diets. *J. Am. Geriat. Soc.*, **33**, 125–32
12. Maeda, H., Gleiser, C. A., Masoro, E. J., Murata, I., McMahan, C. A. and Yu, B. P. (1985). Nutritional influences on aging of Fischer 344 rats: II. Pathology. *J. Gerontol.*, **40**, 671–88
13. McCay, C., Crowell, M. and Maynard, L. (1935). The effect of retarded growth upon the length of life span and upon ultimate size. *J. Nutr.* **10**, 63–79
14. Berg, B. M. and Simms, H. S. (1960). Nutrition and longevity in the rat. II. Longevity and onset of disease with different levels of intake. *J. Nutr.*, **71**, 255–63
15. Bertrand, H. A., Lynd, F. T., Masoro, E. J. and Yu, B. P. (1980). Changes in adipose mass and cellularity through adult life of rats fed *ad libitum* or a life prolonging restricted diet. *J. Gerontol.*, **35**, 827–35
16. Harrison, D. E., Archer, J. K. and Astle, C. M. (1984). Effects of food restriction on aging: separation of food intake and adiposity. *Proc. Natl. Acad. Sci. USA*, **81**, 1835–8
17. Harman, D. (1981). The aging process. *Proc. Natl. Acad. Sci. USA*, **78**, 7124–8
18. McCarter, R., Masoro, E. J. and Yu, B. P. (1985). Does food restriction retard aging by reducing the metabolic rate? *Am. J. Physiol.*, **248**, E488–E490
19. Masoro, E. J., Yu, B. P. and Bertrand, H. A. (1982). Action of food restriction in delaying the aging processes. *Proc. Natl. Acad. Sci. USA*, **79**, 4239–41
20. Everitt, A. V. (1973). The hypothalamic–pituitary control of aging and age-related pathology. *Exp. Geront.*, **8**, 265–77
21. Sapolsky, R., Krey, L. C. and McEwen, B. S. (1986). The neuroendocrinology of stress and aging: the glucocorticoid cascade hypothesis. *Endocrinol. Rev.*, **7**, 284–301
22. Cerami, A. (1985). Hypothesis: glucose as a mediator of aging. *J. Am. Geriatr. Soc.*, **33**, 626–34
23. Cheung, H. T. and Richardson, A. (1982). The relationship between age-related changes in gene expression, protein turnover and the responsiveness of an organism to stimuli. *Life Sci.*, **31**, 605–13
24. Walford, R. L. (1986). *The 120 Year Diet.* (New York: Simon and Schuster)

Section 2
Gut Morphology and Physiology

8
The effects of age on the intestinal epithelium

R. A. GOODLAD, W. LENTON and N. A. WRIGHT

INTRODUCTION

Whilst there is a considerable amount of data published on the development and differentiation of the foetal and neonatal intestine[1-10], there is far less information available concerning the changes associated with aging. The effects of age on the intestine are of some importance in our aging population, especially as some of these effects may have covert clinical manifestations[11].

The effects of age on those less than ideal measures of intestinal function, crypt and villus size[12,13], have given conflicting results. Thrasher[14,15] reported an increase in crypt and villus size with age; however he used 10-day-old mice as his young time point. The intestinal surface area appears to increase with age[16], but it has been reported that the size of the crypts and villi remains fairly constant[17], thus mucosal growth should occur by increasing the number of crypts and villi: however, Clarke[18] reported that the number of villi per intestine reached a maximum after 200 g body weight, and then declined slightly; the number of crypts however increased with age resulting in an increased crypt to villus ratio. Altmann and Enesco[1] also reported an increased crypt to villus ratio in older rats. The effects of crypt fission in the rat has been studied by St Clair and Osborne[19] and although the rate of crypt fission peaks at weaning, there is still a significant basal level in the adult bowel. A low rate of crypt branching also occurs in the adult human gut[20], which increases dramatically in disease.

The effects of age may be confused by some effects only being observed with the onset of senility. In very old rats there appears to be an increase in crypt and villus size in the ileum[21] leading to the suggestion that intestinal function may be impaired and that decreased survival of newly formed crypts is likely.

The ordered pattern of enzyme expression as cells migrate up the villi of aged rats is maintained, but the initiation and duration of enzyme expression appears to be delayed, thus although the villi may be structurally similar to those of young animals, the increase in the proportion of undifferentiated cells would reduce intestinal function[22]. Increased crypt cell population, proliferative indices and growth fractions have also been observed in duodenum, jejunum and ileum of 27-month-old rats[23]. While the uptake of tritiated thymidine per unit tissue in aging mice does not increase, the activity per crypt and the crypt size both increased, especially in the jejunum and ileum (Cullan, Crouse and Sharp, unpublished).

Reduced duodenal and jejunal, but not ileal, intestinal epithelial proliferation, with age, has been reported[24,25]. In very old rats there may be an increase in crypt cell population and in crypt cell production rates; very old animals also seem less able to cope with the strains associated with altered nutrient intake (Holt, unpublished). The effects of age on intestinal epithelial cell proliferation and the cell division cycle have been investigated by Thrasher[14,15] who noted a prolongation of the post-mitotic (G_1) interval; this work was extented by Lesher and Sacher[26] who also reported an increase in cell cycle time, but due to increased durations of the DNA synthesis phase (S) and of G_1. This increase in generation time was not progressive but took place at the end of the growing period and beginning of senility. In this study we report work done on simultaneous measurement of intestinal cell proliferation and absorption in two groups of aged and young rats.

METHODS

Experiment 1

2-week, 10-week and 110-week-old male, Wistar strain rats were housed in groups of four in wire bottomed cages, and were fed a pelleted diet (Labshure P.R.D., Christopher Hill, Poole, Dorset, England). Water was available *ad lib.*

Experiment 2

Male Sprague Dawley rats 3 to 105 weeks of age were kept and fed as described above.

Crypt Cell Production Rate (CCPR)

This was determined in the proximal small intestine by counting the number of vincristine-arrested metaphases per micro-dissected crypt and plotting the mean value against time after vincristine (1 mg/kg) injection. The slope of this line gives the CCPR[13].

Water absorption

The rat was anaesthetised with ether and the intestine from the ligament of Tretz to 5 cm above the ileo-caecal valve was cannulated, rinsed with warm saline and then perfused with a segmental flow of oxygenated medium and warm moist gas (see Figure 8.1). The perfused gut was inflated by a modified Starling resistance, where the outflow from the perfused segment is passed between a rubber bung and a rubber membrane, the other side of which is pressurized (by clamping a sealed silastic tube) until a pressure of 40 mmHg is obtained in the gut. The mesentery was then stripped off and the intestine was placed in a bath permitting the collection of water over timed intervals[27].

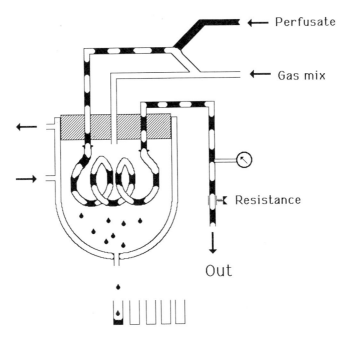

Figure 8.1 Diagram of the perfusion apparatus. Warm perfusate (gassed with 95/5 oxygen/carbon dioxide) is mixed in a 'Y-piece' with warm, moistened gas to generate a segmented flow. The tubing to the gut bath is inside a flexible water jacket (not shown)

Combined techniques

The rats were injected with vincristine at 09.00 and after a 20-min interval the first rat was anaesthetised and prepared for studies of absorption. The time at which the animal was killed was noted to derive time points for the metaphase arrest study. The length of the proximal and distal remnants and of the perfused segment were recorded. The perfused segment was dried at 60°C to a constant dry weight. While the absorption of the first rat was being measured the next rat was prepared and its gut set up in the second bath.

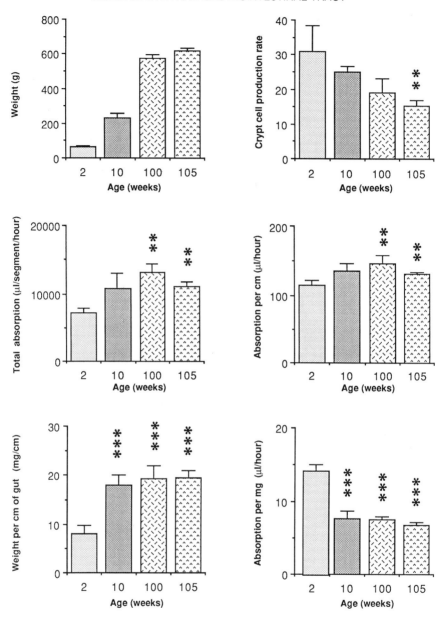

Figure 8.2 The effects of age (in Experiment 1) on body weight, duodenal crypt-cell production rate (cells per crypt per hour), total water absorption per perfused segment, water absorption per unit length, intestinal weight per unit length, and absorption per milligram of intestinal dry weight. The crypt-cell production rate of the oldest rats was significantly less than that of the 2-week and the 10-week groups ($P<0.01$). (** and *** indicate significant difference between the marked groups and the 2-week rats at $P<0.01$ or 0.001, respectively)

Using a two-bath system we were able to study 8–10 rats in the 3 h required for metaphase collection[28].

RESULTS

In the first study the duodenal crypt cell production rate declined with age. (Figure 8.2). The CCPR of the young adult rats (10 weeks) was similar to that reported previously[28,29]. In the oldest rats, the CCPR had decreased and this was statistically significant when compared to the 2-week and the 10-week groups ($P < 0.01$). Water absorption increased with age, principally from increased gut weight.

The absorptive capacity of young rats was less than that of the older groups, but these rats had significantly smaller guts and the absorption rate per unit intestinal weight was significantly ($P < 0.001$) greater.

In the second study, there was an almost linear increase in body weight with age in the first 30 weeks in Sprague-Dawley rats accompanied by a gradual decline in duodenal CCRP (see Figure 8.3). Intestinal length also increased in a similar manner, and then plateaued whilst the weight of intestine continued to increase.

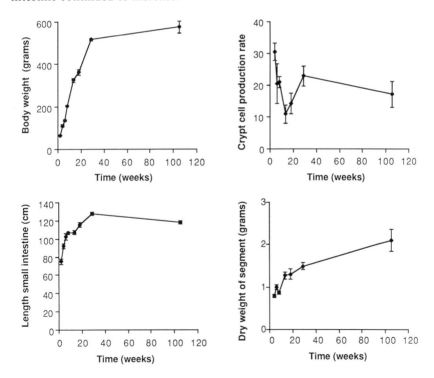

Figure 8.3 The effects of age on body weight, duodenal crypt-cell production (cells per crypt per hour), the total length of the small intestine (perfused segment plus proximal and distal unperfused remnants), and dry weight of the perfused segment

The increase in intestinal weight was associated with a gradual increase in intestinal absorption (Figure 8.4); however water absorption per milligram was considerably more efficient in the young gut than in the adult or old, with no change being seen after 13 weeks.

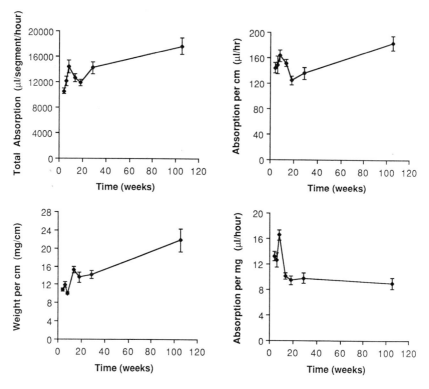

Figure 8.4 The effects of age (in Experiment 2) on total intestinal absorption per perfused segment, absorption per unit length of intestine, the dry weight of the intestine (expressed per unit length), and absorption per milligram of intestinal dry weight

DISCUSSION

The results of the present study illustrate the rapid changes in intestinal epithelial cell proliferation and intestinal mass that occur in early life[2]. The length of the small intestine and net weight of the intestine appears to increase as body weight increases. Absorption rate per centimeter also increases but is less pronounced than the changes in body weight, suggesting that the gut is more developed and has greater absorptive powers in relation to body weight in the young. The young animal has more villi relative to crypts and more villi per unit area[30] which might explain greater absorption rate seen in the young rats. Alternatively change in intestinal permeability may be present. The crypt-cell production rate for young rats also was higher than adult values in both studies, reflecting active proliferation.

As the rats aged there was a gradual increase in absorption resulting from intestinal lengthening and the increase in absorption per centimetre; thus, the absorption per milligram remained constant in old rats, presumably due to the concomitant increase in dry weight per centimetre. Most authors have shown little change in villus height in aging animals. However, changes in villus height as a measure of cell population should be viewed with caution[12,13], particularly since Cheng and Bjerknes[30] have shown that whereas little change in villus height after weaning occurs, there is a progressive increase in villus width.

The observed increase in intestinal mass must have resulted from an increase in the number of crypts and villi[16,19,20] since cell production rate per crypt decreased. Elevation of crypt/villus ratios with age has been reported[1,18,20] thus if more crypts feed a villus each crypt would need to produce less cells to maintain the same villus influx. This is in contrast to the results of Holt[21-23] and Sharp (unpublished), who found increased crypt cell production; however, these workers used considerably older animals. When rats get much older than 2 years of age there is a high mortality rate, thus these very old rats can be considered as 'survivors'.

In this study we only have reported on proliferation rates in the duodenum, and there is evidence to suggest[21-23] that the increase in proliferation in the old rodent is more pronounced in the ileum. Work on the quantification of proliferation in the ileum and colon now is in progress.

In conclusion, important age-related changes in intestinal dynamics and function occur, most of which appear in early life. Whether these are due to 'development' or 'age' is a purely parochial argument: our efforts should be targeted at understanding the mechanisms of these changes.

Acknowledgement

We are pleased to acknowledge the financial assistance of the Cancer Research Campaign.

References

1. Altmann, G. G. and Enesco, M. (1967). Cell number as a measure of distribution and renewal of epithelial cells in the small intestine of growing and adult rats. *Am. J. Anat.*, **121**, 319–36
2. Al-Nafussi, A. I. and Wright, N. A. (1982). Cell kinetics in the mouse small intestine during immediate postnatal life. *Virchows Arch. (B)*, **40**, 51–62
3. Klein, R. M. and McKenzie, J. C. (1983). The role of cell renewal in the ontogeny of the intestine. I. Cell proliferation patterns in adult, foetal and neonatal intestine. *J. Pediat. Gastroenterol.. Nutr.*, **2**, 10–43
4. Potter, G, D, and Lester, R. (1984). The developing colon and nutrition. *J. Pediat. Gastroenterol. Nutr.*, **3**, 484–7
5. Bailey, D. S., Cook, A., McAllister, G., Moss, M. and Mian, N. (1984). Structural and biochemical differentiation of the mammalian intestine during foetal development. *J. Cell Sci.*, **72**, 195–212
6. Wright, N. A. and Alison, M. (1984). *The Biology of Epithelial Cell Populations.* (Oxford: Clarendon Press)

7. Henning, S. J. (1985). Ontogeny of enzymes in the small intestine. *Annu. Rev. Physiol.*, **47**, 231–45
8. Hirano, S. and Kataoka, K. (1986). Histogenesis of the mouse jejunal mucosa with special reference to proliferative and absorptive cells. *Archiv. Histol. Japan*, **49**, 333–48
9. Trahair, J. and Robinson, P. (1986). The development of the ovine small intestine. *Anat. Rec.*, **214**, 294–303
10. Trahair, J., Perry, S., Silver, M. and Robinson, P. M. (1986). Autoradiographic localization of ^{3}H-thymidine incorporation in the small intestinal epithelium of foetal sheep. *J. Pediat, Gastroenterol. Nutr.*, **5**, 648–54
11. Holt, P. R. (1986). Aging changes in the rat small intestine. In Bernardi, M., Facchini, A. and Labo, G. *Nutritional and Metabolic Aspects of Aging.* pp. 41–9. (Eurage)
12. Clarke, R. M. (1973). Progress in measuring epithelial turnover in the villus of the small intestine. *Digestion*, **8**, 161–75
13. Goodlad, R. A. and Wright, N. A. (1982). Quantitative studies on epithelial replacement in the gut. In Titchen, D. A. (ed.) *Techniques in the Life Sciences.* (Ireland: Elsevier)
14. Thrasher, J. D. (1967). Comparison of the cell cycle and cell migration in the intestinal epithelium of suckling and adult mice. *Experientia*, **67**, 1050–1
15. Thrasher, J. D. (1967). Age and the cell cycle of the mouse colonic epithelium. *Anat. Rec.* **157**, 621–6
16. Meshkinpour, H., Smith, M. and Hollander, D. (1981). Influence of aging on the surface area of the small intestine of the rat. *Exp. Gerontol.*, **16**, 399–404
17. Ecknauer, R., Vadakel, T. and Wepler, R. (1982). Intestinal morphology and cell production rate in aging rats. *J. Gerontol.*, **37**, 151–5
18. Clarke, R. M. (1972). The effects of growth and of fasting on the number of villi and crypts in the small intestine of the albino rat. *J. Anat.*, **112**, 27–33
19. St Clair, W. H. and Osborne, J. W. (1985). Crypt fission and crypt number in the small and large bowel of postnatal rats. *Cell Tissue Kinet.*, **18**, 255–62
20. Cheng, H., Bjerknes, M., Amar, J. and Gardiner, G. (1986). Crypt production in normal and diseased human colonic epithelium. *Anat. Rec.*, **216**, 44–8
21. Holt, P. R., Pascal, R. R. and Kotler, D. P. (1984). Effects of aging upon small intestinal structure in the Fischer rat. *J. Gerontol.*, **39**, 642–7
22. Holt, P. R., Tierney, A. R. and Kotler, D. P. (1985). Delayed enzyme expression: a defect of aging rat gut. *Gastroenterology*, **89**, 1026–34
23. Holt, P. R., Yeh, K. Y. and Kotler, D. P. (1988). Altered controls of proliferation in small intestine of senescent rat. *Proc. Natl. Acad. Sci USA*, **85**, 2771–5
24. Lesher, S., Fry, R. J. M. and Kohn, H. I. (1961). Age and the generation time of the mouse duodenal epithelial cell. *Exp. Cell Res.*, **24**, 335–43
25. Fry, R. J. M., Lesher, S. and Kohn, H. I. (1962). Influence of age on the transit time of cells of the mouse intestinal epithelium. III. Ileum. *Lab. Invest.*, **11**, 289–93
26. Lesher, S. and Sacher, G. A. (1968). Effects of age on cell proliferation in mouse duodenal crypts. *Exp. Gerontol.*, **3**, 211–17
27. Fisher, R. B. and Gardner, M. L. G. (1974). A kinetic approach to the study of absorption of solutes by isolated perfusion small intestine. *J. Physiol.*, **241**, 211–34
28. Goodlad, R. A., Plumb, J. A. and Wright, N. A. (1987). The relationship between intestinal crypt cell production and intestinal water absorption measured *in vitro* in the rat. *Clin. Sci.*, **72**, 297–304
29. Goodlad, R. A., Al-Mukhtar, M. Y. T., Ghatei, M. A., Bloom, S. R. and Wright, N. A. (1983). Cell proliferation, plasma enteroglucagon and plasma gastrin levels in starved and refed rats. *Virchows Archiv. (B)*, **45**, 63–73
30. Cheng, H. and Bjerknes, M. (1985). Whole population cell kinetics and postnatal development of the mouse intestinal epithelium. *Anat. Rec.*, **211**, 420–6

9
Aging and small intestinal enzyme activity

P. R. HOLT AND K.-Y. YEH

The process of aging is accompanied in many organs by changes in cell replication and in biochemical or physiological function. The small intestine provides a very special tissue for the study of aging since columnar absorptive cells are produced from crypt progenitor cells continuously throughout life. Thus, the small intestine (and other portions of the gastrointestinal tract) may be affected by factors that alter cell replication during the aging process as described in Chapter 8. Furthermore, crypt cells are immature and undifferentiated. Columnar cells, during their movement from the crypt up the villus, attain differentiated features. These differentiated features include changes in cellular ultrastructure, a loss of proliferative potential and the appearance of expression of many important enzyme activities that are present in 'mature' cells high on the villus. Within epithelial cells, brush border enzymes, such as the disaccharidases, are synthesized within the endoplasmic reticulum and move to their functionally active position in the microvillus membrane. The intestinal crypt–villus column, therefore, is divided into a proliferative zone which comprises the lowest one-half to two-thirds of the crypt, a zone of fully differentiated cells present in the upper two-thirds of the villus, and, between these, a zone of differentiation. Differentiation zone cells gradually develop full expression of the enzyme activity present on the villus.

Only a few studies examining for changes in intestinal enzymes with age have been reported previously (Table 9.1). There has been a notable absence of studies of intestinal enzymes with age in man. The studies of Welsh and co-workers, showing that lactase-specific activity did not fall as a consequence of age, are unique[1]. Studies using experimental animals have shown variable results (Table 9.1). For example, intestinal alkaline phosphatase activity was noted to fall with age when studied biochemically[2] or histochemically[3,4]. On the other hand, the activity of other intestinal enzymes showed no change with age[3,5] or actually were found to be increased[3]. These differences in enzyme activity levels with age in animals might be the result of nutritional differences and disease-free status.

Table 9.1 Effects of age upon intestinal enzyme activity

Author	Reference	Enzyme	Species	Age	Effect
Sayeed	2	Alkaline phosphatase	B6D2F1/j mouse	34 months	Reduction
Leutert	3	Alkaline phosphatase	BD Rat	18 months	Reduction
		Leucine aminopeptidase	BD Rat	18 months	Increase
		α-Glucosidase	BD Rat	18 months	No change
Hohn	4	Acid phosphatase	Rat (Wistar)	24–30 months	No change
Moog	5	Alkaline phosphatase	Mouse (Jackson Lab)	24 months	No change
		Sucrase			No change
		Maltase			No change
Welsh	1	Lactase	Man	80+ years	No change

During the past several years, our laboratory has been studying the effect of aging upon gut enzymes using the barrier-reared, nutritionally defined male Fischer 344 rat as an experimental model. This animal strain has been contracted for by the National Institutes of Aging for gerontological research[6]. The health of this rat colony is monitored closely. We have used mainly the 26–27-month-old rat as a prototype aging animal (since approximately half the Fischer 344 rat colony is dead at this age and animals older than 27 months usually are losing weight) and the 4–5-month-old rat as a young, mature control animal since this rat strain gains little weight after this age. Importantly, food intake is similar in rats at these two ages. In addition, our early studies showed that villus height and epithelial cell number did not differ significantly in the upper intestine of aging rats from that found in young adults[7].

Our initial studies demonstrated a modest reduction in the activity of mucosal enzymes such as the disaccharidases, lactase, sucrase and maltase, in homogenates obtained from mucosal scrapings of the duodenum and jejunum in aging rats[8] (Table 9.2). A simplistic explanation for such lowered

Table 9.2 Effect of aging on intestinal mucosal disaccharidase activity*

Area	Sucrase $\times 10^{-2}$	Maltase $\times 10^{-1}$	Lactase $\times 10^{-3}$
Duodenum			
Young	4.8 ± 0.1	3.51 ± 0.4	10.1 ± 0.8
Aging	3.5 ± 0.1	2.46 ± 0.4	7.3 ± 0.7
p	<0.05	<0.05	<0.05
Jejunum			
Young	6.53 ± 0.8	4.66 ± 0.8	26.4 ± 2.0
Aging	3.68 ± 0.6	3.47 ± 0.2	20.0 ± 2.0
p	<0.02	$= 095$	<0.02

*Enzyme specific activity in International Units shown as mean ± in 5–10 animals in each group

enzyme activity was that intestinal cells of aging animals were unable to synthesize as much enzyme protein as epithelial cells of younger animals. To investigate the mechanism for changes in enzyme expression more fully, we used a method of cryostat slicing of frozen oriented intestinal villus epithelium[8] and then measured the specific activity of several enzymes in tissue slices taken from the villus tip to the crypt base[9]. Peak enzyme activity for duodenal and jejunal sucrase, maltase, alkaline phosphatase and adenosinase deaminase was similar in young and aging rats. However, when enzyme activities from crypt base to villus tip in jejunal and duodenal segments were plotted as a percentage of peak activity, considerable differences became apparent. For example, Figure 9.1 shows changes in the specific activity for jejunal sucrase-isomaltase using sucrase as substrate. Whereas the abrupt increase in sucrase activity from very low crypt levels occurs near the area of the crypt–villus junction in young rats and peak activity is found in cells approximately 40% up the crypt–villus column, the expression of enzyme activity commenced, and peak activity was reached, much further up the crypt–villus column in aging rats. Mathematical calculations of the initiation

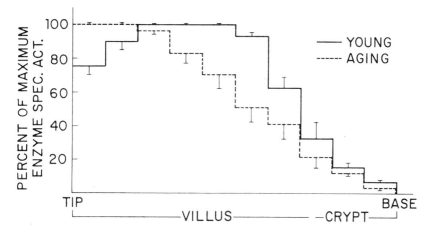

Figure 9.1 Gradients of sucrase-specific activity from sections along the jejunal crypt–villus column in young and aging rats. Data from 11–14 pools of 25 slices, 4-μm thick, normalized to decapercentiles from crypt base to villus tip and presented as mean percent ± SEM of peak specific activity. Approximate proportions of the villus and crypt are indicated on the abscissa.

and duration and point of completion of the expression of duodenal maltase, sucrase, alkaline phosphatase and adenosine deaminase all indicated that they were shifted to a more luminal position[9]. The levels of activity of intestinal enzymes (at least the disaccharidases) of adult rats are believed to be determined by rates of enzyme synthesis, which occurs mainly near the villus base, and the rate of degradation which is maximum at the luminal side[10]. Synthesis has been thought to be controlled by carbohydrate nutrient intake[10] and degradation at least in part by the action of proteases in the intestinal lumen[11,12]. We found that neither bacterial counts nor luminal tryptic activity differed in young and aging rats.

The delay in the expression of intestinal enzymes in aging rats described above could have occurred for at least two different reasons: (1) from a delay in the process of differentiation from undifferentiated crypt cells to fully differentiated villus epithelial cells, or, alternatively, (2) because of differences in the structure or turnover of enzymes present within epithelial cells that otherwise demonstrate well-differentiated villus features. To test the first possibility, both histological and histochemical techniques were used. Our observations on the changes in the initiation of enzyme activity expression indicated that there was a delay in aging rats to a point almost one-third up the villus (Figure 9.1). If this difference was caused by an overall delay in differentiation of epithelial cells, then it might be identifiable morphologically. Under these circumstances, cells in the region of the crypt–villus junction in aging rats should resemble mid-crypt cells in younger animals. By light microscopy, this area of the crypt–villus column did not differ, so that jejunal tissue from two young and two aging rats then was processed for electron microscopy. In both young and aging rats, crypt cells differed from mature villus epithelial cells in the appearance of the microvilli, in nuclear polarity, the abundance of free ribosomes and short endoplasmic reticulum (Figure 9.2)[13] but did not differ from each other. Epithelial cells from the region of the crypt–villus junction and the villus base in young and aging rats showed a similar appearance of gradually increasing microvillus length and density, decreasing free ribosomes (Figures 9.3a and b), and changes in nuclear polarity and in organization of the endoplasmic reticulum. This observation militates against an age-dependent delay of cell maturation during epithelial cell migration up the villus on histologic grounds.

In addition, we used histochemical techniques in an attempt to establish the 'maturation' of intestinal epithelial cells present near the crypt–villus junction in aging rats. In these studies, performed in collaboration with Dr Andrea Quaroni of Cornell University, we sought the presence of antigens that have been shown to be characteristic of epithelial cells present along the crypt–villus column. In three young and aging rats, immunochemical studies were performed using a large number of monoclonal antibodies directed toward antigens present in adult rat intestine[14]. In these studies, 1.0-cm segments of duodenum, jejunum and distal ileum were rinsed, embedded in OCT compound and frozen in liquid nitrogen. Cryostat sections (4–6 μm thick) were allowed to dry, were fixed with 1–2% formaldehyde and incubated with a glycine-containing buffer and stained by an indirect immunofluorescent technique described previously[14]. The antibodies used against 10 gut antigens in these studies are shown in Table 9.3. Only one of the complete range of antigens sought in these studies was found to be specific for the intestine of the Sprague-Dawley rat and was not found in the intestine of Fischer rats. Furthermore, the duodenal–ileal distribution of these antigens appeared to be similar in the two species. These studies were performed to determine whether the region of the crypt–villus junction in aging rats might show a pattern of antigens characteristic of mid-crypt cells. The antibodies specific for antigens present only in crypt cells[15,16] (Table 9.3) showed a very similar distribution of immunofluorescence in the crypt–villus column from duodenum and jejunum of young and aging Fischer animals. Furthermore,

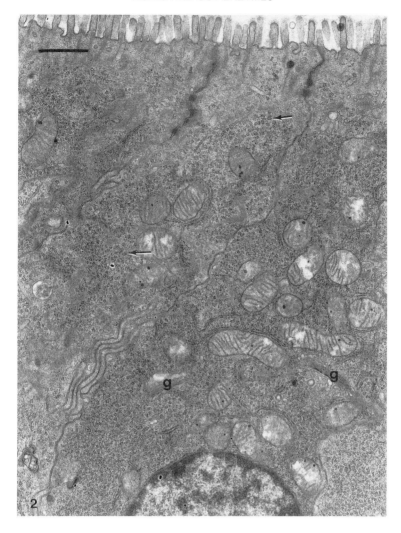

Figure 9.2 Undifferentiated crypt cells in the jejunum of a young Fischer rat characterized by abundant free polyribosomes (arrows), short rough endoplasmic reticulum, short Golgi stacks (g), and short and irregular microvilli. Bar represents 1 μm.

antibodies that specifically detect antigens that occur in the differentiating zone of cells near the crypt–villus junction[15,17] (Table 9.3) also showed no difference in distribution in young and aging rats. Thus, this histochemical pattern permits the conclusion that the process of differentiation of the crypt epithelial cells occurs normally in aging rats. In addition, using a wide range of monoclonal antibodies directed toward antigens usually present in villus epithelial cells[14,16,18] (Table 9.3) we were unable to demonstrate any difference in the distribution in the young and aging rats. These data imply that delayed

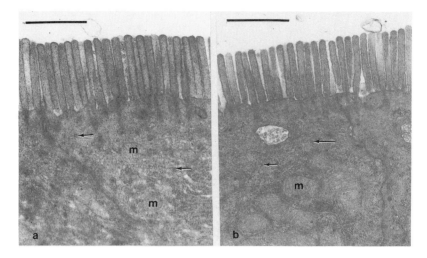

Figure 9.3 Epithelial cells in the differentiating zone of villi near the crypt–villus junction in young (a) and aging (b) rats. No difference in microvillus length or density is seen. Mitochondria (m) in aging rats occasionally (but not consistently) were larger in cells of aging than of young rats. The number of free ribosomes (arrow) decreased similarly at both ages in cells observed higher up the villus. Bar represents 1 μm.

expression of sucrase-isomaltase activity in aging rats does not correlate with expression of sucrase-isomaltase antigen. Alternatively, the immuno-fluorescent method may fail to detect quantitative changes in lower villus cells.

Since aging rats had lower mucosal specific activities of several brush border enzymes and changes in expression of enzyme activities under baseline fed conditions, we decided to test the controls of small intestinal enzyme activities by changing nutritional intake. The response of villus mucosal enzymes to abrupt changes in food intake, starvation or re-feeding after a period of starvation, are well accepted ways of disturbing the homeostatic controls of intestinal function[19].

In our studies, we starved groups of young and aging Fischer 344 rats for a period of 2 or 3 days. Re-feeding was studied in other groups of young and aging rats by using a period of 3 days of starvation followed by 1 day of pelleted chow re-feeding. In these experiments, starvation induced a greater fall in specific or total intestinal activity of duodenal or of jejunal maltase or sucrase in aging than in younger animals. As an example, Table 9.4 demonstrates changes in maltase and sucrase specific activity in the duodenum of young rats and aging rats. The data are presented as enzyme activity as a percentage of activity in fed control animals. Mucosal-specific activity of these enzymes already was significantly lower in the fed aging rats than in young fed control rats in these studies (Table 9.2). Whereas enzyme-specific activity of sucrase in the duodenum of young animals after 3 days of starvation fell by about 30%, sucrase activity fell by about 60% in the aging animals (Table 9.4). One day of chow re-feeding following 3 days of starvation (during which time rats at the two ages showed similar food intake) resulted

Table 9.3 Monoclonal antibodies against epithelial cell antigens used for immunofluorescence studies

Antibody	Ig (sub) type	Antigen specificity	Reference
Antibodies to brush border proteins (enzymes) of villus cells			
BB/34	IgG$_1$	Sucrase-isomaltase	17
BBC1/35	IgG$_1$	Sucrase-isomaltase	14
BB433	IgG$_1$	Aminopeptidase N	14
YBB2/54/3	IgG$_1$	Aminopeptidase N	14
CLB4/40	IgG$_1$	Dipeptidyl-peptidase IV	14
BBC3/BB	IgG$_1$	Maltase-glucoamylase	14
YBB1/57	IgG$_{2A}$	Lactase	14
YBB2/61	IgG$_1$	Lactase	14
FBB3/24	IgG$_1$	Lactase	16
BB4/35	IgG$_1$	Alkaline phosphatase	14
BB5/16	IgG$_1$	Alkaline phosphatase	14
YBB1/83	IgG$_1$	200 + 130 kDa polypeptides	14
BB4/34	IgG$_1$	185 kDa polypeptide	14
BB4/42	IgG$_1$	193 kDa polypeptide	14
Antibodies specific for luminal membrane antigens of crypt and villus cells			
FBB2/28*	IgG$_1$	195 + 185 kDa polypeptides	16
Antibodies specific for crypt and lower villus cells			
CC422	IgG$_1$	28–34 kDa antigen	18
CC4/80	IgG$_1$	28–34 kDa antigen	15
Antibodies specific for crypt cells			
CLB2/33	IgG$_1$	not identified	
YBB3/10	IgM	160 + 135 kDa antigen (CCA)	15
FBB2/29	IgM	160 + 135 kDa antigen (CCA)	16
Antibodies specific for intestinal keratins			
BBC3/40/1	IgG$_1$	53, 48, 46, 42, 40 kDa keratins	
BBC3/48/5	IgG$_1$	48, 46 kDa keratins (specific for differentiated intestinal cells)	

*Did not react with antigens in young or aging Fischer 344 rat intestine, but reacted with intestine from young Sprague-Dawley rats. These antibodies were prepared and characterized as previously described[14]. Negative controls were included and utilized; as first antibody solutions, non-immune mouse serum (diluted 1:25 in PBS + 0.2% BSA), non-immune mouse IgM, or two monoclonal antibodies of the IgM type (CaCo5/37 and CaCo5/75/9)[14] which have failed to stain rat intestinal specimens tested to date. Positive controls were sections stained with monoclonal antibodies to cytokeratins. Stained slides were evaluated independently by at least two investigators within one hour after staining. For immunofluorescence staining, ascites fluids were diluted 1:200 in PBS + 0.2% BSA.

in an abrupt and significant increase in the specific activity of maltase and of sucrase in young animals. The increase in specific activity following 1 day of re-feeding in aging animals far exceeded that found in younger rats (Table 9.4). Changes in the jejunum overall were less dramatic than in the duodenum but showed the same trends. The data imply altered controls of the homeostasis of enzyme activity during the stress of dietary manipulation in the older animals.

Table 9.4 Changes in duodenal mucosal enzyme specific activity of young and aging rats during starvation and re-feeding (mean of 7–9 animals in each group)

Rat	Percentage change from control fed rats			
	Sucrase	Maltase	Lactase	Alkaline phosphatase
Starved				
Young	− 30	− 33	+ 16	− 5
Aging	− 62*	− 52*	+ 56	− 35*
Re-fed				
Young	+ 33	+ 30	+ 40	+ 51
Aging	+ 77*	+ 66*	+ 106*	+ 44*

* Significantly different from control fed rats at $p < 0.05$

Altered enzyme activity in aging rats could result from a change in the synthesis or turnover of the enzyme or to a change in enzyme structure in aging rat intestine. We have recently performed preliminary studies on the structure and function relationships of one intestinal brush border enzyme, sucrase-isomaltase (S-I). To this end, we have purified brush border S-I using as starting material a mucosal preparation derived from young rats. Purity was established by polyacrylamide gel electrophoresis and isoelectric focusing. We have prepared a polyclonal antibody of high specificity by the injection of this purified S-I into New Zealand rabbits. To seek changes in the protein composition of the epithelium of aging rats, homogenates of mucosal scrapings were extracted with Triton X-100 and 2% SDS, and the extracts were subjected to SDS polyacrylamide gel electrophoresis. No major changes in the patterns of Coomassie blue stained proteins were observed between young and aging Fischer animals. The Western blot immunoblotting patterns shown in Figure 9.4, from young and aging animals, indicate that the mobility of S-I subunits appear to be essentially identical. These studies would suggest that there are no major differences in the structure of S-I from the jejunum of young and aging Fischer rats.

We also have performed preliminary studies of the relationship of sucrase enzyme activity to the content of S-I protein present in young and aging small intestine. Mucosal homogenates were extracted with 0.5% Triton X-100. S-I protein was quantitated by rocket immunoelectrophoresis, using 0.5% antiserum against S-I in 1.0% agarose gel with 0.5% Triton X-100. Sucrase-specific activity as a function of S-I protein was lower in aging than in young rats (Table 9.5). This was seen in fed, 3-day starved and 1-day refed animals. In addition, this preliminary data clearly show that starvation reduced S-I specific activity and re-feeding increased specific activity in both young and aging animals. This latter observation is similar to those presented by Quan and Gray[20]. The data support the concept that enzyme protein is preserved during starvation and may be available in a more active form during the re-feeding period. These observations imply that there is a minor alteration in sucrase-isomaltase protein structure which appears to be adaptable to changes in nutrient availability. It is conceivable that the altered specific activity found

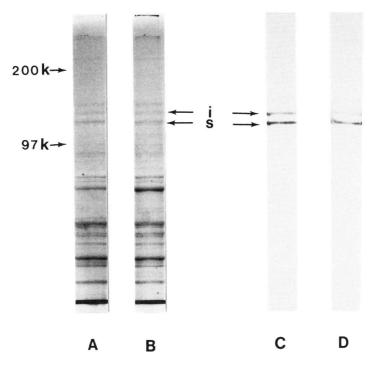

Figure 9.4 Protein profile and sucrase-isomaltase mobility of jejunal mucosa from young and aging rats by SDS polyacrylamide gel (7.5%) electrophoresis and immunoblotting. Mucosal proteins visualized by Coomassie blue staining in young (lane A) and aging (lane B) rats. The mobility of sucrase (s) and isomaltase (i) subunits in young (lane C) and aging (lane D) rats are identified by immunoblotting.

in the proximal intestine of aging rats, may be due in part to a defect in the conversion of inactive S-I molecules to an enzymatically active form.

Numerous observations have been made on enzyme changes that accompany the aging process in other organs, particularly the liver. From these studies, several general conclusions have been reached[21]. It is clear that the specific activity of some enzymes falls with age whereas others are unaltered or actually are increased. When a fall in enyzme activity occurs, examination of the protein molecule usually has revealed few major structural changes. Thus, no differences in molecular weight, charge, K_m or behaviour toward inhibitors were observed in the enzymes studied to date. On the other hand, changes in heat stability occur[22] and some enzymes from aging rodents have shown a lower specific activity (as a function of immunoprecipitable protein content) (see Chapter 5). Generally, the adaptive responses of enzyme action have been blunted in aging animals[23]. Often, minor physical treatment has changed an 'old' to a 'young' enzyme[24]. These observations suggest some minor changes in conformation between such enzymes. It seems likely, therefore, that any changes that occur in aging enzymes are due to post-translational alterations rather than changes in amino acid sequence[25]. The

Table 9.5 Effect of age and changes in diet on jejunal sucrase-isomaltase (S-I)* activity and content (per gram mucosa)

Rat†	Enzyme activity (μmoles/min)	S-I protein (mg)	Specific activity
Control			
Y ($n=7$)	8.0 ± 0.7	0.24 ± 0.02	34 ± 2
A ($n=7$)	6.6 ± 0.9	0.25 ± 0.03	27 ± 2
$p=$	0.066	NS	0.03
Starved			
Y ($n=3$)	4.4 ± 0.4	0.22 ± 0.02	20 ± 3
A ($n=3$)	3.8 ± 0.8	0.24 ± 0.05	16 ± 1
$p=$	NS	NS	NS
Re-fed			
Y ($n=6$)	8.0 ± 0.7	0.24 ± 0.02	35 ± 5
A ($n=6$)	6.0 ± 0.4	0.22 ± 0.02	28 ± 3
$p=$	0.004	NS	0.05

* Sucrase activity determined by standard methods. Sucrase-isomaltase protein determined by rocket immunoelectrophoresis. Data presented as mean ± SEM in the number of animals shown in parentheses. Differences determined by one-tailed paired t-tests
† Y = young; A = aging

present preliminary observations on sucrase-isomaltase are in accord with these general phenomena described previously in enzymes from lower animal species or in the rodent liver. Our future studies aim to pursue these preliminary observations of rodent intestinal sucrase-isomaltase from aging rats by purifying the enzyme from young and from aging intestine and conducting experiments with such 'pure' enzymes. In addition, we plan to relate changes in enzyme structure and function with any associated changes in enzyme protein synthesis and turnover.

Acknowledgments

This work was supported in part by NIH grants AG 01625, AM 33916, AM 32656 and CA 44714 and by the Overseas Shipholding Corporation. The excellent technical assistance of A. Dominguez and A. Washington and the participation of Drs A. Quaroni and D. Kotler are gratefully acknowledged.

References

1. Welsh, J. D., Poley, J. R., Bhatia, M. and Stevenson, D. E. (1978). Intestinal disaccharidase activities in relation to age, race and mucosal damage. *Gastroenterology*, **75**, 847–55
2. Sayeed, M. M. and Blumenthal, H. T. (1968). Age difference in the intestinal phosphomonoesterase activity of mice. *Proc. Soc. Exp. Biol. Med.*, **129**, 1–3
3. Leutert, V. G., Jahn, K. and Weise, K. (1973). Altersabhängige Veränderungen der Enzymaktivität von Enterozyten – histochemische Untersuchungen. *Z. Alternsforsch.* **26**, 375–8

4. Hohn, P., Gabbert, H. and Wagner, R. (1978). Differentiation and aging of the rat intestinal mucosa. II. Morphological, enzyme histochemical and disc electrophoretic aspects of the aging of the small intestinal mucosa. *Mech. Age. Dev.*, **7**, 217–26

5. Moog, F. (1977). The small intestine in old mice: Growth, alkaline phosphatase and disaccharidase activities, and deposition of amyloid. *Exp. Gerontol.*, **12**, 223–35

6. Coleman, G. L., Barthold, S. W., Osbaldiston, G. W., Foster, S. J. and Jonas, A. M. (1977). Pathological changes during aging in barrier-reared Fischer 344 male rats. *J. Gerontol.*, **32**, 258–78

7. Holt, P. R., Pascal, R. R. and Kotler, D. P. (1984). Effect of aging upon small intestinal structure in the Fischer rat. *J. Gerontol.*, **29**, 642–47

8. Holt, P. R., Kotler, D. P. and Pascal, R. R. (1983). A simple method for determining epithelial cell turnover in small intestine: Studies in young and aging rat gut. *Gastroenterology*, **84**, 69–74

9. Holt, P. R., Tierney, A. R. and Kotler, D. P. (1985). Delayed enzyme expression: A defect of aging rat gut. *Gastroenterology*, **89**, 1026–34

10. Riby, J. E. and Kretchmer, N. (1984). Effect of dietary sucrose on synthesis and degradation of intestinal sucrase. *Am. J. Physiol.*, **246**, 6757–63

11. Alpers, D. H. and Tedesco, F. J. (1975). The possible role of pancreatic proteases in the turnover of intestinal brush border proteins. *Biochim. Biophys. Acta*, **401**, 28–40

12. Riepe, S. P., Goldstein, J. and Alpers, D. H. (1980). Effect of secreted *Bacteroides* proteases on human intestinal brush border hydrolases. *J. Clin. Invest.*, **66**, 314–22

13. Madara, J. L. and Trier, J. S. (1987). Functional morphology of the mucosa of the small intestine. In Johnson, L. R. (ed.) *Physiology of the Gastrointestinal Tract*. pp. 1209–49 (New York: Raven Press)

14. Quaroni, A. and Isselbacher, K. J. (1985). Study of intestinal cell differentiation with monoclonal antibodies to intestinal cell surface components. *Dev. Biol.*, **111**, 267–79

15. Quaroni, A. (1985). Crypt cell development in newborn rat small intestine. *J. Cell Biol.*, **100**, 1601–10

16. Quaroni, A. (1986). Fetal characteristics of small intestinal crypt cells. *Proc. Natl. Acad. Sci. USA*, **83**, 1723–7

17. Quaroni, A. (1985). Pre- and postnatal development of differentiated functions in rat intestinal epithelial cells. *Dev. Biol.*, **111**, 280–92

18. Hauri, H. P., Quaroni, A. and Isselbacher, K. J. (1980). Monoclonal antibodies to sucrase-isomaltase: Probes for the study of postnatal development and biogenesis of the intestinal microvillus membrane. *Proc. Natl. Acad. Sci. USA*, **77**, 6629–33

19. Deren, J. J., Broitman, S. A. and Zamcheck, N. (1967). Effect of diet upon intestinal disaccharidases and disaccharide absorption. *J. Clin. Invest.*, **46**, 189–95

20. Quan, R. and Gray, G. (1987). Sucrase-alpha-dextrinase reduction by carbohydrate-free (CF) diet: Conversion of active to inactive enzyme. *Gastroenterology*, **92**, 1585

21. Makrides, S. C. (1983). Protein synthesis and degradation during aging and senescence. *Biol. Rev.*, **58**, 343–422

22. Rothstein, M. (1979). The formation of altered enzymes in aging animals. *Mech. Age. Dev.*, **9**, 197–202

23. Adelman, R. C. (1979). Loss of adaptive mechanisms during aging. *Fed. Proc.*, **38**, 1968–71

24. Sharma, H. K. and Rothstein, M. (1978). Age-related changes in the properties of enolase from *Turbatrix aceti*. *Biochemistry*, **17**, 2869–76

25. Richardson, A. (1981). The relationship between aging and protein synthesis. In Florini, J. R. (ed.) *CRC Handbook of Biochemistry in Aging*. pp. 79–101 (Boca Raton, Florida: CRC Press)

10
Age-related alterations in the lipid dynamics and lipid–protein interactions of intestinal and hepatic membranes

T. A. BRASITUS

INTRODUCTION

Cellular membranes clearly are involved in many critical functions of the cell[1,2]. Alterations in the structure of these membranes during the aging process could, therefore, have important consequences in terms of cellular functions. Recently, it has been postulated that changes in cell-membrane structure–function play a crucial role in the aging of cells[3,4]. This 'membrane hypothesis of aging' is supported by a number of theoretical considerations and by experimental testing[3,4].

Several excellent reviews concerned with changes in cell membranes during aging have been published[1,4]. In this review, a general overview of the topic will not be attempted but will focus on the changes in intestinal and liver membranes that have been described during aging, with particular emphasis on lipid–protein interactions, lipid dynamics and lipid compositional alterations previously shown to occur in the membranes of enterocytes and hepatocytes.

ALTERATIONS IN ENTEROCYTE MEMBRANES DURING AGING

Plasma Membranes

The major cell type lining the mucosa of the small intestine, the enterocyte, is involved and responsible for many important functions[5]. Functions include: nutrient absorption; absorption and/or secretion of water and electrolytes; digestion of substances such as peptides and disaccharides; and synthesis of compounds, such as lipoproteins, for transport from intestinal cells to the extracellular spaces[5]. In order to perform these various functions, the enterocyte is highly specialized and its plasma membrane differentiated into luminal (brush-border) and contraluminal (basolateral) regions. To date, studies concerned with alterations in lipid–protein interactions and lipid dynamics in the membranes of enterocytes during aging have been sparse and limited to brush-border membranes.

In this regard, recent studies by Pang et al.[6] and Schwarz et al.[7,8] have demonstrated a decrease in small intestinal brush-border membrane 'lipid fluidity'* during postnatal development in rats and rabbits. Pang et al.[6], utilizing electron spin resonance techniques, demonstrated that the spin label, 5-doxylstearic acid appeared to be in a more 'disordered environment' in brush-border membrane of newborn rabbits than in membranes from their adult counterparts. Moreover, experiments utilizing cholera toxin as an external stimulus to test for structural responses in these membrane preparations, also suggested that the luminal membranes from newborns were inherently more disordered than membranes prepared from adult animals[6]. Based on these observations, Pang et al.[6] suggested that the mucosal barrier to foreign materials may be incomplete in the newborn period.

Similarly Schwarz et al.[7], using steady-state fluorescence polarization techniques, found that the fluorescence anisotropy of the probe diphenylhexatriene (DPH) increased during the weaning period in rabbit jejunal and ileal luminal membranes, indicating a decreased membrane lipid fluidity. Furthermore, an increased cholesterol/phospholipid molar ratio (0.56 for 14–21-day-old versus 0.83 for adult rabbit jejunum) appeared, at least in part, to be responsible for this difference in fluidity[7].

Recently, Schwarz et al.[8] have also shown that brush-border membranes from jejunum and ileum of suckling 14–20-day-old rats were more fluid than their membrane counterparts prepared from mature post-weaning rats (28–49 days' old). These alterations in fluidity appeared to be secondary to a higher total lipid and total phospholipid content per milligram of protein in the plasma membranes of suckling rats compared to membranes from post-weaning rats. In agreement with these latter findings, Neu et al.[9] have shown a decrease in the fluidity of small intestinal luminal membranes of 'mature' rats (30 days' old) compared to membranes prepared from younger animals (22-day foetus or 5 days' old), using fluorescence polarization techniques. Taken together these studies indicate that during development, the small intestinal luminal membranes of rats and rabbits become less fluid, as assessed by electron spin resonance and steady-state fluorescence polarization techniques.

To determine whether these fluidity and compositional differences were due to a developmental trend with age, rather than from dietary and/or other

---

* The term 'lipid fluidity' as applied to model bilayer and natural membranes is used throughout this chapter to express the relative motional freedom of the lipid molecules or substituents thereof. More detailed descriptions have been published[28]. Briefly, as evaluated by steady-state fluorescence polarization of lipid fluorophores, fluidity is assessed by the parameters of the modified Perrin equation[28]. An increase in fluidity corresponds to a decrease in either the correlation time, T_c, or the hindered anisotropy, r_∞, of the fluorophore, thereby combining the concepts of the 'dynamic' and 'static' (lipid order) components of fluidity.

factors associated with weaning, our laboratory examined and compared these membrane parameters in young, adult and old animals[10]. In these studies the lipid fluidity of proximal and distal small intestinal brush-border membranes prepared from Fischer 344 rats 6, 17 and 117 weeks' old was measured using steady-state fluorescence polarization techniques and the DPH probe. In agreement with the previous findings of others[8,9], the lipid fluidity of both proximal and distal brush-border membranes of rats aged 6 weeks was found to be significantly greater compared to membranes of rats aged 17 weeks. Interestingly, however, there was no significant differences in the fluidity of membranes prepared from animals aged 17 and 117 weeks. Moreover, a lipid thermotropic phase transition was observed at $17.5 \pm 1.3°C$ in the proximal membranes of the youngest group, approximately 5–6°C lower than that of older animals (Figure 10.1). The latter finding would be in keeping with the greater fluidity of the younger animals' membranes[10].

The difference in lipid composition which accounted for the higher fluidity of the youngest preparations included a decreased cholesterol/phospholipid molar ratio in both the proximal and distal halves of the small intestine and, in the proximal half alone, an increased lipid/protein ratio (w/w) and double-bond index. The foregoing reduction in the cholesterol/phospholipid molar ratio was secondary to a higher content of total phospholipid, whereas, the increment in double-bond index resulted from an increase in arachidonic acid ($C_{20:4}$) residues in the youngest membranes compared to adult and old membranes. These findings suggested that an age-dependent decrease in fluidity of intestinal proximal and distal luminal membranes occurs in the early post-weaning period in the rat. It does not appear, however, that this trend in membrane fluidity to decrease continues to occur during the aging process but rather reaches a plateau. This pattern of fluidity, moreover, was unlike that of the brush-border membrane's p-nitrophenyl phosphatase (alkaline phosphatase), whose specific activity was found to decline progressively in the older age group[10].

Earlier studies by our laboratory had operationally classified rat small intestinal brush-border membranes into two groups[11]. The first group consisted of the digestive enzymes sucrase, lactase, maltase, γ-glu-tamyltranspeptidase and leucine aminopeptidase. Each of these activities yielded a single slope in their respective Arrhenius plot in the range of 10–40°C and did not appear to functionally experience the effects of the lipid thermotropic transition[11]. Each member of the second group including alkaline phosphatase, magnesium- and calcium-dependent adenosine triphosphatase, and D-glucose transport, however, did demonstrate changes in the slope of their respective Arrhenius plots, i.e. a change in the energy of activation in the range 25–30°C, which corresponded to the lower region of the lipid transition[11]. These groups have been termed 'extrinsic' and 'intrinsic' activities, respectively. Given the disparate patterns of fluidity and alkaline phosphatase activity in the brush-border membranes during aging (see above), it would appear unlikely, therefore, that these two parameters were related in this instance. Rather, as previously suggested[12], the decrease in alkaline phosphatase activity seen with age more likely represents a decrease in protein synthesis.

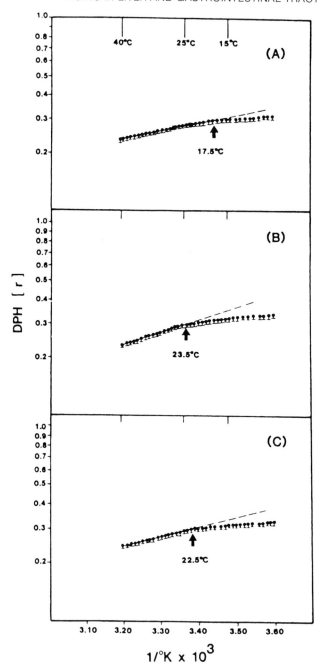

Figure 10.1 Arrhenius plots of the fluorescence anisotropy (r) of diphenylhexatriene (DPH) in proximal microvillus membranes of rats aged 6 weeks (A), 17 weeks (B) and 117 weeks (C). (Reproduced with permission of *Biochimica Biophysica Acta*, Elsevier Science Publishers BV)

Similarly, it should be noted, based on previous observations in a number of other membranes[13-15], that the plateau in fluidity values of intestinal membranes seen during these studies was somewhat surprising. In this regard, prior studies in the membrane of lymphocytes[13], platelets[14] and even rose petals[15] had suggested an inverse relationship between fluidity and aging, i.e. fluidity decreased with increased age. The small intestinal fluidity data would, therefore, suggest that generalizations concerning the relationship between membrane fluidity and aging cannot easily be made and must be experimentally determined for each individual membrane.

ALTERATIONS IN HEPATOCYTE MEMBRANES DURING AGING

Plasma membranes

In 1975, Hegner and Platt[16] reported that the fluidity of rat hepatic plasma membranes was lower in old rats compared to young rats. More recently, Nokubo[17] found that the fluidity of rat hepatocyte plasma membranes, as assessed by steady-state fluorescence polarization using the DPH probe, decreased progressively with age after 2 months in male rats, whereas, in female rats the fluidity of these plasma membranes only began to decrease after 24 months. Taken together, these studies suggest that, in general, rat hepatocyte membrane fluidity decreases with age but may be influenced by such factors as hormones related to the sex of the animals.

It should be noted that while these studies are interesting, they suffer from two major problems. First, analyses of the lipid composition of these membranes, which might have been useful in elucidating the factor responsible for their fluidity differences, were not performed; and second, these plasma membranes undoubtedly contained both canalicular and sinusoidal fractions. Given the availability of newer methodologies[18], it might be useful to examine each of these regions of the plasma membrane separately during aging. Further studies will, therefore, be necessary to examine the lipid dynamics of hepatocyte plasma membranes during aging.

Conclusions reached concerning plasma membrane enzyme activities and their relationship with changes in fluidity during the aging process are difficult to interpret[16,17], given the likelihood that the preparations examined may have differed with respect to their relative percentages of canalicular and sinusoidal regions.

Hepatocyte intracellular membranes

The effect of aging on the lipid composition and fluidity of hepatic mitochondrial membranes of female Fischer 344 rats recently has been determined by Vorbeck et al.[19]. These investigators have shown a progressive age-dependent increase in the cholesterol/phospholipid molar ratio of mitochondrial membranes, secondary to progressive increases and decreases, respectively, in their cholesterol and phospholipid contents. Furthermore, steady-state fluorescence polarization studies utilizing DPH revealed a highly significant age-dependent increase in the lipid structural order parameter of these membranes, which was consistent with their increased molar ratio of cholesterol/phospholipid.

In contrast to these findings of Vorbeck et al.[19], Grinna[20], using male Sprague-Dawley rats, reported no significant changes in total phospholipids of mitochondrial membranes during aging. A significant age-related increase in total cholesterol content and cholesterol/phospholipid molar ratio was noted[20]. More recently, Horton and Spencer[21] also have reported an increased cholesterol content of hepatic mitochondrial membranes isolated from aged Wistar rats. Taken together these studies indicate that the cholesterol/phospholipid molar ratio of rat hepatic mitochondrial membranes increases during aging which, in turn, leads to a decrease in their lipid fluidity. Further studies will be necessary to examine the mechanism(s) responsible for these age-related compositional and fluidity alterations as well as to elucidate their functional significance in rat hepatocyte mitochondrial membranes. Based on the observations noted above, any such studies should consider sex and strain of the animals as important variables.

In 1979, Kapitulnik et al.[22] reported an increase in rat hepatic microsomal membrane fluidity at birth and a continued increase in fluidity to 3 months of age. More recently, Armbrecht et al.[23], utilizing electron paramagnetic resonance techniques and the spin labels 5-nitroxide and 16-nitroxide stearic acid, extended these observations to show a further increase in fluidity from 3 to 25–27 months of age in microsomal membranes. Since the increase in fluidity with age was seen with both spin labels, the results suggest that the increased fluidity extended from the surface of the membrane into its interior.

Armbrecht et al.[23] also noted the absence of a break in Arrhenius plots of these spin label probes in young membranes whereas a break was seen in old membranes at 24°C. These data would be consistent with an absence of a lipid-phase transition in the younger membranes, while the older membranes appeared to possess such a transition. These findings again would support structural changes in the microsomal membranes with age. Unfortunately, Armbrecht et al.[23] did not examine the lipid compositional parameters responsible for these age-related fluidity differences, but suggested, based on prior studies by Grinna[24], that they might be secondary to an overall age-related increase in the degree of unsaturation of the major membrane fatty acids. However, Grinna[24] also has previously shown that a significant age-related increase in the cholesterol/phospholipid molar ratio was seen in microsomal membranes which theoretically should lead to decreased membrane fluidity. Based on these disparate observations, therefore, the compositional alterations underlying the fluidity changes seen by Armbrecht et al.[23] are unclear at this time and will require further study.

Additional support for age-related structural changes in the membrane lipids of rat hepatic microsomes has been provided by Grinna and Barber[25–27]. These investigators have shown that the kinetic parameters as well as the energies of activation and discontinuities seen in Arrhenius plots of various microsomal enzymatic activities changed with age[25–27]. These results again strongly suggest that the interactions of microsomal membrane components are altered during aging.

SUMMARY AND COMMENTS

Intestinal and hepatic cellular membranes are useful experimental preparations to examine age-related alterations of their lipid dynamics and protein–lipid interactions. The plasma membranes of these cells, in particular, offer a number of advantages including their high degree of functional specialization of luminal and contraluminal regions, as well as the feasibility of preparing sufficient quantities of relatively purified preparations for examination by a variety of experimental techniques, including steady-state fluorescence polarization and electron spin resonance.

Studies conducted, to date, suggest that age-related changes in the lipid composition and physical state of the lipid occur in every plasma and intracellular membrane of enterocytes and hepatocytes thus far examined. In this regard, however, it is important to realize that each cellular membrane appears to have its own distinct pattern of age-related alterations in these biochemical and biophysical parameters. At present, therefore, it is difficult to make generalizations concerning these membrane parameters in relationship to the process of aging. It would seem reasonable to suggest, however, that these structural changes should, at least in part, be responsible for many of the functional alterations present in these membranes during the aging process.

Future studies in this area should provide interesting and potentially important information on structure–function relationships during aging. Investigators should, however, realize that an integrated approach in which the lipid dynamics, lipid composition as well as lipid–protein interactions in these membranes are all simultaneously examined would yield the most useful information in terms of mechanism(s) responsible for age-related membrane changes.

Lastly, investigators should focus on specific regions of plasma membranes, utilize several different experimental probes for biophysical analyses, and consider such variables as sex and animal strain when studying age-related alterations in the physical state of the lipid and lipid–protein interactions in intestinal and hepatic membranes.

References

1. Grinna, L. S. (1977). Changes in cell membranes during aging. *Gerontology*, **23**, 452–64
2. Bangham, A. D. (1972). Lipid bilayers and biomembranes. *Annu. Rev. Biochem.*, **41**, 753–66
3. Zs.-Nagy, I. (1978). A membrane hypothesis of aging. *J. Theor. Biol.*, **75**, 189–95
4. Zs.-Nagy, I. (1979). The role of membrane structure and function in cellular aging: a review. *Mech. Age. Dev.*, **9**, 237–46
5. Schachter, D. (1985). Lipid dynamics and lipid–protein interaction in intestinal plasma membranes In Watts & Depont (eds.) *Progress in Protein–Lipid Interactions*. pp. 231–58. (Amsterdam: Elsevier Science Publishers)

6. Pang, K. Y., Bresson, J. L. and Walker, W. A. (1983). Development of the gastrointestinal barrier. III. Evidence for structural differences in microvillus membranes from newborn and adult rabbits. *Biochim. Biophys. Acta*, **727**, 201–8
7. Schwarz, S. M., Ling, S., Hostetler, B., Draper, J. P. and Watkins, J. B. (1984). Lipid composition and membrane fluidity in the small intestine of the developing rabbit. *Gastroenterology*, **86**, 1544–51
8. Schwarz, S. M., Hostetler, B., Ling, S., Mone, M. and Watkins, J. B. (1985). Intestinal membrane lipid composition and fluidity during development in the rat. *Am. J. Physiol.*, **248**, G200–G207
9. Neu, J., Ozaki, C. K. and Angelides, K. J. (1986). Glucocorticoid-mediated alterations in the fluidity of brush-border membrane in rat small intestine. *Pediat. Res.*, **20**, 79–82
10. Brasitus, T. A., Yeh, K. Y., Holt, P. R. and Schachter, D. (1984). Lipid fluidity and composition of intestinal microvillus membranes isolated from rats of different ages. *Biochim. Biophys. Acta*, **778**, 341–8
11. Brasitus, T. A., Schachter, D. and Mamouneas, T. G. (1979). Functional interactions of lipids and proteins in rat intestinal microvillus membranes. *Biochemistry*, **18**, 4136–44
12. Dice, J. F. (1985). Cellular theories of aging as related to the liver. *Hepatology*, **5**, 508–13
13. Rivnay, B., Globerson, A. and Shinitzky, M. (1979). Viscosity of lymphocyte plasma membrane in aging mice and its possible relation to serum cholesterol. *Mech. Age. Dev.*, **10**, 71–9
14. Cohen, B. M. and Zubenko, G. S. (1985). Aging and the biophysical properties of cell membranes. *Life Sci.*, **37**, 1403–9
15. Borochov, A., Halevy, A. and Shinitzky, M. (1976). Increase in microviscosity with aging in protoplast plasmalemma of rose petals. *Nature (London)*, **263**, 158–9
16. Hegner, D. and Platt, D. (1975). Effect of essential phospholipids on the properties of ATPase of isolated rat liver plasma membranes of young and old animals. *Mech. Age. Dev.*, **4**, 191–200
17. Nokubo, M. (1985). Physicalchemical and biochemical differences in liver plasma membranes in aging F-344 rats. *J. Gerontol.*, **40**, 409–14
18. Storch, J., Schachter, D., Inoue, M. and Wolkoff, A. W. (1983). Lipid fluidity of hepatocyte plasma membrane subfractions and their differential regulation by calcium. *Biochim. Biophys. Acta*, **727**, 209–12
19. Vorbeck, M. L., Martin, A. P., Long, J. W. Jr., Smith, J. M. and Orr, R. R. (1982). Aging-dependent modification of lipid composition and lipid structural order parameter of hepatic mitochondria. *Arch. Biochem. Biophys.*, **217**, 351–61
20. Grinna, L. S. (1977). Age related changes in the lipids of the microsomal and the mitochondrial membranes of rat liver and kidney. *Mech. Age. Dev.*, **6**, 197–205
21. Horton, A. A. and Spencer, J. A. (1981). Reversal of age-dependent decline in respiratory control ratio by hepatic regeneration. *FEBS Lett.*, **133**, 139–41
22. Kapitulnik, J., Tshershedsky, M. and Barenholz, Y. (1979). Fluidity of the rat liver microsomal membrane increases at birth. *Science*, **206**, 843–4
23. Armbrecht, H. J., Birnbaum, L. S., Zenser, T. V. and Davis, B. B. (1982). Changes in hepatic microsomal membrane fluidity with age. *Exp. Gerontol.*, **17**, 41–8
24. Grinna, L. S. (1976). Effects of dietary α-tocopherol on liver microsomes and mitochondria of aging rats. *J. Nutr.*, **106**, 918–29
25. Grinna, L. S. and Barber, A. A. (1972). Age-related changes in membrane lipid content and enzyme activities. *Biochim. Biophys. Acta*, **288**, 347–53
26. Grinna, L. S. and Barber, A. A. (1975). Kinetic analyses of the age-related differences in glucose-6-phosphatase activity. *Exp. Gerontol.*, **10**, 319–23
27. Grinna, L. S. (1977). Age-related alterations in membrane lipid and protein interactions: Arrhenius studies of microsomal glucose-6-phosphatase. *Gerontology*, **23**, 342–9
28. Brasitus, T. A. and Dudeja, P. K. (1985). Correction of abnormal lipid fluidity and composition of rat ileal microvillus membranes in chronic streptozotocin-induced diabetes by insulin therapy. *J. Biol. Chem.*, **260**, 12405–9

11
Aging and lipid absorption

A. B. R. THOMSON, M. KEELAN, M. L. GARG and M. T. CLANDININ

INTRODUCTION

Nam et ipsa scientia potestas est – Knowledge is power
Francis Bacon, *Meditationes Sacrae,* 1597

A number of clear, succinct and scholarly articles have been written over the past five years on the topic of the digestion, absorption and intestinal metabolism of lipids[1-18]. The micellar hypothesis of fat absorption has been re-examined[19]. The role of diet fat in subcellular structure and function has been examined in detail[20], and the importance of membrane lipid composition on cellular function has been carefully reviewed[21]. The approach of this review article will be to focus on the effects of aging.

AGING

Overview, from crib to adolescence

What is the signal for the changes in aging? Is the adaptation of intestinal function advantageous to the older animal, or a deterrent to longevity? Is intestinal aging a process of 'running down' or 'running up' to counter potentially adverse metabolic changes? Aging may be viewed as a continuation of some processes begun at an earlier period of development, and a return of other processes to a condition observed in youth (Figure 11.1). For example, mucosal surface area falls with aging, but only when compared with youth, not with birth. The *in vitro* uptake of lipids continues to fall and unstirred layer resistance continues to rise progressively, whereas the uptake of glucose and amino acids falls away from the high levels of youth, back to the lower levels at birth. The factors responsible for the 'breaking' of some changes and the acceleration of others, remain to be determined. Is aging a reversion of some processes to the perinatal state? Of greater importance is the answer to the question: 'are the adaptations occurring with aging a benefit to the continued well-being of the individual, or do these changes contribute

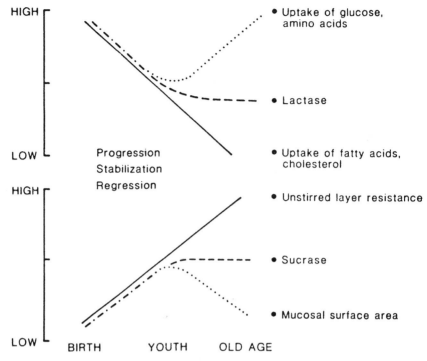

Figure 11.1 Patterns of intestinal development at different ages. At birth and up until weaning, there are only two patterns which are apparent, but with further aging, six different patterns emerge. (From Ref. 22)

to the age-associated processes of degeneration?' Is the effect of aging on the intestinal tract (or liver, or any other organ, for that matter) a beneficial or a detrimental adaptive process? Were we to know the answer, then we might better attempt to influence these three distinct patterns of progression, plateau and reversal[22], and thereby prevent or reverse the detrimental effects of aging on intestinal function.

The initiation of the post-natal ontogenic events in the rat gastrointestinal tract is probably determined by the animal's genetic program, while the terminal phase of intestinal development seems to be influenced more by environmental factors such as nutrients, hormones and other mediators. From the time of birth to senescence, there are alterations in the digestive and transport function of the intestine. Many of these investigations have been performed in rodents and have shown, for example, a reduction in the carrier-mediated absorption of valine and lysine[23] suggesting that the number of carrier molecules for absorption of these amino acids declines with aging. The transport of phosphate across the small intestine consists of two components, a saturable electroneutral sodium-dependent component, and an unsaturable sodium-independent component. The energy driving the first component is provided by an extracellular to intracellular sodium gradient maintained by the Na^+–K^+-ATPase at the basolateral membrane (BLM).

Both components of phosphate uptake decline with aging[24]. The effect of aging on the absorption of some nutrients is likely a specific effect on the uptake mechanisms rather than any effect on the morphology of the small bowel[25].

There is increased intestinal permeability to PEG-400 in old as compared with young rats[26], suggesting that the intestinal protective barrier to the absorption of potentially harmful environmental substances may be less efficient in aging animals. However, the absorption of some solutes such as xylose is unaffected by aging[27]. Thus, there are likely to be specific signals influencing the transport of specific nutrients.

What are the factors possibly responsible for the ontogenic expression of intestinal digestive and transport function? Regulatory factors that may initiate maturational changes include the pituitary–adrenal–thyroid secretion. While these hormones may modulate the developmental changes, the initiation of intestinal maturation is not dependent upon these factors. For example, studies using a transplantation technique in which jejunal isographs from newborn rats are implanted under the skin of newborn hosts have demonstrated an ontogenic timing mechanism in the jejunum which initiates the expression of sucrase activity[28]. The cellular basis for the timing of the expression of sucrase activity is unknown but may be mediated by the number of cell divisions. This activity is modulated by extrinsic systemic and luminal factors, but the timing for sucrase activity expression appears to be a stringent inherent property of the tissue itself. It is unknown whether age-associated intestinal changes are themselves also an inherent property of the tissue.

While post-natal ontogenic events may be an inherent property of the tissue, modulated by dietary constituents, pituitary–adrenal–thyroid axis and gastrointestinal peptides, what is the mechanism of the effect of aging on the intestine? Is this a process of beneficial adaptation (not to be tampered with), or detrimental running down, which should be modified? Clearly, dietary signals influence the intestinal adaptive process, at least at one end of the age spectrum: the weaning period is characterized by a shift from a liquid fat-rich, low-iron diet supplied by the mother to a solid diet rich in carbohydrates and iron. The proportion of carbohydrate relative to fat and the iron content of the weaning diet are critical for the maturation of intestinal microvillus enzymes but not for the ontogenic changes in DNA synthesis. However, initiation of changes in intestinal cell proliferation, DNA synthesis and mucosal enzymes are not diet-dependent, but may be triggered by the inter-action of the genetic program and hormonal mediators. The protein content of the weaning diet modulates the ontogenic changes in DNA synthesis and appears to be a factor in the completion of the growth of the gastrointestinal tract[29]. The exact mechanism by which luminal nutrients modify this devel-opmental process remains an enigma. However, the practical impact of, for example, the use of total parenteral nutrition for nutritional support of infants with disorders of the gastrointestinal tract is clear, with reduced development of stomach, small bowel and pancreatic growth[30]. Thus, despite normal weight gain, total serum protein and hematocrit concentrations, intravenous-fed animals failed to develop normally.

Membrane composition and function

The topic of the 'aging gut' has recently been reviewed[31]. Membrane function may be influenced by the membrane composition and physical properties[32-39], and there are several studies of change of brush-border membrane (BBM) or BLM fluidity[40-43] or of composition[44-50] in health and disease. What information that is available suggests that altered membrane transport function is associated with changes in BBM phospholipids and/or fatty acyl constituents, such as occurs with ileal resection, chronic ethanol ingestion, abdominal radiation or diabetes mellitus. What is the effect of aging?

Aging influences the composition and function of a number of different cell membranes[51-59]. Glycoproteins synthesized by rat small intestine change with age[60]. Differences in glycoprotein metabolism exist throughout the rat intestine and may play a role in the process of differentiation[61,62], although the importance of glycoprotein metabolism in the aging process is unknown.

Lipid peroxidation by free radicals, such as superoxide, give rise to changes in membrane properties and functions[63]. Aging increases the amount of superoxide radicals, resulting in reduced membrane fluidity in rat liver plasma membrane[64].

It has been proposed that the fluidity of membranes in general may decrease progressively with age, and may thereby account for certain of the concomitants of senescence[52,53]. In both rats and rabbits, there are increases in the BBM cholesterol:phospholipid ratio (owing to cholesterol content rising while the phospholipid content remains unchanged) and a corresponding decrease in membrane fluidity in ileal BBM at the time of weaning[65]. Pang and co-workers[66] used electron spin resonance to detect decreased order in BBM prepared from the intestines of newborn as compared with adult rabbits. Schwarz et al.[67] studied the fluorescence polarization of diphenylhexatriene (DPH) and they also observed greater fluidity of BBM of suckling rats and rabbits as compared with adults.

The differences in lipid composition which accounted for the higher fluidity of the preparations from younger animals included a decreased cholesterol:phospholipid molar ratio in both the proximal and distal halves of the small intestine, a lower sphingomyelin:phosphatidylcholine ratio and, in the proximal half alone, increases in the lipid:protein ratio and double-bond index. The reduction in cholesterol:phospholipid ratio derived mainly from a higher content of total phospholipid, and the increment in double-bond index resulted from an increase in arachidonic acid residues. Greater fluidity in the brush-border membrane of 6-week as compared with 17-week Fischer 344 rats was determined by fluorescence anisotropy of DPH[68]. However, between 17 and 117 weeks of age, the fluidity of the BBM increased rather than decreased with age. Both kinds of changes were observed only in the proximal and not in the distal intestine. Thus, part of the dilemma of establishing the effects of aging on the intestine, let alone in any other tissue, relates to the definition of 'old', for the changes observed with a 'young–old' may be very different from true senescence.

Certain of these compositional changes with aging rat intestine have been reported for other tissues: for example, decreases in total lipid or phospholipid were observed in rat liver[69,70], kidney[70] and pancreas[71]. Increases in the cholesterol:phospholipid ratio have been noted in rat erythrocytes[72], skeletal muscle[69] and in microsomal and mitochondrial fractions of rat liver[73]. A tendency for the fatty acids of some membranes to become more saturated with age has also been noted[53]. Moreover, age-related changes in essential fatty acid metabolism have also been reported[54]. The reduced activities of some BBM enzymes from aging rats may be owing to an increase in the proportion of relatively undifferentiated villus epithelial cells[74]. Thus, the process of aging clearly alters the structure and function of the small intestine.

It is assumed that changes in bulk membrane fluidity, as measured by membrane probes, reflect alterations in membrane lipid in the immediate microenvironment of specific membrane functions. However, it is possible that changes in the boundary lipids may not necessarily be concurrent with alterations in bulk phase lipids. Furthermore, changes in fluidity do not necessarily result in alterations in enzyme activities, and enzyme activity may change without alterations in the membrane fluidity. For example, another argument suggesting a dissociation between membrane fluidity and enzyme activity comes from the work of Brasitus et al.[68], comparing microvillus membranes of rat enterocytes from 17 versus 117-week-old rats showed a significant increase in fluidity in the older group, although there was a progressive decrease in the specific activity of p-nitrophenyl phosphatase. Finally, the finding that a given experimental manipulation may alter the activity of only some membrane enzymes on transport carriers raises the possibility that a given signal will be targeted to only certain boundary lipids.

Morphology

Conflicting reports on age-related changes in mucosal surface area are observed in rats[75,76]. In mature 1-year-old animals, there was a decline in villus height, number of cells per villus and mucosal surface area when compared with young animals, so that the jejunal characteristics of mature animals resembled those of weaning rabbits[77]. Also, the mucosal surface area of the ileum was similar in weaning, young and mature rabbits. The effective surface area of the unstirred water layer is increased with aging in rats and rabbits. Studies on epithelial cell turnover in the small intestine reveal similar rates of cell migration in young and aging rats[78]. In weaning pigs, amino acid transport sites are distributed along the length of the villus, whereas in mature rodents, most of the transport sites are located in the upper third of the villus[79–81]. It remains to be established, in a given animal species, whether the total number of transporting enterocytes lining the villus is affected by the aging process. Thus, it is not yet established whether the pool of functioning transport enterocytes is altered by aging, and it is this pool rather than just the total mucosal surface area or total number of enterocytes which is important in maintaining normal levels of intestinal transport.

Both the BBM sucrase (Suc) and alkaline phosphatase (AP) increase in young as compared with weaning rabbits, but the ratio of AP:Suc remains unchanged[77]. The Suc remains high in the mature rabbits but AP declines so that the ratio of AP:Suc falls. In weaning rabbits, the total BBM phospholipid content and the ratio of total phospholipid:total cholesterol are lower in the ileum than in the jejunum. The jejunal BBM total phospholipids and total cholesterol are higher in the mature than in the weanling animal jejunum when expressed as nmol/mg protein, but the ratio of total phospholipid:total cholesterol is unaffected by aging. The greatest percentage of jejunal BBM phospholipid is comprised of phosphatidylcholine (PC) and phosphatidylethanolamine (PE). The increased BBM total phospholipid content in mature animals is associated with a higher amount and lower proportion of PC, but a higher proportion of sphingomyelin and phosphatidylserine. The reduced value of the incremental change in free energy associated with aging reflects a lower relative permeability to fatty acids. Thus, aging of the intestine represents a continuum of morphological, functional and biochemical changes. The alterations in intestinal absorption are therefore not owing to major age-related changes in mucosal surface area or cell turnover, but are more likely related to alterations in the BBM lipid composition.

Plasma lipid concentrations

Stange and Dietschy[82] have compared plasma cholesterol levels and lipoprotein profiles, absolute rates of sterol synthesis and low-density lipoprotein (LDL) uptake in various organs of immature (4 weeks) and mature (15 weeks) rats. The plasma cholesterol level and its distribution among the major lipoprotein density fractions were similar in both groups. This finding is consistent with previous reports that plasma cholesterol levels in the rat are stable during the first 6 months of life and, thereafter, increase only to a variable degree in different strains of rat[83,84] or remain unchanged, even in old rats 22 months of age[85]. Plasma lipoproteins may serve as one of the regulators of sterol synthesis[86] and, possibly, receptor-mediated LDL uptake in various extrahepatic tissues[87]. The content of newly-synthesized cholesterol was several-fold higher in all tissues of young as compared to old rats, but the whole body content of cholesterol was identical.

The changes in rates of sterol synthesis observed in the various organs of the older rats thus cannot be attributed to a concomitant alteration in plasma cholesterol levels[82], but rather are probably a response to the diminished demand for cellular cholesterol as the rate of tissue growth diminishes. This age-related decline in sterol synthesis has been described previously in tissues such as liver[88,89] and skin[90]. The importance of different organs to total-body sterol synthesis remains similar with increasing age, although the skin (11% versus 24% of total) rather than the small bowel (15% versus 8%) becomes the second-most important organ after the liver (49% versus 45%) in older animals.

The rates of LDL cholesterol uptake are the same in liver and gastrointestinal tract of young and old animals. The calculation of absolute rates of tissue cholesterol acquisition from both sources indicated that, in most organs, the majority of tissue cholesterol was derived from local synthesis rather than from LDL uptake in both age groups. Indeed, with increasing age, total cholesterol acquisition decreases several-fold, primarily as a consequence of the diminished rate of sterol synthesis. With the 80% decline in body synthesis of cholesterol with aging, despite an essentially constant rate of LDL uptake, it is clear that there is independent regulation of rates of tissue cholesterol synthesis and LDL uptake. These data also suggest that the number of LDL receptors per gram of tissue remains constant during the transition from rapid to slow growth[91].

The reciprocal changes in rates of cholesterol synthesis with unchanged rates of LDL uptake despite marked changes in cholesterol balance across the intestine[92], liver[93] and other tissues may account for the observation that in many species, including man, the plasma LDL cholesterol levels remain remarkably constant under conditions where marked changes in cholesterol balance have been induced by dietary, surgical or dietary manipulations[94-96]. Only under circumstances where adaptive responses of the biosynthetic pathway are exceeded or blocked are changes in tissue LDL uptake and, hence, levels of circulating LDL cholesterol found[97,98].

Vitamins A and D

Aging is also associated with changes in the intestinal absorption of cholesterol[99,100], vitamin A[101], amino acids[102] and glucose[100,103]. Serum levels of vitamin A have been found to be reduced in older women, despite apparently adequate nutritional intake of the vitamin[104]. *In vivo* perfusion studies in groups of rats varying in age from 1.5 to 39 months have demonstrated that the absorption of radiolabelled vitamin A increased in a linear fashion with the age of the animals. The continued progressive increase in the total surface area and size of the small bowel observed in this study, could not account for the observations of enhanced vitamin A uptake[101].

While the exact mechanism which accounts for the observed increase in vitamin A absorption with aging remained unexplained, this increased uptake was paralleled by increased efficiency of absorption of other lipids or lysophylic compounds such as lipid-soluble drugs, fatty acids and other fat-soluble vitamins. For example, vitamin D_3 absorption increased between 9 and 41 weeks of age in rats and remained relatively constant thereafter up to 101 weeks of age[105]. This finding is surprising since metabolic bone disease, bone fragility and pathological fractures are common in aging individuals[106]. Thus, explanations such as impaired conversion of vitamin D to its active metabolites rather than impaired intestinal absorption must represent the explanation for these clinical findings.

These findings are different in some aspects from those of Holt and Dominguez[107]. These workers demonstrated that 5-month-old rats absorbed more vitamin D_3 than did 21-month-old animals. Differences in experimental design may account for the discrepancies: in the studies of Holt and Dominguez, vitamin D was infused into the proximal duodenum and neither endogenous biliary or pancreatic secretions were excluded from the perfused intestine, as was performed in the experiments of Hollander and Tarnawski[105]. Also, in these latter studies, the vitamin D was infused at 250 nM, a physiological concentration, as compared to the higher concentrations perfused in the studies of Holt and Dominguez. Holt and Dominguez solubilized vitamin D in an artificial detergent, pluronic F68 and lecithin, both of which may change intestinal absorption of fat-soluble vitamins[107]. Also, when absorption was expressed as total animal absorption, then the data of Holt and Dominguez demonstrated that there was no difference in amount absorbed per young versus old animal. Thus, variations in experimental design, perfusion, and analysis of data may well explain the differences between these two studies. Nonetheless, taking all these considerations into account, it would appear that a given dose of vitamin D is apparently not malabsorbed, at least in old animals.

TRIACYLGLYCEROL, CHOLESTEROL AND FATTY ACIDS

The absorption of long-chain triacylglycerols may be impaired with aging[108], possibly owing to impaired secretion of pancreatic lipase[109,110]. There is a 61% increase in oleic acid absorption as rats age between 6 and 138 weeks of age. This enhanced uptake of this fatty acid is due to an increase in the effective surface area of the unstirred water layer, a decrease in the effective thickness of this diffusion barrier, and a resulting decrease in diffusion resistance[105–107].

An increase in the age of animals from 3 to 21 months results in a decrease in oleic acid exsorption. The exsorption of oleic acid into the intestinal perfusate is not simply a process of 'leakiness' of the intestinal epithelium; rather, exsorption of this fatty acid is modified by factors that change the characteristics of the perfusate, the intestinal epithelium or the unstirred water layer.

The effect of aging on lipid uptake depends upon the lipophilicity of the probe, the effective resistance of the unstirred water layer, the permeability of the BBM, and the species of the animal. The overall absorption rate of compounds with higher diffusion coefficients and greater aqueous solubility (such as medium-chain alcohols and fatty acids) decreases with aging. On the other hand, absorption of compounds such as cholesterol and vitamin A with relatively low diffusion coefficients and minimal aqueous solubility is greater in older animals, especially in the presence of high unstirred water layer resistance. For example, *in vitro* studies have also shown that when the unstirred water layer resistance is high, the uptake of a homologous series of short- and medium-chain fatty acids is greater in older than in younger animals (Figure 11.2). In contrast, when unstirred layer resistance is low, uptake is higher in suckling and mature rather than in old rabbits[111]. The incremental free energy change associated with the addition of each CH_2 group to the fatty acid chain was 50% higher in the suckling and mature animals than in the old animals, and the estimated functional morphological surface area of the jejunal membrane was also higher in the suckling and mature animals.

Cholesterol uptake *in vitro* is greater in suckling than in older rabbits (Figure 11.3) over a wide range of durations of incubation, varying con-

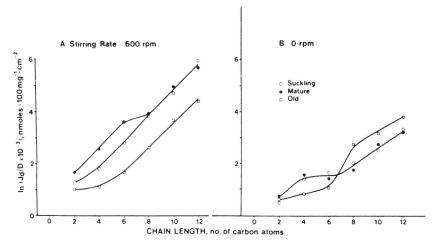

Figure 11.2 Relationship between rates of uptake of a homologous series of saturated fatty acids and number of carbon atoms in each compound. (From Ref. 111)

centrations of cholesterol or bile acid and at low or high values of unstirred layer resistance[112]. Thus, the differences in the *in vitro* uptake of cholesterol into the jejunum of rabbits of varying ages is owing to the lower passive permeability properties of the BBM and to higher effective resistance of the overlying unstirred water layer (Figure 11.4). In rabbits, the resistance of this diffusion barrier increases with aging[112], whereas in rats the resistance falls or remains unchanged[105,106].

When unstirred water layer resistance is high, such as occurs *in vivo*[100] or *in vitro* with no stirring of the bulk phase, then the uptake of cholesterol and fatty acids is higher in older than in younger animals. For example, as rats age, their maximal capacity to absorb linoleic acid increased 5-fold both in the jejunum and ileum. Changes in the dimensions and characteristics of the unstirred water layer with aging may again have accounted for the increase in the capacity of the small bowel to absorb linoleic acid. In other studies, resistance of the unstirred water layer has been shown to remain relatively stable at all ages studied[106].

However, the reason for the discrepancy between the *in vivo* results showing increased cholesterol uptake and the *in vitro* studies showing reduced cholesterol uptake with aging cannot be explained only on the basis of differences in unstirred layer resistance. Explanations for the variations in the reported effects of aging on cholesterol uptake may have been related to mild distension of the intestine during the *in vivo* perfusion studies; even the mild distension of the intestine associated with the formation of everted intestinal sacs results in an alteration in the permeability properties of the jejunum and a marked increase in the rate of uptake of fatty acid[113,114] and cholesterol. Indeed, the quantitative values for uptake of lipid *in vivo* are 10-fold greater than those observed *in vitro*[115]. Finally, there are marked differences in cholesterol uptake between species, with a much higher rate of uptake in the rat than in the

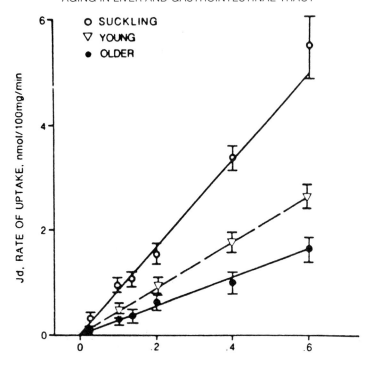

Figure 11.3 Effect of varying concentrations of cholesterol on the *in vitro* rate of jejunal cholesterol uptake in rabbits of different ages. (From Ref. 99)

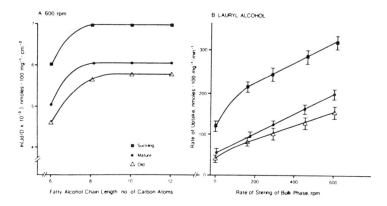

Figure 11.4 Effect of stirring and chain length on *in vitro* uptake of fatty alcohols into jejunum of rabbits of different ages. (From Ref. 99)

rabbit[116]. Thus, it is possible that there are true species-related differences in the rate of uptake of cholesterol in animals of different ages with an increase in cholesterol uptake in rats and a decrease in cholesterol uptake in rabbits.

Alternatively, the metabolism of lipids once they have been taken up by the enterocytes, and their exit across the basolateral membrane into the lymphatics or portal circulation, may vary with aging. These processes, rather than the initial uptake of lipid from the lumen, may be the important factors in the modulation of lipid absorption with aging. Thus, differences between *in vivo* and *in vitro* results (increased cholesterol uptake in older rats *in vivo* versus decreased cholesterol uptake in older rabbits *in vitro*) may be related to the contribution to absorption *in vivo* of enterocyte metabolism and exit across the BLM. It remains unknown whether the enterocyte microsomal enzyme activities change with aging, or whether the permeability properties of the basolateral membrane change with aging. However, based on the lower *in vitro* uptake of lipids yet high *in vivo* absorption which occurs with aging, it may be speculated that the exit of lipids from the enterocyte is greater in older than in younger animals.

Bile acids

The enterohepatic circulation of bile salts is important for the maintenance of a bile salt pool of sufficient size and concentration to permit absorption of dietary lipid. The factors involved in the maintenance of this ideal bile salt pool include the rate of hepatic bile salt synthesis, the concentration of bile salts by the gall bladder and efficient re-absorption of bile salt conjugates in the intestine. The bile salt pool size in newborn infants is decreased when compared with body surface area-matched healthy adults. Bile salt transport is mediated by a sodium-dependent co-transport system that is similar to that described for glucose, amino acids and inorganic phosphates. Taurocholate (TC) transport into rat ileal brush border membrane vesicles is incompletely developed in 2-week-old suckling rats but becomes fully expressed by the time of weaning at 3 weeks of age[117]. Kinetic analysis suggests that maturation of the taurocholate carriers occurs near weaning, primarily through an increase in functional bile acid carriers within the ileal brush-border membrane[118]. Using brush-border membrane vesicles, sodium-enhanced uptake of TC appeared abruptly and was first apparent on day 17 and an overshoot uptake was demonstrated on day 18. The lower maximal transport rate and higher apparent Michaelis constant in young as compared with adult rats likely reflected a difference in the number of functional bile acid carriers or developmental alterations in the physical character of the membrane itself, with subsequent enhancement of carrier–substrate interaction. Maturation of the rabbit from weaning to adulthood does not influence the relative passive permeability of the jejunum or colon to bile acids, but does increase active ileal uptake of conjugated and unconjugated cholic acid and deoxycholic acid, but not chenodeoxycholic acid[113].

Development of active ileal transport of bile acids parallels other developmental changes such as increasing plasma levels of endogenous corticosteroid and thyroxine, alterations in membrane microenvironment and expansion of the bile acid pool (resulting from co-existent maturation of hepatic uptake, synthesis and excretion). Glucocorticoids, already known to mediate several intestinal changes at the time of weaning in the rat, may play a role in the maturation of the bile salt pool, although the importance of glucocorticoids in the development of ileal active bile salt transport has been questioned. Thus, while glucocorticoid treatment promotes precocious development of some intestinal transport systems such as magnesium, calcium and glucose-dependent sodium transport and vitamin B_{12} absorption, this effect is not uniform. Pre-term infants whose mothers received dexamethasone or phenobarbital have been found to have larger bile salt pools, increased bile salt synthesis and reduced turnover rates for cholate and chenodeoxycholate compared to similarly aged infants of untreated mothers; an influence of dexamethasone on the intestinal contribution to the maintenance of bile salt pool size appears unlikely.

With increasing post-natal age, the microvillus membrane cholesterol content rises while the phospholipid content remains unchanged. Simultaneously, the microvillus membrane fatty acid composition changes from predominantly saturated to unsaturated species in both jejunum and ileum[65]. However, the absence of fluidity change at 37°C suggests that the association of alterations in active ileal bile salt transport and microvillus membrane lipid composition and fluidity may not be physiologically significant or interrelated. It remains unknown whether these same signals play any role in the changes in bile acid absorption which occur with aging.

Possible signals

Dietary insult at an early age may affect the normal development of some of the functional properties of the gastrointestinal tract. These effects may continue into later life and may impair the subsequent development of the intestinal tract. For example, a 2-week period of under-nutrition in the rat followed by nutritional rehabilitation is associated with significantly elevated intestinal lactase activity as compared with a well-nourished control group[119]. The early feeding of a high- or a low-cholesterol diet may alter the normal age-associated changes in intestinal transport of nutrients[120]. Thus, there may be late effects of early nutrition, and some of the changes observed with aging may be owing to factors exerting their influence in youth.

While diet plays an important role in maintaining intestinal lactase activity during the suckling period[121], such luminal factors likely have a limited temporal role. The proportion of carbohydrate relative to fat and iron content of the weaning rat diet is critical for maturation of intestinal microvillus enzymes, but not for the ontogenic changes in DNA synthesis. The protein content of the weaning diet modulates the ontogenic changes in DNA synthesis and may be a factor in the completion of the growth of the gastrointestinal tract[29].

Is intestinal transport of sugars and amino acids subject to critical-period programing? The brilliant pioneering work of Karasov, Diamond and co-workers[122] has raised this important question. Critical-period phenomena are events in which a biological mechanism is turned irreversibly on or off only once during an individual's lifetime in response to conditions prevailing at some critical stage. Early diet changes in the carbohydrate:protein ratio have irreversible effects on gut and body size, but these early changes in dietary composition of these macronutrients did not exert specific irreversible effects on the transport of glucose, choline, leucine, lysine or aspartate. Nonetheless, in old animals, active and passive glucose transport increases reversibly on a high-carbohydrate diet, whereas amino acid transport increases reversibly on a high-protein diet[122]. It is unclear why early diet had irreversible anatomic effects which persisted when mice were switched to the same or opposite rations at an early age, but did not have a specific effect on glucose transport independent of the effect on intestinal mass. However, the presence of critical period phenomena on specific transport effects, independent of changes in intestinal morphology, may be demonstrated by early feeding of diets varying in their content of saturated versus polyunsaturated fatty acids (unpublished observations, 1987). Thus, the age-associated changes in intestinal transport function may be influenced by conditions which were present at an early age, even as early as at weaning.

THE HUMAN CONDITION

Our understanding of the regulatory mechanism of intestinal differentiation originates mainly from studies on rat and mouse. However, the morphological and functional development of the human intestine is unlike that of the rat and mouse: the foetal human intestine organizes villi covered with well-differentiated enterocytes during the end of the first term *in utero*. By 12 weeks of gestation, maltase and sucrase show an activity about half of that of a young child. Alkaline phosphatase is present at 10 weeks and rises until week 23 of gestation. Lactase activity remains low during the entire gestational period and increases during the last weeks of pregnancy. Using organ culture of human foetal small intestine, specific increases of lactase and alkaline phosphatase activities is induced by the addition of hydrocortisone to the culture medium. DNA synthesis is increased as well, together with an increase in the labelling index of the epithelial cells[123].

Factors controlling enzymatic maturation during ontogenesis of the gut are now being examined in human foetal intestine maintained in organ culture[124]. The addition of dexamethasone, insulin or amniotic fluid to the culture medium did not further enhance brush-border enzyme activities, except for lactase whose levels were doubled by dexamethasone. Thus, in addition to the differences which exist among mammalian species in the timing of enzyme development, there may be a species specificity in the factors involved in foetal enzymatic maturation.

Human small bowel biopsy specimens have been shown to absorb fatty acids from micellar lipid solutions and to synthesize triglyceride (TG) during organ culture[125]. TG synthesis was influenced by micellar bile salt concentration as well as by micellar concentration of oleate and mono-olein. Organ cultured human intestinal mucosa is also capable of TG secretion.

Orally administered stable isotope-labelled substrates have been used to measure glucose oxidation, protein turnover and fat malabsorption in humans. The rate of $^{13}CO_2$ appearance in breath after substrate administration reflects the extent of endogenous metabolism. The absorption of stable-isotope labelled fatty acids in humans[126] has demonstrated a much higher efficiency for the absorption and subsequent oxidation of oleic and linoleic acid than for stearic acid (97.2%, 99.9% and 78.0%, respectively). In man a significant amount of ingested long-chain fatty acids (e.g. $C_{16:0}$) may be rapidly oxidized by extra-mitochondrial routes that are known to be active in liver in animal models (unpublished observations, 1987). Thus, it is apparent that selective compartmentalization of products of fatty acid absorption from the enterocyte may in part pre-determine the peripheral versus hepatic utilization of dietary fatty acid. Clearly, further information is required to understand the regulation by the enterocyte of the traffic of dietary fatty acids through lipid pools. But even more importantly, this stable isotope technology must be extended to studies of older humans.

SUMMARY AND FUTURE DIRECTIONS

The current state of knowledge of lipid absorption has been reviewed in this chapter. Aging appears to be associated with no change in the uptake of some nutrients, and an increase or decrease in the absorption of others. The altered uptake of lipids which may accompany the aging process appears to occur as a result of complex and multi-factorial interacting factors acting in concert with contributions from villus morphology, membrane composition, cellular metabolism and lipoproteins. Many aspects of lipid absorption and aging have not yet been explored.

It is unknown whether the established alterations in lipid absorption are the result of the aging process itself, or whether the alterations in lipid absorption represent an adaptation from a signal arising from some other component of the aging process. It is unknown whether these age-related changes in lipid uptake are detrimental to the animal, or represent a beneficial adaptation. If the intestinal adaptation is in fact detrimental to the animal, then can the aging of the intestine be prevented by dietary means aimed at altering the lipid changes in the brush border membrane?

Cui bono? Cui – each and every one of us who walks this earth. New insights into the mechanisms of aging must be gained, and a better understanding of the pathogenesis of disease processes will emerge. A unique approach must be taken, one marrying the multi-disciplinary cooperative interactions of nutritionists, physiologists, biochemists, immunologists and care-givers. The techniques must be admirably sophisticated, and the enthusiasm for the goals must be flambuoyant. Yet we must not be captivated by technology at the expense of science. Fresh, imaginative and achievable goals must be set for highly focused research efforts. All of us interested in this process of aging must contribute to this citizenship of knowledge in the global academic environment.

'... old age in this universal man ought not to be sought in the times nearest his birth, but in those most remote from it.'

Pascal (1623–1662), *Preface to the Treatise on Vacuum*

References

1. Thomson, A. B. R. and Dietschy, J. M. (1981). Intestinal lipid absorption: major extracellular and intracellular events. In (ed.) Johnson, L. R. *Physiology of the Gastrointestinal Tract*. pp. 1147–220 (New York: Raven Press)
2. Carey, M. C., Small, D. M. and Bliss, C. M. (1983). Lipid digestion and absorption. *Annu. Rev. Physiol.*, **45**, 651–77
3. Tso, P. and Simmonds, W. J. (1984). The absorption of lipid and lipoprotein synthesis. *Lipid Res. Method.*, 191–216
4. Grundy, S. M. (1983). Absorption and metabolism of dietary cholesterol. *Annu. Rev. Nutr.*, **3**, 71–96
5. Green, P. H. R. and Glickman, R. M. (1981). Intestinal lipoprotein metabolism. *J. Lipid Res.*, **22**, 1153–73
6. Mahley, R. W. and Innerarity, T. L. (1983). Lipoprotein receptors and cholesterol homeostasis. *Biochim. Biophys. Acta*, **737**, 197–222
7. Norum, K. R., Berg, T., Helgerud, P. and Drevon, C. A. (1983). Transport of cholesterol. *Physiol. Rev.*, **63**, 1343–419
8. Bisgaier, C. L. and Glickman, R. M. (1983). Intestinal synthesis, secretion, and transport of lipoproteins. *Annu. Rev. Physiol.*, **45**, 625–36
9. Watkins, J. B. (1985). Lipid digestion and absorption. *Pediatrics*, **75**, 151–6
10. Tso, P. (1985). Gastrointestinal digestion and absorption of lipid. In Paoletti, R. and Kritchevsky, D. (eds.) *Advances in Lipid Research*. (New York: Academic Press Inc.)
11. Shiau, Y.-F. (1987). Lipid digestion and absorption. In Johnson, L. R. (ed.) *Physiology of the Gastrointestinal Tract*. 2nd ed. (New York: Raven Press)
12. Chapman, M. J. (1980). Animal lipoproteins: chemistry, structure and comparative aspects. *J. Lipid Res.*, **21**, 789–853
13. Brown, M. S. and Goldstein, J. L. (1979). Receptor-mediated endocytosis: insights from the lipoprotein receptor system. *Proc. Natl. Acad. Sci. USA*, **76**, 3330–7
14. Eisenberg, S. (1984). High density lipoprotein metabolism. *J. Lipid Res.*, **25**, 1017–58
15. Friedman, H. I. and Nylund, B. (1980). Intestinal fat digestion, absorption and transport. A review. *Am. J. Clin. Nutr.*, **33**, 1108–39
16. Patton, J. S. (1981). Gastrointestinal lipid digestion. In Johnston, L. R. (ed.) *Physiology of the Gastrointestinal Tract*. Vol. 2, pp. 1123–46 (New York: Raven Press)
17. Boucrot, P. (1983). Phosphatidylcholines – Digestion and intestinal absorption. *Reprod. Nutr. Dev.*, **23**, 943–58
18. Hauton, J. C., Domingo, N., Mortigne, M., Lafont, H., Nalbone, G., Chanussot, F. and Lairon, D. (1986). A quantitative dynamic concept of the interphase partition of lipids: application to bile salt–lecithin–cholesterol mixed micelles. *Biochimie*, **68**, 275–85
19. Borgstrom, B. (1985). The micellar hypothesis of fat absorption: must it be revisited? (review). *Scand. J. Gastroenterol.*, **20**, 389–94
20. Clandinin, M. T., Field, C. J., Hargreaves, K., Morson, L. and Zsigmond, E. (1985). Role of diet fat in subcellular structure and function. *Can. J. Physiol. Pharmacol.*, **63**, 546–56
21. Spector, A. A. and Yorek, M. A. (1985). Membrane lipid composition and cellular function. *J. Lipid Res.*, **26**, 1015–35
22. Thomson, A. B. R. and Keelan, M. (1986). The development of the small intestine. *Can. J. Physiol. Pharmacol.*, **64**, 13–29
23. Younoszai, M. K., Smith, C., Finch, M. H. (1985). Comparison of *in vitro* jejunal uptake of L-valine and L-lysine in the rat during maturation. *J. Pediatr. Gastroenterol. Nutr.*, **4**, 992–7
24. Borowitz, S. M. and Ghishan, F. K. (1985). Maturation of jejunal phosphate transport by rat brush border membrane vesicles. *Pediatr. Res.*, **19**, 1308–12
25. Corazza, G. R., Frazzoni, M., Gatto, M. R. A. and Gasbarrini, G. (1986). Ageing and small-bowel mucosa: a morphometric study. *Gerontology*, **32**, 60–5
26. Hollander, D. and Tarnawski, H. (1985). Aging-associated increases in intestinal absorption of macromolecules. *Gerontology*, **31**, 133–7
27. Johnson, S. L., Mayersohn, M. and Conrad, K. A. (1985). Gastrointestinal absorption as a function of age: xylose absorption in healthy adults. *Clin. Pharmacol. Ther.*, **38**, 331–5
28. Yeh, K-Y. and Holt, P. R. (1986). Ontogenic timing mechanism initiates the expression of rat intestinal sucrase activity. *Gastroenterology*, **90**, 520–6

29. Buts, J. P. and Nyakabasa, M. (1985). Role of dietary protein adaptation at weaning in the development of the rat gastrointestinal tract. *Pediatr. Res.*, **19**, 857–62
30. Goldstein, R. M., Hebiguchi, T., Luk, G. D., Taqi, F., Guilarte, T. R., Franklin, R. A., Niemiec, P. W. and Dudgeon, D. L. (1985). The effects of total parenteral nutrition on gastrointestinal growth and development. *J. Pediatr. Surg.*, **20**, 785–91
31. Thomson, A. B. R. and Keelan, M. (1986). The aging gut. *Can. J. Physiol. Pharmacol.*, **64**, 30–8
32. Cooper, R. A., Arner, C., Wiley, J. S. and Shattil, S. J. (1975). Modification of red cell membrane structure by cholesterol rich lipid dispersions. *J. Clin. Invest.*, **55**, 115–26
33. Cooper, R. A. (1977). Abnormalities of cell-membrane fluidity in the pathogenesis of disease. *New Engl. J. Med.*, **297**, 371–7
34. Cooper, R. A. and Shattil, S. J. (1981). Membrane cholesterol – is enough too much? *N. Engl. J. Med.*, **302**, 49–51
35. Grunge, M. and Deuticke, B. (1974). Changes of membrane permeability due to extensive cholesterol depletion in mammalian erythrocytes. *Biochim. Biophys. Acta*, **356**, 125–30
36. Kroes, J. and Ostwald, R. (1971). Erythrocyte membranes – effect of increased cholesterol content on permeability. *Biochim. Biophys. Acta*, **249**, 647–50
37. Read, B. D. and McElhaney, R. N. (1976). Influence of membrane lipid fluidity on glucose and uridine facilitated diffusion in human erythrocytes. *Biochim. Biophys. Acta*, **419**, 331–41
38. Shattil, S. J. and Cooper, R. A. (1976). Membrane microviscosity and human platelet functional. *Biochemistry*, **15**, 4832–7
39. Van Deenan, L. L. M., De Gier, J. and Demel, R. A. (1972). Relation between lipid composition and permeability of membranes. In *Current Trends in the Biochemistry of Lipids*. p. 377. (New York: Academic Press)
40. Brasitus, T. A. and Schachter, D. (1982). Cholesterol biosynthesis and modulation of membrane cholesterol and lipid dynamics in rat intestinal microvillus membranes. *Biochemistry*, **21**, 2241–6
41. Brasitus, T. A. and Schachter, D. (1980). Lipid dynamics and lipid–protein interactions in rat enterocyte basolateral and microvillus membranes. *Biochemistry*, **19**, 2763–9
42. Brasitus, T. A., Tall, A. R. and Schachter, D. (1980). Thermotropic transitions in rat intestinal plasma membranes studied by differential scanning calorimetry and fluorescence polarization. *Biochemistry*, **19**, 1256–61
43. Brasitus, T. A., Schachter, D. and Mamouneas, T. G. (1979). Functional interactions of lipids and proteins in rat intestinal microvillus membranes. *Biochemistry*, **18**, 4136–44
44. Hauser, H., Howell, K., Dawson, R. M. C. and Bowyer, D. E. (1980). Rabbit small intestinal brush border membrane preparation and lipid composition. *Biochim. Biophys. Acta*, **602**, 567–77
45. Forstner, G. G., Tanaka, K. and Isselbacher, K. J. (1968). Lipid composition of the isolated rat intestinal microvillus membrane. *Biochem. J.*, **109**, 51–9
46. Kawai, K., Fujita, M. and Nakao, M. (1974). Lipid components of two different regions of an intestinal epithelial cell membrane of mouse. *Biochim. Biophys. Acta*, **369**, 222–33
47. Bloj, B. and Zilversmith, D. B. (1982). Heterogeneity of rabbit intestine brush border plasma membrane cholesterol. *J. Biol. Chem.*, **257**, 7608–14
48. Millington, P. F. and Gritchley, D. R. (1968). Lipid composition of the brush borders of rat intestinal epithelial cells. *Life Sci.*, **7**, 839–45
49. Penzes, L. (1970). Data on the chemical composition of the aging intestine. *Digestion*, **3**, 174–8
50. Profirov, Y. I. (1981). *In vitro* modifications of cholesterol/phospholipid ratio of enterocytes brush border membrane and its effect on L-leucine accumulation. *Int. J. Biochem.*, **13**, 875–7
51. Grinna, L. S. (1977). Age-related changes in the lipids of the microsomal and the mitochondrial membranes of rat liver and kidney. *Mech. Age. Dev.*, **6**, 197–205
52. Zs-Nagy, I. (1979). The role of membrane structure and function in cellular aging: A review. *Mech. Age. Dev.*, **9**, 237–46
53. Grinna, L. S. (1977). Changes in cell membranes during aging. *Gerontology*, **23**, 452–64
54. Rivnay, B., Bergman, S., Shinitzky, M. and Globerson, A. (1980). Correlations between

membrane viscosity, serum cholesterol, lymphocyte activation and aging in man. *Mech. Age. Dev.*, **12**, 119–26

55. Rubin, M. S., Swislocki, N. I. and Sonnenberg, M. (1973). Changes in rat liver plasma membrane phospholipids during aging. *Proc. Soc. Exp. Biol. Med.*, **142**, 1008–10

56. Hawcroft, D. M. and Martin, P. A. (1974). Studies on age-related changes in the lipids of mouse liver microsomes. *Mech. Age. Dev.*, **3**, 121–30

57. Hohn, P., Gabbert, H. and Wagner, R. (1978). Differentiation and aging of the rat intestinal mucosa. II. Morphological, enzyme histochemical and disc electrophoretic aspects of the aging of the small intestinal mucosa. *Mech. Age. Dev.*, **7**, 217–26

58. Wilson, P. D. (1983). The histochemistry of aging. *Histochem. J.*, **15**, 393–410

59. Tiwari, R. K., Clandinin, M. T. and Cinader, B. (1986). Effect of high/low dietary linoleic acid feeding on mouse splenocytes: modulation by age and influence of genetic variability. *Nutr. Res.*, **6**, 1379–87

60. Shub, M. D., Pang, K. Y., Swann, D. A. and Walker, W. A. (1983). Age-related changes in chemical composition and physical properties of mucus glycoproteins from rat small intestine. *Biochem. J.*, **215**, 405–11

61. Weiser, M. M. (1973). Intestinal epithelial cell surface membrane glycoprotein synthesis. I. An indicator of cellular differentiation. *J. Biol. Chem.*, **248**, 2536–41

62. Brasitus, T. A. and Keresztes, R. S. (1983). Glycoprotein metabolism in rat colonic epithelial cell populations with different proliferative activities. *Differentiation*, **24**, 239–44

63. Sun, G. Y. and Sun, A. Y. (1984). Dietary antioxidants, membrane lipids and aging. In Armbrecht, H. J., Prendergast, J. M. and Coe, R. M. (eds.) (New York: Springer-Verlag)

64. Hegner, D. (1980). Age-dependence of molecular and functional changes in biological membrane properties. *Mech. Age. Dev.*, **14**, 101–18

65. Heubi, J. E. and Fellows, J. L. (1985). Postnatal development of intestinal bile salt transport. Relationship to membrane physicochemical changes. *J. Lipid Res.*, **26**, 797–805

66. Pang, K.-Y., Bresson, J. L. and Walker, W. A. (1983). Development of the gastrointestinal mucosal barrier. Evidence for structural differences in microvillus membranes from newborn and adult rabbits. *Biochim. Biophys. Acta*, **727**, 201–8

67. Schwarz, S. M., Hostetler, B., Ling, S., Lee, L. and Watkins, J. B. (1982). Fluorescence polarization studies of the small intestinal microvillus membrane during development. *Gastroenterology*, **82**, 1174 (Abstract)

68. Brasitus, T. A., Yeh, K-Y, Holt, P. R. and Schachter, D. (1984). Lipid fluidity and composition of intestinal microvillus membranes isolated from rats of different ages. *Biochim. Biophys. Acta*, **788**, 341–8

69. Carlson, L. A., Froberg, S. O. and Nye, E. R. (1968). Effect of age on blood and tissue lipid levels in the male rat. *Gerontologia*, **14**, 65–79

70. Grinna, L. S. and Barber, A. A. (1973). Lipid peroxidation in livers and kidneys from young and old rats. *Biochem. Biophys. Res. Commun.*, **55**, 773–9

71. Prasannan, K. G. (1972). Influence of age on the total lipid, phospholipid and cholesterol contents of pancreas and liver of albino rats. *Experientia*, **29**, 946–7

72. Malhotra, S. and Kritchevsky, D. (1975). Cholesterol exchange between the red blood cells and plasma of young and old rats. *Mech. Age. Dev.*, **4**, 137–45

73. Grinna, L. S. and Barber, A. A. (1976). Lipid changes in the microsomal and mitochondrial membranes of rat liver during aging. *Fed. Proc.*, **35**, 1425E (Abstract)

74. Holt, P. R., Tierney, A. R. and Kotler, D. P. (1985). Delayed enzyme expression: a defect of aging rat gut. *Gastroenterology*, **89**, 1026–34

75. Penzes, L. and Skala, J. (1977). Changes in the mucosal surface area of the small gut of rats of different ages. *J. Anat.*, **127**, 217–22

76. Meshkinpour, H., Smith, M. and Hollander, D. (1981). Influence of aging on the surface area of the small intestine in the rat. *Exp. Gerontol.*, **16**, 399–404

77. Thomson, A. B. R. and Rajotte, R. V. (1984). Insulin and islet cell transplant – effect on intestinal uptake of lipids. *Am. J. Physiol. (Gastrointest. Liver Physiol., 9)*, **246**, G627–G633

78. Holt, P. R., Kotler, D. P. and Pascal, R. R. (1983). A simple method for determining epithelial cell turnover in small intestine. Studies in young and aging rat gut. *Gastroenterology*, **84**, 69–74

79. Smith, M. W. (1981). Autoradiographic analysis of alanine uptake by newborn pig intestine. *Experientia*, **37**, 868–70

80. Smith, M. W., Peterson, J. Y. F. and Peacock, M. A. (1984). A comprehensive description of brush border membrane development applying to enterocytes taken from a wide variety of mammalian species. *Comp. Biochem. Physiol.,* **77A,** 655–62

81. Cheeseman, C. I. (1986). Expression of amino acid and peptide transport systems in rat small intestine. *Am. J. Physiol.,* **251,** G636–G641

82. Stange, E. F. and Dietschy, J. M. (1984). Age-related decreases in tissue sterol acquisition are mediated by changes in cholesterol synthesis and not low density lipoprotein uptake in the rat. *J. Lipid Res.,* **25,** 703–13

83. Uchida, K., Nomura, Y., Kadowaki, M., Takase, H., Takano, K. and Takeuchi, N. (1978). Age-related changes in cholesterol and bile acid metabolism in rats. *J. Lipid Res.,* **19,** 544–52

84. Liepa, G. U., Masoro, E. J., Bertrand, H. A. and Yu, B. P. (1980). Food restriction as a modulator of age-related changes in serum lipids. *Am. J. Physiol.,* **238,** E253–E257

85. Van Lenten, B. J. and Roheim, P. S. (1982). Changes in the concentrations and distributions of apolipoproteins of the aging rats. *J. Lipid Res.,* **23,** 1187–95

86. Andersen, J. M. and Dietschy, J. M. (1977). Regulation of sterol synthesis in 15 tissues of rat. II. Role of rat and human high and low density plasma lipoproteins and of rat chylomicron remnants. *J. Biol. Chem.,* **252,** 3652–9

87. Goldstein, J. L. and Brown, M. S. (1977). The low-density lipoprotein pathway and its relation to atherosclerosis. *Annu. Rev. Biochem.,* **46,** 897–930

88. Shefer, S., Hauser, S., Lapar, V. and Mosbach, E. H. (1972). HMG CoA reductase of intestinal mucosa and liver of the rat. *J. Lipid Res.,* **13,** 402–12

89. Takeuchi, N., Yamamura, Y., Katayama, Y., Hayashi, C. and Uchida, K. (1976). Impairment of feedback control and induction of cholesterol synthesis in rat by aging. *Exp. Gerontol.,* **11,** 121–26

90. Trout, E. C., Kato, K. Y. T., Hizer, C. A. and McGavack, T. H. (1962). *In vitro* synthesis of free and ester cholesterol in various tissues of young and old rats. *J. Gerontol.,* **17,** 363–8

91. Dietschy, J. M., Spady, D. K. and Stange, E. F. (1983). Quantitative importance of different organs for cholesterol synthesis and low density lipoprotein degradation. *Biochem. Soc. Trans.,* **11,** 639–41

92. Stange, E. F. and Dietschy, J. M. (1983). Cholesterol synthesis and low density lipoprotein uptake are regulated independently in rat small intestine epithelium. *Proc. Nat. Acad. Sci. USA,* **80,** 5739–43

93. Dietschy, J. M., Turley, S. D. and Spady, D. K. (1983). The role of the liver in lipid and lipoprotein metabolism. In Bianchi, L., Gerok, W., Lanadmann, L., Sickinger, K. and Stalder, G. A. (eds.) *Liver in Metabolic Diseases.* (Lancaster: MTP Press)

94. Weis, H. J. and Dietschy, J. M. (1974). Adaptive responses in hepatic and intestinal cholesterogenesis following ileal resection in the rat. *Eur. J. Clin. Invest.,* **4,** 33–41

95. Ginsberg, H., Le, N. A., Mays, C., Gibson, J. and Brown, W. V. (1981). Lipoprotein metabolism in nonresponders to increased dietary cholesterol. *Arteriosclerosis,* **1,** 463–70

96. Kesaniemi, Y. A. and Grundy, S. M. (1984). Turnover of low density lipoproteins during inhibition of cholesterol absorption. *Arteriosclerosis,* **4,** 41–8

97. Kovanen, P. T., Bilheimer, D. W., Goldstein, J. L. Haramillo, J. J. and Brown, M. S. (1981). Regulatory role for hepatic low density lipoprotein receptors *in vivo* in the dog. *Proc. Nat. Acad. Sci. USA,* **78,** 1194–8

98. Bilheimer, D. W., Grundy, S. M., Brown, M. S. and Goldstein, J. L. (1983). Mevinolin and colestipol stimulate receptor-mediated clearance of low density lipoprotein from plasma in familial hypercholesterolemia heterozygotes. *Proc. Nat. Acad. Sci. USA,* **80,** 4124–8

99. Thomson, A. B. R. (1981). Aging and cholesterol uptake in the rabbit jejunum. Role of the bile salt micelle and the unstirred water layer. *Dig. Dis. Sci.,* **26,** 890–6

100. Hollander, D. and Morgan, D. (1979). Increase in cholesterol intestinal absorption with aging in the rat. *Exp. Gerontol.,* **14,** 201–4

101. Hollander, D. and Morgan, D. (1979). Aging: its influence on vitamin A intestinal absorption *in vivo* by the rat. *Exp. Gerontol.,* **14,** 301–5

102. Winter, D., Dobre, V. and Oeriu, S. (1971). Cysteine-^{35}S absorption in old rats. *Exp. Gerontol.,* **6,** 367–71

103. Freeman, H. J. and Quamme, G. A. (1986). Age-related changes in sodium-dependent glucose transport in rat small intestine. *Am. J. Physiol.,* **251,** G208–G217

104. Harril, I. and Cervone, N. (1977). Vitamins status of older women. *Am. J. Clin. Nutr.*, **30**, 431–40

105. Hollander, D. and Tarnawski, H. (1984). Influence of aging on vitamin D absorption and unstirred water layer dimensions in the rat. *J. Lab. Clin. Med.*, **103**, 462–9

106. Gallagher, J. C., Riggs, B. L., Eisman, J., Hamstra, A., Arnaud, S. B. and DeLuca, H. F. (1979). Intestinal calcium absorption and serum vitamin D metabolites in normal subjects and osteoporotic patients: effect of age and dietary calcium. *J. Clin. Invest.*, **64**, 729–36

107. Holt, P. R. and Dominguez, A. A. (1981). Intestinal absorption of triglyceride and vitamin D_3 in aged and young rats. *Dig. Dis. Sci.*, **26**, 1109–15

108. Webster, S. G. P., Wilkinson, E. M. and Gowland, E. (1977). A comparison of fat absorption in young and old subjects. *Age Ageing*, **63**, 113–17

109. Montgomery, R. D., Haeney, M. R., Ross, I. N., Sammons, H. G., Barford, A. V., Balakrishnan, S., Mayer, P. P., Culank, L. S., Field, J. and Gosling, P. (1978). The ageing gut: A study of intestinal absorption in relation to nutrition in the elderly. *Q. J. Med.*, **47**, 197–211

110. Price, H. L., Gazzard, B. G. and Dawson, A. M. (1977). Steatorrhoea in the elderly. *Br. Med. J.*, **1**, 1582–4

111. Thomson, A. B. R. (1980). Effect of age on uptake of homologous series of saturated fatty acids into rabbit jejunum. *Am. J. Physiol.*, **39**, G363–G371

112. Thomson, A. B. R. (1979). Unstirred water layer and age-dependent changes in rabbit jejunal D-glucose transport. *Am. J. Physiol. (Endocrin. Metab. Gastrointest. Physiol.)*, **236**, E685–E691

113. Thomson, A. B. R. and O'Brien, B. D. (1981). Uptake of cholesterol into rabbit jejunum using three *in vitro* techniques: importance of bile acid micelles and unstirred layer resistance. *Am. J. Physiol.*, **241**, G270–G274

114. Thomson, A. B. R. and O'Brien, B. D. (1980). Uptake of a homologous series of saturated fatty acids into rabbit intestine using three *in vitro* techniques. *Dig. Dis. Sci.*, **25**, 209–15

115. Hotke, C., McIntyre, Y. and Thomson, A. B. R. (1985). Jejunal uptake of sugars, cholesterol, fatty acids and fatty alcohols *in vivo* in diabetic rats. *Can. J. Physiol. Pharm.*, **63**, 1356–61

116. Thomson, A. B. R. and Rajotte, R. (1983). Effect of dietary modification on the uptake of glucose, fatty acids and alcohols in diabetic rats. *Am. J. Clin. Nutr.*, **39**, 394–403

117. Barnard, J. A., Ghishan, F. K. and Wilson, F. A. (1985). Ontogenesis of taurocholate transport by rat ileal brush border membrane vesicles. *J. Clin. Invest.*, **75**, 869–73

118. Moyer, M. S., Heubi, J. E., Goodrich, A. L. Balistreri, W. F. and Suchy, F. J. (1986). Ontogeny of bile acid transport in brush border membrane vesicles from rat ileum. *Gastroenterology*, **90**, 1188–96

119. Majumdar, A. P. N. (1986). Effects of undernutrition and subsequent nutritional rehabilitation or hydrocortisone administration on growth and function of the gastrointestinal tract in rats. *Nutr. Rep. Int.*, **33**, 187–98

120. Thomson, A. B. R. (1986). Early nutrition and intestinal transport function: effect of low-cholesterol diet. *J. Lab. Clin. Med.*, **107**, 365–77

121. Karasov, W. H., Solberg, D. H., Chang, S. D., Hughes, M., Stein, E. D. and Diamond, J. M. (1985). Is intestinal transport of sugars and amino acids subject to critical-period programming? *Am. J. Physiol.*, **249**, G770–G785

122. Karasov, W. H. and Diamond, J. M. (1987). Adaptation of intestinal nutrient transport. In Johnson, L. R. (ed.) *Physiology of the Gastrointestinal Tract*. 2nd edn. (New York: Raven Press)

123. Arsenault, P. and Menard, D. (1985). Influence of hydrocortisone in human fetal small intestine in organ culture. *J. Pediatr. Gastroenterol. Nutr.*, **4**, 893–901

124. Simon-Assmann, P., Lacroix, B., Kedinger, M. and Haffen, K. (1986). Maturation of brush border hydrolases in human fetal intestine maintained in organ culture. *Early Human Develop.*, **13**, 65–74

125. Zimmerman, J., Gati, I., Eisenberg, S. and Rachmilewitz, D. (1985). Fat absorption and triglyceride synthesis and secretion by cultured human intestinal mucosa. *Isr. J. Med. Sci.*, **21**, 962–7

126. Jones, P. J. H., Pencharz, P. B. and Clandinin, M. T. (1985). Absorption of ^{13}C-labeled stearic, oleic, and linoleic acids in humans: application to breath tests. *J. Lab. Clin. Med.,* **105,** 647–52

12
Influence of aging on dietary lipid absorption by the small intestine

D. HOLLANDER

INTRODUCTION

Attempts at understanding the aging process are ultimately directed at manipulating the process in order to prolong life and maintain physical and mental health. So far, the only successful experimental manipulation which accomplished these aims has been dietary caloric restriction. By restricting dietary caloric intake, numerous investigators have been able to prolong the life of mice, rats and some non-mammalian species. This experimental manipulation did not only prolong the life span of animals, but also resulted in decreased incidence of neoplasia, renal failure and other degenerative or aging associated disorders.

The mechanisms by which dietary caloric restriction influences the life-span and health of animals are not known. It is clear, however, that dietary intake of nutrients also could be modulated and modified by the process of intestinal nutrient absorption. A change in intestinal absorptive capacity or efficiency might modify the nutrient and/or caloric load available for metabolic processes. We, therefore, embarked on a series of experiments designed to examine the interaction between nutrient absorption and aging. Because of our extensive experience and expertise in studying intestinal absorption of lipids we concentrated on the interaction between aging and the absorption of lipid nutrients.

Dietary lipids present a major physical and biochemical challenge to their absorption by the gastrointestinal tract. Lipids require lumenal processing with pancreatic enzymes and bile acids before they can be absorbed. Once they enter the absorptive cells, lipids require a complicated transport system in the absorptive cells for their transfer from the intestine to the general circulation. Because of the pivotal role that lipids play in normal nutrition we examined the influence of aging on dietary lipid absorption in male Sprague-Dawley rats varying in age from 1 to 30 months.

RESULTS

Pancreatic functions

Pancreatic enzyme hydrolysis is essential for conversion of dietary tri-glycerides to monoglycerides and free fatty acids. When we examined the influence of aging on pancreatic secretory capacity, we found that under basal conditions both protein and amylase output were maximal at 3 months

Table 12.1 Amylase secretion

Age (months)	Number of animals	Basal		Stimulated	
		Concentration (Units/ml)	Output (Units/h)	Concentration (Units/ml)	Output (Units/h)
3	5	2050 6 ± 238.7	896 9 ± 145.5	1743 3 ± 82.1	1558 5 ± 120.9
4	3	2243.8 ± 78.7	1042 2 ± 92.1	1259 5 ± 212.2	1101 0 ± 392.6
13	3	2209 9 ± 371.1	1144 7 ± 222.9	3332 4 ± 297.2	3317 1 ± 251.3
24	3	1759 6 ± 94.2*	808 7 ± 70.0	1115 7 ± 120.6*†	949 2 ± 178.0*†
27	4	429 4 ± 14.3*	80 4 ± 4.7*	1076 2 ± 179.2*†	288 8 ± 57.8*†

All values are expressed as mean ± SEM
* $p < 0.05$ difference between the experimental value and the value at 3 months of age (maturity)
† $p < 0.05$ difference between the experimental value and the value at 13 months of age when peak stimulated secretory activity occurred

of age, but decreased to less than 20% of their maximal values by 27 months[1]. When we stimulated pancreatic secretions with secretin (18 units/kg/h), aging (27 months) rats had showed a major reduction in secretory volume, bicar-bonate output, protein output and amylase output (Table 12.1)[2]. Decreased pancreatic secretion would cause poor hydrolysis which in turn would diminish the overall absorptive efficiency of dietary lipids.

Intestinal perfusion methods

In order to study the influence of aging on the maximal absorptive capacity of the small intestine, we perfused selected lipid nutrients through the proxi-mal or distal small intestine *in vivo* in restrained rats of varying ages (3–30 months). We used a standardized well-delineated perfusion technique which measures the disappearance rate of lumenal lipids after correction for fluid shifts. The lipid nutrients were solubilized in a physiological micellar solution and presented as a 'pre-digested' mixture to the absorptive surface, thereby, bypassing the pancreatic and biliary steps of the absorptive pathway.

Fatty acids absorption

Dietary fatty acids are not only a major caloric source but some are essential for prostaglandin production and normal metabolism[4,5]. The major human dietary essential fatty acid is linoleic and both jejunal and ileal absorptive

Table 12.2 Linoleic acid absorption

Age (months)	Absorption (μmol/100 cm per hour)	
	Jejunum	Ileum
1	7.7 ± 0.9	5.5 ± 0.9
3	22.6 ± 1.7*	8.7 ± 1.0*
12	27.7 ± 2.1	10.9 ± 1.2
28	40.0 ± 5.7*	24.2 ± 3.6*

Values are mean $\pm$ SEM. Number of animals of each age group as indicated in Table 12.1
* Denotes significant ($p < 0.05$) difference from the value at the next lower age group

Table 12.3 Intestinal wall and liver content of linoleic acid

Age (months)	Jejunum (nmol/100 mg)	Ileum (nmol/100 mg)	Liver (nmol/liver)
1	488.6 ± 62.7	851.5 ± 28.4	61.1 ± 5.6
3	612.1 ± 58.4	846.9 ± 28.9	232.6 ± 24.7*
12	544.9 ± 99.8	783.9 ± 81.7	242.0 ± 14.4
28	577.9 ± 12.4	797.2 ± 12.7	249.8 ± 15.6

Values are mean $\pm$ SEM. The number of animals of each age group is indicated in Table 12.1
* Denotes significant ($p < 0.05$) change from the value at the next lower age group

capacity for linoleic acid was found to increase with aging (Table 12.2). In parallel, the intestinal wall and liver content of linoleic acid also increased in aging experimental animals (Table 12.3)[6]. We found a somewhat similar increase in the maximal small intestinal absorptive capacity for oleic acid[7]. Thus, it appears that the maximal efficiency of intestinal absorption of long chain fatty acids is increased with aging.

Lipid soluble vitamins

Using the same *in vivo* perfusion method described above[3] we investigated the influence of aging on the maximal intestinal capacity to absorb lipid soluble vitamins. We found that 24.8% of infused vitamin A (retinol) was absorbed at 1.5 months of age as compared to 37.7% at 30 months of age[8]. These results represent a 50% aging-associated increase of vitamin A absorptive capacity by the small intestine. Using the same method we found a similar increase in vitamin D_3 absorption with aging (Table 12.4).

Table 12.4 Vitamin D_3 absorption

Age (weeks)	No. rats	Absorption (pmol/100 cm/h)	p*
9	4	1209.1 ± 108.5	—
20	3	1896.1 ± 132.7	<0.01
41	4	2114.2 ± 138.7	<0.01
70	3	2370.8 ± 941.0	>0.05
101	4	2355.4 ± 494.0	>0.05

Single-pass method. Perfusate: pH 6.5, 250 nM vitamin D_3, 10 mM sodium taurocholate, 2.5 mM oleic acid, and 2.5 mM mono-olein. Flow rate 0.5 ml/min. Six 20-min collections per animal. Values are mean ± SE
* Absorption rates compared with that of the next younger age group using Student's test and analysis of variance

Unstirred water layer dimensions

One factor which controls the absorption rate of lipids by the small intestine is the unstirred water layer (UWL). Lipids must diffuse through this layer to reach the lumenal cell membrane and be absorbed. The greater the thickness and resistance of the UWL, the more likely it is to become a rate-limiting step in the absorption of lipid nutrients[10]. Conversely, the greater the surface area of the UWL, the faster lipids diffuse through it. We used a modified version of the method described by Diamond[11] to assess the thickness of the UWL *in vivo*, and the methods described originally by Wilson and Dietschy[12] to assess the surface area and resistance of the UWL with aging. We found that the thickness of the UWL decreased from 318 to 268 μm between 1 and 29 months of age[13]. When linoleic acid was used as the probe molecule, we found that the surface area of the UWL increased with aging, while its resistance decreased (Tables 12.5 and 12.6)[6]. Similar age-related changes in the dimensions of the UWL were found when vitamin D_3 was used as the probe[9].

The decreased thickness and resistance of the UWL and increased total surface area would facilitate the absorption of lipids by the aging small intestine. These changes could be owing to alterations in the rigidity or compliance of the aging small intestine. Perhaps these changes which increase the maximal absorption of lipids compensate for the decrease in pancreatic functions with aging.

DISCUSSION

The rate and maximal capacity of the small intestine to absorb dietary nutrients could determine what fraction of ingested nutrients would eventually be available for metabolism. Intestinal absorptive capacity could be very important during aging since metabolic needs of nutrients depend so much on their dietary availability and intestinal absorption rate. Moreover, since dietary caloric restriction is a potent experimental tool in increasing the life

Table 12.5 Resistance of unstirred water layer

	R = (d)/(Sw)(D) (mm/ml per 100 cm length)	
Age (months)	Jejunum	Ileum
1	3.89	5.45
3	1.33*	3.46*
12	1.08	2.75
28	0.75*	1.24*

Values are mean for each age group. Number of rats at each age is indicated in Table 12.1
* Denotes significant ($p < 0.05$) difference from the next lower age

Table 12.6 Surface area of unstirred water layer

	Surface area of $UWL = (Jd)(d)/(C_1)(D)$ (cm^2/100 cm length)	
Age (months)	Jejunum	Ileum
1	68.1	48.6
3	163.0*	63.1*
12	200.8	78.7
28	297.7*	180.2*

Values are means for each age of animals. The number of animals in each age group in indicated in Table 12.1
* Denotes a significant ($p = 0.05$) difference from the value of the next lower age group

span of animals, the interaction between aging and intestinal absorptive capacity is of crucial importance.

Many physiological functions decrease during aging. Examples of such a general trend include decreased renal, pulmonary and cardiovascular functions. Therefore, when we planned to measure the influence of aging on the intestinal absorptive capacity of nutrient lipids, we expected to find an aging associated decline in absorptive capacity as well. Indeed, pancreatic secretory functions declined with aging (Table 12.1). The decline in secretory volume and enzymes output was in concert with some isolated clinical observations of pancreatic insufficiency with aging[14]. Since pancreatic insufficiency would result in malabsorption of complex dietary carbohydrates, proteins and lipids this finding could suggest that aging may be associated with general nutrient malabsorption of ingested nutrients. However, we must remember that pancreatic secretory capacity has an enormous reserve and, even an 80–90% decrease in enzyme output does not necessarily result in clinically significant malabsorption. The reserve capacity of the small intestine also may compensate for impaired pancreatic enzyme secretion and nutrient maldigestion. Therefore, the clinical significance of our findings is not clear. Careful human studies will be needed to determine whether pancreatic insufficiency exists in aging individuals, and if so, to what extent it may influence absorption.

When we removed the pancreatic factor and assessed lipid absorption from a 'pre-digested' mixture we found that aging is associated with increased intestinal capacity to absorb lipids. Intestinal absorption of linoleic acid, vitamin A, vitamin D_3 and oleic acid increased with aging (Tables 12.2–12.4). It appears that the increased absorptive capacity for lipids is due, at least in part, to a decrease in the resistance of the unstirred water layer (UWL). This layer covers the lumenal surface of the absorptive cell membrane and is a major barrier for the diffusion of lipids[10–13]. The resistance of the UWL is inversely proportional to the surface area of the layer which appears to be increased with aging[6,9,13]. The increased total surface area of the UWL could be due to greater utilization of the lateral surface of the intestinal villi for absorption. This change with aging would result in decreased overall resistance to lipid absorption but not to protein or carbohydrate absorption which are not regulated by the UWL resistance. Thus, our findings of increased lipid absorptive capacity with aging are not in conflict with the general trend of decreased intestinal absorption of non-lipid nutrients[15]. In addition, our findings of increased absorptive capacity of lipids may not necessarily mean that net lipid absorption would be increased in aging individuals when lipids are ingested orally. Our experiments using a 'pre-digested' lipid mixture are a measure of the small intestinal maximal capacity to absorb lipids and not the entire chain of events which includes biliary and pancreatic digestion. It is possible that the increase in intestinal capacity to absorb lipids is an adaptation of the bowel to decreased pancreatic and hepatic digestive functions[15]. If so, the net result of these processes might be to normalize lipid absorption in aging individuals. Clearly, we need additional information in aging humans and in aging animals to resolve these questions.

Acknowledgement

These studies were supported by Grant AG 2767 from the National Institutes on Aging.

References

1. Hollander, D. and Dadufalza, V. D. (1984). Aging association pancreatic exocrine insufficiency in the unanesthetized rat. *Gerontology*, **30**, 218–222
2. Pelot, D., LaRusso, J. V. and Hollander, D. (1987). The influence of aging on basal and secretin stimulated pancreatic exocrine secretion in the unanesthetized rat. *Age*, **10**, 1–4
3. Hollander, D. (1981). Intestinal absorption of vitamins A, E, D and K. *J. Lab. Clin. Med.*, **97**, 449–62
4. Hwang, D. H., Mathias, M. M., Dupont, J. and Meyer, D. L. (1975). Linoleate enrichment of diet and prostaglandin metabolism in rat. *J. Nutr.*, **105**, 995–1002
5. Crawford, M. A. (1983). Background to essential fatty acids and their prostanoid derivatives. *Br. Med. Bull.*, **39**, 210–13
6. Hollander, D., Dadufalza, V. D. and Sletten, E. G. (1984). Does essential fatty acid absorption change with aging? *J. Lipid Res.*, **25**, 129–34
7. Hollander, D. and Dadufalza, V. D. (1983). Increase intestinal absorption of oleic acid with aging in the rat. *Exp. Gerontol.*, **18**, 287–92

8. Hollander, D. and Morgan, D. (1979). Aging: its influence on vitamin A intestinal absorption *in vivo* by the rat. *Exp. Gerontol.*, **14** (6), 301–5

9. Hollander, D. and Tarnawski, H. (1984). Influence of aging on vitamin D absorption and unstirred water layer dimensions in the rat. *J. Lab. Clin. Med.*, **103,** 462–9

10. Thomson, A. B. R. (1980). Effect of age on uptake of homologous series of saturated fatty acids into rabbit jejunum. *Am. J. Physiol.*, **239,** G363–G371

11. Diamond, J. M. (1962). The mechanism of solute transport by the gallbladder. *J. Physiol. (London)*, **161,** 474–502

12. Wilson, F. A. and Dietschy, J. M. (1974). The intestinal unstirred layer: its surface area and effect on active transport kinetics. *Biochim. Biophys. Acta*, **363,** 112–26

13. Hollander, D. and Dadufalza, V. D. (1983). Aging: its influence on the intestinal unstirred water layer thickness, surface area and resistance in the unanesthetized rat. *Can. J. Physiol. Pharmacol.*, **61,** 1501–8

14. Becker, G. H., Meyer, J. and Necheles, H. (1950). Fat absorption in young and old. *Gastroenterology*, **14,** 80–92

15. James, O. F. W. (1983). Gastrointestinal and liver functions in old age. *Clin. Gastroenterol.*, **12,** 671–91

13
Intestinal absorption of sugars: effect of aging

G. ESPOSITO, A. FAELLI, C. LINDI, M. TOSCO, P. MARCIANI, M. N. ORSENIGO AND G. MONTICELLI

INTRODUCTION

Studies of intestinal sugar transport during ageing have received more attention recently than in the past. However, the results obtained to date have been contradictory, presumably because of the different animal species and strains used, the different methodologies employed and the different ages of animals studied which makes a direct comparison of the results more difficult. Nevertheless, some findings deserve attention because they have been repeatedly confirmed.

Studies of the ageing gut involve differing fields of investigation including morphology and morphometry, studies of chemical composition and physical properties, qualitative and quantitative enzyme activity of enterocytes and their plasma membranes and characteristics of transport mechanisms and permeability. Recent reviews have highlighted different aspects of gut physiology and biochemistry during ageing[1-5].

The present report includes studies perfected in the past few years in our laboratory on effects of ageing on the transport of sugars, Na^+ and fluid in the rat jejunum and ileum. Initially our studies were done in an integrated system, under *in vivo* conditions and subsequently in the everted, cannulated and perfused gut *in vitro*. Finally studies were performed on the brush-border membrane (BBM), which controls the entry of solutes into the cell.

MATERIALS AND METHODS

Albino male Wistar strain (Charles River Italiana) rats were fed a rodent laboratory chow. They were divided into four groups according to age: very young (35–45 days old), young (2 months old), adult (7 months old) and old animals (approximately 20 months old). Animals were fasted 16 h before study but with free access to water. The techniques that were used for the *in vivo* experiments, for everted gut studies and brush-border membrane vesicles' (BBMV) uptake observation have been described previously[6-8].

The incubation and perfusion fluid used was Krebs–Ringer–bicarbonate solution gassed with 95% O_2–5% CO_2 and re-circulated by a peristaltic pump. When intracellular concentrations of sugars and electrolytes and cell volumes were estimated, the extracellular space was studied at all four ages[8-10].

The D-glucose and the non-metabolizable 3-O-methyl-D-glucose (3MG) were used at concentrations shown in the legends of figures and tables. Transport rates are given in μmoles, μequivalents or ml per gram of dry weight of scraped mucosa per hour. Solute concentrations are expressed in mmoles per litre of intracellular water. The tissue/mucosal (T/M) ratio was defined as the ratio of cellular and either mucosal or lumenal fluid sugar concentrations. All values are reported as means ± S.E. Significance of differences among groups was assayed with Student's *t* test.

RESULTS AND DISCUSSION

In vivo experiments

D-Glucose and 3MG which share the same transport system at the level of the lumenal membrane of the enterocyte were used.

D-glucose

Sugar concentration in the three main compartments, namely lumen, cell and blood was estimated (Table 13.1). Cell D-glucose concentrations either were undetectable or very low but always lower than that in the blood as shown previously[6-11].

Studies with 3MG (Table 13.2) showed the presence of this sugar within the cell but at a concentration always lower than in the blood; in all age groups of animals no evidence for cell accumulation occurs as was found previously[6,11,12].

Cell electrolyte concentration and cell volume was not affected by ageing. However, net D-glucose transport was lower in old rats than other age groups (Table 13.1) and net Na^+ and fluid transport were constant in all groups. These observations indicate that electrolyte transport, and fluid transport are more strictly preserved than glucose movement. It must be pointed out that some of these experimental data are affected by large standard errors owing to the biological variability among animals.

3-O-methyl-D-glucose

Since 3MG is a non-metabolizable sugar it was found intracellulary during its trans-intestinal transport. Cell accumulation, however, did not occur (Table 13.2). As in the case of D-glucose, cell K^+ concentration and cell

Table 13.1 Studies of glucose transport in *in vivo* perfused rat jejunum at differing ages

	D-glucose (mM)			T/M	Cell Na^+ (mEq)	Cell K^+ (mEq)	Cell water (ml/g)	Net D-glucose transport (μmol g$^{-1}\cdot$h^{-1})	Net Na^+ transport (μequiv. g$^{-1}\cdot$h^{-1})	Net fluid transport (ml g$^{-1}\cdot$h^{-1})	Wet wt/dry wt
	Lumen	Cell	Blood								
Very young rats	3.6±0.2	—	8.3±0.7	—	14±1	157±7	3.3±0.2	167±28	1575±265	10.9±1.7	5.1±0.1†
Young rats	3.1±0.2	—	7.9±0.3	—	15±2	149±6	2.9±0.2	169±13	966±189	6.8±1.3	4.3±0.1
Adult rats	3.3±0.1	—	6.6±0.4**	—	10±1	148±10	2.8±0.1	150±11	684±257	4.8±1.8	4.6±0.1
Old rats	3.2±0.3	—	6.8±0.8	—	9±3	131±21	2.2±0.1	92±3*	643± 4	4.5±0.1	3.9±0.1**

Initial D-glucose concentration in the lumenal perfusing fluid is 5.56 mM.
Values are means ± SE of 3–8 experiments. P values are versus those of the young rat group.
* $P<0.01$; ** $P<0.05$; † $P<0.001$

Table 13.2 Studies of 3-O-methyl-D-glucose transport in *in vivo* perfused rat jejunum at different ages

	3-O-Methyl-D-glucose (mM)			T/M	Cell Na^+ (mEq)	Cell K^+ (mEq)	Cell water (ml/g)	Net 3-O-Methyl-D-glucose transport (μmol g$^{-1}\cdot$h^{-1})	Net Na^+ transport (μequiv. g$^{-1}\cdot$h^{-1})	Net fluid transport (ml g$^{-1}\cdot$h^{-1})	Wet wt/dry wt
	Lumen	Cell	Blood								
Very young rats	4.3±0.1	3.1±0.1	10.1±0.5*	0.74±0.02	4±1*	142±2	3.0±0.1	64± 6	677±108	4.7±0.8	4.9±0.1
Young rats	4.3±0.1	2.9±0.3	4.7±0.4	0.68±0.04	15±1	145±2	3.0±0.2	62± 6	791± 76	5.5±0.5	4.6±0.2
Adult rats	4.4±0.1	4.2±0.1†	7.8±0.9**	0.97±0.04*	10±1**	147±4	2.3±0.1**	59± 7	1033±201	7.0±1.0	3.9±0.2
Old rats	4.5±0.2	4.2±1.3	7.7±1.9	0.94±0.30	8±2**	144±4	2.3±0.4	63±10	728±137	5.1±1.0	3.9±0.5

Initial 3-O-methyl-D-glucose concentration in the lumenal perfusing fluid is 5.15 mM.
Values are means ± SE of 3–5 experiments. P values are versus those of the young rat group.
* $P<0.01$; ** $P<0.05$; † $P<0.02$

119

volumes were almost unaffected by ageing during 3MG transport. Cell Na^+ concentration changed to a small extent. Unlike D-glucose, net trans-intestinal transport of 3MG was not altered with age but the amounts transported were quite low at all ages. Net Na^+ and fluid transports also were unaffected by ageing.

In conclusion, most of the properties of the enterocyte are not affected to a major extent by ageing. Sugar transport *in vivo* is determined as the amount disappearing from the lumen; therefore, unlike 3MG, D-glucose transport might be obscured in part by metabolism. Unstirred water layers as well might obscure sugar transport differences in the four age groups of animals[14,15]. *In vivo*, only D-glucose absorption is reduced in old animals. Such a reduced *in vivo* sugar transport in old rats was also reported by others[16,17].

In vitro experiments

Net trans-intestinal D-glucose and 3MG transport was determined in the everted, cannulated and perfused jejunum and ileum in the same four age groups of animals that were studied *in vivo*. This preparation is useful since it allows easy access to the main three compartments involved in transport processes without the influence of the nervous, hormonal and vascular systems.

D-Glucose: jejunum and ileum

Higher D-glucose (Table 13.3) and 3MG cell (Table 13.4) accumulation were found in the jejunum of young rats which declined with age; in old rats sugar accumulation did not occur (Table 13.3). In the ileum, however, sugar accumulation was observed only in very young animals whereas it was absent in the other three age groups (Table 13.4).

Cell electrolyte concentrations were unchanged in all age groups except for a reduction in Na^+ and K^+ in the jejunal enterocytes of old rats. Overall, the data indicate that the cellular electrolyte homeostasis is effectively maintained.

A reduction in cell volume was consistently observed in both jejunum and ileum. The wet-to-dry weight ratio of scraped mucosa was lower in old rats indicating that total tissue water had decreased; since the extracellular space had relatively increased, intracellular water was reduced. In addition, old animals have similar cellular electrolyte concentrations to that of other ages but with reduced cell water suggesting that aged enterocytes are smaller and consequently more numerous. Some morphological studies showed that the number of epithelial cells in the particular intestinal length considered, increased with age[18].

Net trans-intestinal transport of D-glucose increased from very young to young rats but then was lower in adult and old rats. In contrast, net Na^+ and fluid transport was similar in the first three age groups but decreased in old rats. In the ileum, sugar transport declined from younger to older animals with almost no D-glucose transport in adult and old rats suggesting that the ileum was unable to compensate for decreased sugar transport in the jejunum.

Table 13.3 Cellular sugar and electrolyte concentration and trans-intestinal transport in everted and perfused rat jejunum

	D-glucose (mM)				Cell Na⁺ (mEq)	Cell K⁺ (mEq)	Cell water (ml/g)	Net D-glucose transport (μmol g⁻¹·h⁻¹)	Net Na⁺ transport (μequiv. g⁻¹·h⁻¹)	Net fluid transport (ml g⁻¹·h⁻¹)	Wet wt/dry wt
	Mucosal	Cell	Serosal	T/M							
Very young rats	4.3±0.4	5.5±1.7	5.0±0.3	1.3±0.4	46±4	98±4	4.4±0.1	88±24†	1196±221	8.3±1.5	6.4±0.2
Young rats	4.6±0.2	14.3±2.9	8.4±0.7	3.1±0.7	36±2	123±7	4.2±0.1	278±25	1744±231	12.5±1.7	6.4±0.3
Adult rats	5.0±0.2	8.2±1.6	6.6±0.3	1.6±0.2	36±4	103±4	4.7±0.2	155±29**	1279±176	8.9±1.2	7.1±0.3
Old rats	5.4±0.4	6.6±0.3*	5.6±0.4	1.2±0.6*	45±4	96±4†	2.9±0.2†	73±10†	547±78†	3.5±0.7†	4.7±0.4*

D-glucose concentration in 50 ml mucosal and 5 ml serosal fluid is 5.56 mM. The experimental temperature is 28°C.
Values are means ± SE of 5–7 experiments. P values are versus those of the young rat group.
* $P < 0.05$; ** $P < 0.02$; † $P < 0.001$

Table 13.4 Cellular sugar and electrolyte concentration and trans-intestinal transport in everted and perfused rat ileum

	D-glucose (mM)				Cell Na⁺ (mEq)	Cell K⁺ (mEq)	Cell water (ml/g)	Net D-glucose transport (μmol g⁻¹·h⁻¹)	Net Na⁺ transport (μequiv. g⁻¹·h⁻¹)	Net fluid transport (ml g⁻¹·h⁻¹)	Wet wt/dry wt
	Mucosal	Cell	Serosal	T/M							
Very young rats	4.3±0.3	16.3±4.8**	5.1±0.5	4.0±1.3**	41± 4	102±5	4.3±0.1	151±33	1896±355	13.0±1.9	6.5±0.2
Young rats	5.3±0.1	4.7±0.8	5.6±0.2	0.9±0.1	32± 4	118±7	4.1±0.2	100±10	2195±445	13.7±2.0	6.8±0.3
Adult rats	5.3±0.1	4.1±0.9	4.4±0.2	0.8±0.2	34±10	113±6	3.7±0.1	−6±16†	1007±128**	7.8±1.3**	7.7±0.6
Old rats	5.3±0.2	5.5±2.4	5.8±0.5	1.0±0.4	37± 8	98±9	2.2±0.3†	61±32	912±260**	6.0±1.9**	4.1±0.4*

D-glucose concentration in 50 ml mucosal and 5 ml serosal fluid is 5.56 mM. The experimental temperature is 28°C.
Values are means ± SE of 6 experiments. P values are versus those of the young rat group.
* $P < 0.01$; ** $P < 0.05$; † $P < 0.001$

121

Table 13.5 Cellular sugar and electrolyte concentration and trans-intestinal transport in everted and perfused rat jejunum

	3-O-methyl-D-Glucose (mM)						Cell water (ml/g)	Net 3-O-methyl-D-glucose transport (μmol g⁻¹·h⁻¹)	Net Na⁺ transport (μequiv. g⁻¹·h⁻¹)	Net fluid transport (ml g⁻¹·h⁻¹)	Wet wt/dry wt
	Mucosal	Cell	Serosal	T/M	Cell Na⁺ (mEq)	Cell K⁺ (mEq)					
Very young rats	4.7 ± 0.1	9.4 ± 0.9	5.5 ± 0.1	2.1 ± 0.2†	43 ± 4	103 ± 4	4.5 ± 0.1	123 ± 24	1066 ± 300	5.5 ± 0.8	6.5 ± 0.1
Young rats	4.7 ± 0.1	7.3 ± 0.6	5.1 ± 0.1	1.5 ± 0.1	55 ± 5	107 ± 4	4.1 ± 0.2	80 ± 10	1249 ± 269	8.6 ± 1.8	6.0 ± 0.3
Adult rats	4.6 ± 0.1	8.2 ± 1.7	5.2 ± 0.1	1.8 ± 0.4	40 ± 7	111 ± 3	3.7 ± 0.1	98 ± 20	1549 ± 337	9.8 ± 1.0	5.7 ± 0.1
Old rats	4.7 ± 0.1	7.7 ± 0.8	4.9 ± 0.1	1.6 ± 0.5	55 ± 2	103 ± 6	2.5 ± 0.5*	37 ± 12**	601 ± 169	4.1 ± 1.2	4.3 ± 0.6†

3-O-methyl-D-glucose concentration in 50 ml mucosal and 5 ml serosal fluid is 5.15 mM. The experimental temperature is 28°C.
Values are means ± SE of 4–9 experiments. P values are versus those of the young rat group.
* $P<0.01$; ** $P<0.05$; † $P<0.02$

Table 13.6 Cellular sugar and electrolyte concentration and trans-intestinal transport in everted and perfused rat ileum

	3-O-methyl-D-glucose (mM)						Cell water (ml/g)	Net 3-O-methyl-D-glucose transport (μmol g⁻¹·h⁻¹)	Net Na⁺ transport (μequiv. g⁻¹·h⁻¹)	Net fluid transport (ml g⁻¹·h⁻¹)	Wet wt/dry wt
	Mucosal	Cell	Serosal	T/M	Cell Na⁺ (mEq)	Cell K⁺ (mEq)					
Very young rats	4.9 ± 0.1	5.7 ± 0.4*	4.8 ± 0.1	1.2 ± 0.1†	43 ± 3††	109 ± 4	4.2 ± 0.1*	11 ± 4	768 ± 269	5.2 ± 2.0	6.2 ± 0.2
Young rats	4.7 ± 0.1	3.9 ± 0.4	4.8 ± 0.1	0.8 ± 0.1	22 ± 3	113 ± 4	3.4 ± 0.2	7 ± 2	708 ± 153	4.3 ± 1.0	5.7 ± 0.2
Adult rats	4.8 ± 0.2	5.2 ± 1.5	4.9 ± 0.1	1.1 ± 0.3	26 ± 3	136 ± 3††	2.7 ± 0.3	4 ± 1	675 ± 182	4.3 ± 1.3	5.3 ± 0.4
Old rats	4.8 ± 0.1	6.6 ± 0.7*	4.9 ± 0.2	1.4 ± 0.1*	21 ± 6	125 ± 8	2.3 ± 0.5**	4 ± 2	91 ± 65***	0.6 ± 0.4**	4.7 ± 0.8

3-O-methyl-D-glucose concentration in 50 ml mucosal and 5 ml serosal fluid is 5.15 mM. The experimental temperature is 28°C.
Values are means ± SE of 4–9 experiments. P values are versus those of the young rat group.
* $P<0.01$; ** $P<0.05$; † $P<0.02$; †† $P<0.001$

122

In both jejunum and ileum, Na^+ transport was significantly less in the oldest group of animals but otherwise was maintained.

3-O-methyl-D-glucose: jejunum and ileum

3MG accumulation did not occur in either jejunum or ileum (Tables 13.5 and 13.6) except in the jejunum of very young rats. This occurred probably from a lower affinity of the sugar carrier for 3MG. The sugar concentrations used in these experiments are appropriate for transport studies but less for accumulation experiments.

Cell electrolyte concentrations were similar in jejunum and ileum at all four ages and are also close to those noted with D-glucose (Table 13.3). However, also in the case of 3MG, cell volumes were consistently lower in jejunum and ileum of old rats.

It must be noted that *in vivo* experiments showed a much lower cell Na^+ and a higher cell K^+ concentration, as always found in *in vivo* vs. *in vitro* experiments (Tables 13.1 and 13.2), probably owing to a better Na^+-K^+-ATPase activity under the former condition.

Net trans-intestinal 3MG transport was lower than D-glucose transport under the same experimental conditions. However, the pattern of 3MG transport in rat jejunum is different; in fact there is a statistically significant decrease only in old animals, the other age groups displaying a similar (lower in the ileum) transport activity.

Net trans-intestinal Na^+ transport behaves approximately as that in the presence of D-glucose with the same amount of Na^+ transport in the first three age groups of animals and a drop in old rats, in both jejunum and ileum.

It must be noted that in 3MG experiments, sugar and Na^+ transports are lower than in D-glucose experiments in both jejunum and ileum; this is probably owing to the lower energy available when glucose is absent.

3MG transport *in vitro* is somewhat higher than *in vivo*; a possible explanation is that under *in vivo* conditions the sugar moves from lumen to blood and from cell to blood against a higher chemical potential gradient. An approximately similar situation occurs for D-glucose experiments.

Finally, by comparing net D-glucose and 3MG jejunal transport *in vitro* in the first two age groups of animals, namely very young and young rats, a much higher D-glucose transport can be found in young animals while 3MG transport is similar, or somewhat higher, in very young and young rats (Tables 13.3 and 13.5). The basal lactic acid production, however, is similar

Table 13.7 Lactate production by mucosal scrapings

Animal	Lactate (μmoles/g/30 min)*	Wet weight/ dry weight
Very young rats ($n=8$)	185 ± 28	6.41 ± 0.3
Young rats ($n=10$)	173 ± 23	6.43 ± 0.2

*Lactate production is given in μmoles per gram of dry weight of scraped mucosa. Lactic acid was determined by an enzymatic method[19]

in the two age groups of rats (Table 13.7). Therefore, the different D-glucose transport can not be explained in terms of different metabolic rate. The higher D-glucose transport activity in the jejunum of young rats might be explained by the brush-border membrane properties of the enterocyte of young animals (see later).

EXPERIMENTS WITH BRUSH-BORDER MEMBRANE VESICLES (BBMV)

This technique is very useful to study the properties of the membrane involved in sugar entry into the cell. In fact, it is possible to elucidate the characteristics of transport processes without being influenced by cellular metabolism.

We have shown that D-glucose uptake into BBMV is affected by ageing[8,21]. In fact, in the first three age groups of animals there is an overshoot owing to the presence of a Na^+ gradient (Na^+ outside, no Na^+ inside the vesicle); this overshoot is higher in young rats and lower but similar in very young and adult animals. Old rats do not show any overshoot. This pattern parallels that observed in the everted intestine for net trans-intestinal transport of D-glucose. In very young rats the low sugar uptake might indicate the presence of a Na^+-dependent mechanism of sugar entry which is not completely developed yet, while in adult rats this mechanism begins to be less efficient. In old animals sugar entry mechanism seems to have changed completely as if the nature of sugar movement had changed as well. In fact, the typical overshoot is no longer present while there is a continuous increase in sugar entry.

To study the influence of membrane electrical potential difference between the inside and the outside of the vesicle (internal side negative), the vesicles were short-circuited with valinomycin[21]. For very young animals the over-shoot did not change; this might indicate that the main driving force for sugar entry is the chemical potential gradient of Na^+.

Young animals showed a reduced, but not abolished, overshoot, thus indicating that both the chemical and electrical potential gradients played a role in sugar accumulation.

In adult animals the overshoot disappeared; this might suggest that the electrical potential gradient is the main driving force. Finally, old animals were affected neither by the electrical nor by the chemical potential gradient, thus indicating that sugar uptake into vesicles seems to be Na^+-independent. Moreover, sugar uptake in old rats was similar when the ion gradient was generated by NaCl or KCl.

In a set of experiments the kinetic parameters for D-glucose uptake into BBMV from rats of the four age groups, were also determined. The uncor-rected uptake rates were fitted by non-linear regression analysis to an equation implicating one diffusional and two saturable terms[20] (Table 13.8 and Figures 13.1–13.4).

The purpose of this approach was to verify whether one or more saturable components of Na^+-dependent D-glucose transport were present in the lumenal membrane of the enterocyte, namely one with low affinity and high

Table 13.8. Kinetic parameters for D-glucose uptake in BBM vesicles of rats of different ages

Animal	J_{max}	K_M	J'_{max}	K'_M	P
Very young	308	1.94	24	0.06	17.5
Young	241	1.28	27	0.12	73.8
Adult	318	0.58	0	0	3.5
Old	521	3.16	51	0.05	15.2

Uptake: pmoles/mg protein/sec. K_M in mM. P in nl/mg protein/sec

capacity and the other with high affinity and low capacity, and in addition, whether a passive diffusional component might also exist.

As summarized in Table 13.8 it seems that, by fitting the experimental points, two saturable and one diffusional components are present in animals of different ages except for adult rats where only one saturable and a very small passive diffusional component occur.

The low-affinity–high-capacity component is present, in decreasing order, in old, adult, very young and young rats while the high-affinity–low-capacity component is present in old, young and very young animals; in adult rats it is absent. It is interesting to observe that the passive diffusional component is very high in young rats, lower but similar in very young and old animals and almost absent in adult rats. Figures 13.1 to 13.4 show in detail the different components present in the four age groups of animals. These three components, even if in a different order of location and distribution in the four age groups of animals, have also been found recently in rat small intestine[22].

An analysis of the results obtained in kinetic experiments seems, on the whole, to be in agreement with that of the results obtained in everted sac experiments. Young rats possess the highest transport activity, intracellular sugar accumulation, overshoot phenomenon, apparent permeability coefficient in spite of a lower J_{max} as compared, for instance, with adult animals. These findings might be interpreted in part as the result of a reduced sugar backflux from the cell to the lumen with a consequent cellular sugar accumulation which in turn is responsible for an increased sugar exit across the basolateral membrane of the enterocyte resulting in an increased net trans-intestinal transport. In fact, K_M value for sugar backflux across the lumenal membrane, calculated from the experimental data obtained in everted sac and BBMV experiments, is much greater than the influx value. Moreover, this K_M value for sugar backflux in young rats is higher than in the other age groups of animals.

What we need is more information on the membrane properties and driving forces responsible for sugar movement across the basolateral membrane of the enterocyte.

It must be pointed out here that data obtained under *in vivo* experiments are the result of many homeostatic processes addressed to regulate, modulate and finalize the activity of a cell or of an organ. The *in vitro* preparations usually select and sometimes highlight one or more properties of the activity

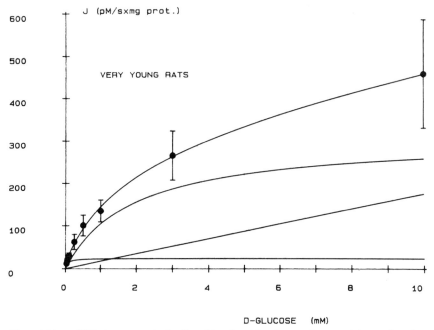

Figure 13.1   D-[^{14}C]-glucose uptake (ordinate) into brush border membrane vesicles as a function of different sugar concentrations (abscissa). D-Glucose concentrations (in mM) in the external medium were 0.03, 0.05, 0.10, 0.25, 0.50, 1.0, 3.0, 5.0 and 10.0, respectively. Each point with S.E. (vertical bar) is a mean of at least 4 different animals (every determination in triplicate). Experiments were carried out at room temperature. Uncorrected uptakes were fitted by nonlinear regression analysis to an equation involving one diffusional and two saturable terms[20].

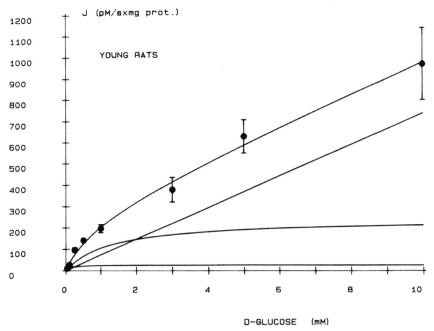

Figure 13.2   See Figure 13.1

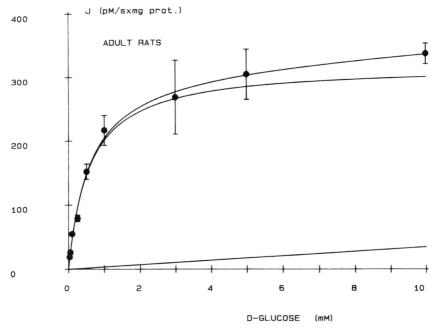

Figure 13.3 See Figure 13.1

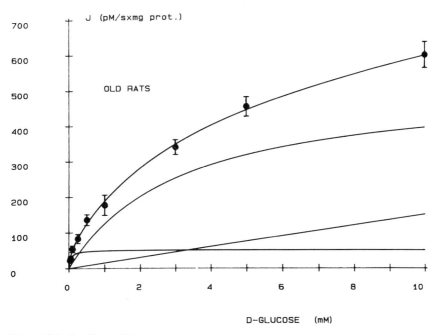

Figure 13.4 See Figure 13.1

of a cell or of an organ. Membrane preparations are useful tools for the understanding of a single property of a single function of the cell. Therefore, whenever possible, it is highly desirable to study the function of an organ by using different methods and techniques in order to get more and more information necessary for a complete understanding of its role in the general economy of the organism.

Acknowledgements

This work was supported by a research grant from the Consiglio Nazionale delle Ricerche, Special Project: Preventive and Rehabilitative Medicine-Mechanisms of Aging (C.T. 86.01761.56), and by a grant from Ministero Pubblica Istruzione, Rome (40%).

References

1. Penzes, L. (1980). Intestinal absorption in the aged. *Acta Med. Acad. Sci. Hung.*, **37**, 203–209
2. Holt, P R. (1985). The small intestine. *Clin. Gastroenterol*, **14**, 689–723
3. Keelan, M., Walker, K. and Thomson, A. B. R. (1985). Intestinal morphology, marker enzymes and lipid content of brush border membranes from rabbit jejunum and ileum: effect of aging. *Mech. Age. Dev.*, **31**, 49–68
4. Thomson, A. B. R. and Keelan, M. (1986). The aging gut. *Can. J. Physiol. Pharmacol.*, **64**, 30–38
5. Vinardell, M. P. (1987). Age influences on intestinal sugar absorption. *Comp. Biochem. Physiol.*, **86**, 617–23
6. Esposito, G., Faelli, A. and Capraro, V. (1973). Sugar and electrolyte absorption in the rat intestine perfused *in vivo*. *Pflüg. Arch.*, **340**, 335–48
7. Faelli, A., Esposito, G., Tosco, M. and Capraro, V. (1981). Cell bicarbonate and chloride in the jejunum of rat and hamster incubated *in vitro*. *J. Physiol. (Paris)*, **77**, 845–9
8. Esposito, G., Faelli, A., Tosco, M., Orsenigo, M. N. and Batistessa, R (1985). Age-related changes in rat intestinal transport of D-glucose, sodium and water. *Am. J. Physiol.*, **249**, G328–G334
9. Esposito, G., Faelli, A., Tosco, M., Burlini, M. and Capraro, V. (1979). Extracellular space determination in rat small intestine by using markers of different molecular weights.. *Pflüg. Arch.*, **382**, 67–71
10. Esposito, G. and Csaky, T. Z. (1974). Extracellular space in the epithelium of rats' small intestine. *Am. J. Physiol.*, **226**, 50–55
11. Esposito, G., Faelli, A. and Capraro, V. (1977). A critical evaluation of the existence of an outward sugar pump in the basolateral membrane of the enterocyte. In Kramer, M. and Lauterbach, F. (eds.) *Intestinal Permeation*. pp. 107–113. (Amsterdam: Excerpta Medica)
12. Esposito, G. (1984). Intestinal permeability of water-soluble non-electrolytes: sugars, amino acids, peptides. In Csaky, T. Z. (ed.). *Handbook of Experimental Pharmacology*. pp. 567–611. (Berlin: Springer-Verlag)
13. Esposito, G., Faelli, A., Tosco, M., Orsenigo, M. N. and Capraro, V. (1982). *In vivo* and *in vitro* sugar transport in frog intestine. *Biochim. Biophys. Acta*, **688**, 798–802
14. Thompson, A. B. R. (1979). Unstirred water layer and age-dependent changes in rabbit jejunal D-glucose transport. *Am. J. Physiol.*, **236**, E685–E691
15. Hollander, D. and Dadufalra, V. D. (1983). Aging: its influence on the intestinal unstirred water layer thickness, surface area, and resistance in the unanesthetized rat. *Can. J. Physiol. Pharmacol.*, **61**, 1501–8
16. Feibusch, J. M. and Holt, P. R. (1982). Impaired absorptive capacity for carbohydrate in the aging human. *Dig. Dis. Sci.*, **27**, 1095–100

17. Vinardell, M. P. and Bolufer, J. (1984). Age-dependent changes on jejunal sugar absorption by rat *in vivo*. *Exp. Gerontol.,* **19,** 73–8

18. Altmann, G. G. and Enesco, M. (1967). Cell number as a measure of distribution and renewal of epithelial cells in the small intestine of growing and adult rats. *Am. J. Anat.,* **121,** 319–36

19. Scholz, R., Schmitz, H., Bücher, T. and Lampen, J. O. (1959). Ueber die Wirkung von Nystatin auf Backerhefe. *Biochem. Z.,* **331,** 71–86

20. Brot-Laroche, E., Serrano, M.-A., Delhomme, B. and Alvarado, F. (1986). Temperature sensitivity and substrate specificity of two distinct Na^+-activated D-glucose transport systems in guinea pig jejunal brush border membrane vesicles. *J. Biol. Chem.,* **261,** 6168–76

21. Lindi, C., Marciani, P., Faelli, A. and Esposito, G. (1985). Intestinal sugar transport during ageing. *Biochim. Biophys. Acta,* **816,** 411–14

22. Freeman, H. J. and Quamme, G. A. (1986). Age-related changes in sodium-dependent glucose transport in rat small intestine. *Am. J. Physiol.,* **251,** G208–G217

14
Changes in the components of the intestinal calcium transport system with age

H. J. ARMBRECHT

Calcium (Ca^{2+}) absorption declines markedly with age in humans. In addition, older persons tend to consume less Ca^{2+} in their diet. This combination of decreased Ca^{2+} absorption and decreased dietary Ca^{2+} may contribute to the decrease in bone mass seen in the elderly. Therefore, it is important to understand the mechanisms responsible for decreased Ca^{2+} absorption with age. Knowledge of the mechanisms responsible for decreased Ca^{2+} absorption may suggest ways of improving Ca^{2+} absorption and preserving bone mass in the elderly.

AGE-RELATED CHANGES IN CALCIUM ABSORPTION IN MAMMALS

A number of human studies have demonstrated that there is a decrease in the absorption of Ca^{2+} with age[1-3]. The exact relationship of this decrease to chronological age is uncertain owing to the inherent variability of human studies. One study reported that intestinal absorption declined as a negative exponential function of age[3]. In this study, there was a more rapid decline in intestinal absorption in the younger population than in the older population. A second study, which used different experimental techniques, fit their absorption data to a linear least squares model. They reported a linear decline in intestinal absorption with age[1]. However, the data also could have been fit to a negative exponential function. A third study, which measured Ca^{2+} absorption in a predominantly older population, reported a decrease in absorption after 60 years of age[2].

In order to study the mechanism of the decline in Ca^{2+} absorption, we have used the Fischer 344 rat as an animal model. This rat shows an age-related decrease in the absorption of Ca^{2+} that is similar to that seen in humans[4,5]. This decreased Ca^{2+} absorption results in negative Ca^{2+} balance when adult rats are fed diets which maintain positive Ca^{2+} balance in young rats[6]. The F344 rat also demonstrates significant bone loss later in its life span[7].

Ca^{2+} absorption declines as a negative exponential function of age in the

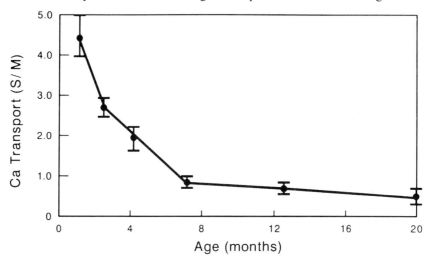

Figure 14.1 Changes in Ca^{2+} transport with age. Ca^{2+} transport was measured using everted duodenal sacs incubated with radiolabelled Ca^{2+} for 1.5 h. Ca^{2+} transport is expressed as the ratio of radioactivity on the serosal compared to the mucosal side (S/M). Data points are the mean ± SEM of 4–8 rats

Fischer 344 rat (Figure 14.1). Ca^{2+} absorption was measured *in vitro* using everted intestinal segments from the proximal duodenum[4,5]. Everted segments were incubated with radioactive Ca^{2+} on both sides for 1.5 h. At the end of the experiment, the ratio of Ca^{2+} on the outside (serosal) to Ca^{2+} on the inside (mucosal) of the sac was calculated. This technique measures primarily active, energy-dependent absorption of Ca^{2+}. In Figure 14.1, Ca^{2+} transport, as measured by the serosal to mucosal ratio (S/M), is plotted as a function of age of the rat. There is a marked decline in active Ca^{2+} transport between 1 and 4 months of age. This is followed by a much shallower decline between 4 and 7 months of age with little change thereafter. A similar pattern is seen when intestinal Ca^{2+} uptake rather than trans-epithelial Ca^{2+} transport is measured[8]. Sprague-Dawley rats show similar changes in Ca^{2+} absorption with age[9].

MECHANISM OF CALCIUM ABSORPTION BY THE SMALL INTESTINE

Figure 14.2 shows the pathway of Ca^{2+} across the intestinal epithelial cell and the stimulation of that pathway by 1,25-dihydroxyvitamin D. 1,25-Dihydroxyvitamin D is the hormonal form of vitamin D which has the most biological activity in the intestine[10]. Luminal Ca^{2+} enters the intestinal absorptive cell by crossing the brush-border membrane via a carrier-mediated mechanism. This is thought to be a passive process, since the luminal Ca^{2+} concentration is much higher than the intracellular Ca^{2+} concentration. Ca^{2+} entry may be facilitated by a cluster of integral brush-border membrane proteins known collectively as the particulate Ca^{2+}-binding complex $(CaBC)$[11].

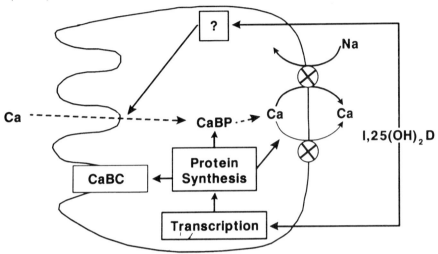

Figure 14.2 Effect of 1,25-dihydroxyvitamin D on intestinal absorption of calcium. Ca^{2+} crosses the brush-border membrane, is translocated across the cell in conjunction with calcium-binding protein (CaBP), and is actively extruded across the basal-lateral membrane by either an ATP-requiring pump or a Na^+–Ca^{2+} counter-transport system. Ca^{2+} movement across the brush-border membrane may be facilitated by a Ca^{2+}-binding complex (CaBC) and changes in membrane composition. 1,25-Dihydroxyvitamin D enhances Ca^{2+} movement across the cell by increasing brush-border permeability to Ca^{2+}, increasing cytoplasmic CaBP, and increasing the activity of the basolateral membrane pump

Ca^{2+} then moves across the absorptive cell to the basal lateral surface of the cell. The specific pathway by which Ca^{2+} transverses the cell is not known, but it is thought that the Ca^{2+} is either sequestered by intracellular organelles or bound to cytosolic proteins. One cytosolic protein which may play a role in the translocation of Ca^{2+} is the vitamin D-dependent Ca^{2+}-binding protein (CaBP). This soluble protein binds Ca^{2+} with a high affinity, is markedly stimulated by 1,25-dihydroxyvitamin D, and correlates well with Ca^{2+} absorption[12].

At the basal lateral surface of the cell, Ca^{2+} is translocated out of the cell and into the blood. Ca^{2+} is actively transported across the basal lateral membrane by either an ATP-dependent pump and/or by a Na^+–Ca^{2+} exchange mechanism[13]. Quantitatively, the Ca^{2+} pump is probably the more important mechanism.

1,25-Dihydroxyvitamin D, whose mechanism of action is similar to that of the steroid hormones, acts at several subcellular sites to stimulate Ca^{2+} absorption in young animals. 1,25-Dihydroxyvitamin D acts at the brush-border membrane to enhance Ca^{2+} entry into the cell. The mechanism for this rapid action of 1,25-dihydroxyvitamin D is unknown, but it may involve alteration in the lipid composition of the brush-border membrane. 1,25-Dihydroxyvitamin D also increases the amount of $CaBC^{11}$. In the cytoplasm, 1,25-dihydroxyvitamin D increases the amount of $CaBP^{12}$. At the basal lateral membrane, 1,25-dihydroxyvitamin D increases the capacity of the basal lateral membrane to actively pump Ca^{2+} [14]. These long-term effects of 1,25-dihydroxyvitamin D are mediated by transcription and synthesis of new proteins.

In terms of the age-related decline in Ca^{2+} absorption, we have been interested in three questions. First, what changes take place in the components of the Ca^{2+} transport system with age? Second, what changes take place in the serum levels of 1,25-dihydroxyvitamin D with age? Third, what changes take place in the responsiveness of the intestine to 1,25-dihydroxyvitamin D with age?

AGE-RELATED CHANGES IN COMPONENTS OF THE CALCIUM TRANSPORT SYSTEM

The first component of the Ca^{2+} transport system which we studied is the active pumping of Ca^{2+} by the basal lateral membrane. We were particularly interested in studying the active component of Ca^{2+} transport since the intestinal sac experiments suggested that there was a large decrease in the active transport of Ca^{2+} with age. Basal lateral membrane vesicles (BLMV) were isolated by differential and gradient centrifugation from young (2 month) and adult (12 month) rats. Uptake of Ca^{2+} by BLMV was measured using radioactive Ca^{2+} and Millipore filtration[13]. In vesicles isolated from

Table 14.1 Calcium uptake by brush-border and basal-lateral membrane vesicles

	Ca^{2+} uptake (pmoles/mg protein/20 min)		
Age	Basal lateral membranes		Brush border membranes
	$(-ATP)$	$(+ATP)$	
Young	0.8 ± 0.1	36.7 ± 1.7	2775 ± 21
Adult	0.8 ± 0.1	8.0 ± 0.3	3234 ± 46
Old	—	—	2905 ± 32

Entries are the mean ± S.E.M. of triplicate determinations from a single experiment. Young, adult, and old rats were 2–3, 12–14, and 22–24 months old, respectively

young animals, ATP markedly stimulated Ca^{2+} uptake (Table 14.1). However, in vesicles isolated from adult animals, ATP-stimulated Ca^{2+} uptake was only 22% of the level seen in the young. There was no difference in Ca^{2+} uptake with age in the absence of ATP. The ATP-dependent Ca^{2+}

uptake by BLMV from young rats was inhibited by vanadate and osmotic shock (data not shown). This suggests that under these experimental conditions uptake is owing to Ca^{2+} pumping into an osmotic space.

To further characterize the age-related changes in BLMV Ca^{2+} transport, we performed kinetic studies of Ca^{2+} transport. The uptake of Ca^{2+} was measured after 10 s at Ca^{2+} concentrations ranging from 0.02 to 1.0 μM. For the young animals, the apparent affinity of the Ca^{2+} transport system was 0.27 μM. For the adults, the apparent affinity was 0.25 μM, which was not significantly different from the young. However, there was a large difference in the maximal velocity of the two transport systems. For the young, the maximal velocity of the transport system, was 3.76 nmoles/min/mg. For the adult, the maximal velocity was only 0.75 nmoles/min/mg. These findings suggest that there is a decreased number of Ca^{2+} transporters in BLMV from the adult rats. However, the Ca^{2+} transporters that are present in the adult rats are fully functional in terms of their affinity for Ca^{2+}.

The second component of the Ca^{2+} transport system which we studied is the movement of Ca^{2+} across the brush-border membrane. We isolated brush-border membrane vesicles (BBMV) by differential centrifugation and magnesium precipitation, and we studied Ca^{2+} uptake by Millipore filtration[15]. Ca^{2+} uptake by BBMV did not change significantly with age (Table 14.1). In contrast to the BLMV, Ca^{2+} uptake by the BBMV was not inhibited by vanadate or osmotic shock. In addition, Ca^{2+} uptake by BBMV was about 100 times greater per mg protein than Ca^{2+} uptake by BLMV. This suggests that Ca^{2+} uptake by BBMV probably represents binding to the membrane itself rather than transport into a vesicular space. Parallel studies of glucose transport have demonstrated that these brush-border membrane preparations do form osmotically-active vesicles[15]. These experiments provide no evidence for age-related changes in Ca^{2+} entry into the cell across the brush-border membrane. On the other hand, the large amount of non-specific binding to the membrane surface in this experimental system may mask possible age-related changes.

Finally, we studied age-related changes in a cytosolic component of the Ca^{2+} transport system – the vitamin D-dependent Ca^{2+}-binding protein (CaBP). The amount of this protein was quantitated in intestinal supernatants prepared from the proximal duodenum. The protein was quantitated immunologically using antiserum kindly provided by Dr Elizabeth Bruns (University of Virginia, Charlottesville, VA, USA)[4]. In Figure 14.3, the concentration of CaBP was plotted as a function of age. There was a large decrease in the concentration of CaBP between 2 and 6 months. There was a further decrease between 6 and 15 months and only a slight change thereafter. These changes in CaBP closely parallel the age-related decrease in active transport seen in everted intestinal segments (Figure 14.1).

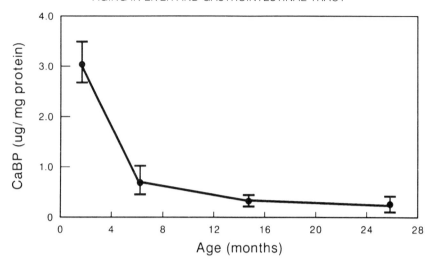

Figure 14.3 Changes in intestinal CaBP with age. CaBP was quantitated immunologically in supernatants prepared from the proximal duodenum. Data points are the mean ± SEM of 4–5 rats

AGE-RELATED CHANGES IN SERUM 1,25-DIHYDROXYVITAMIN D

We next examined serum levels of 1,25-dihydroxyvitamin D to determine if age-related changes in the Ca^{2+} transport system were explainable in terms of changes in serum 1,25-dihydroxyvitamin D. Serum 1,25-dihydroxyvitamin D was measured by a competitive binding assay which utilized the calf thymus receptor[16]. In F344 rats, serum 1,25-dihydroxyvitamin D decreased markedly between 1 and 5 months of age, showed less of a decline between 5 and 13 months of age, and demonstrated a shallow linear decline thereafter (Figure 14.4).

To determine the degree of correlation of serum 1,25-dihydroxyvitamin D with Ca^{2+} absorption and intestinal CaBP, we plotted these parameters along with serum 1,25-dihydroxyvitamin D (Figure 14.4). To a first approximation, all the parameters show a similar decrease with age. These data suggest that the age-related decline in Ca^{2+} absorption can be explained in terms of the age-related decrease in serum 1,25-dihydroxyvitamin D. At the subcellular level, the decrease in CaBP with age could account for the decline in Ca^{2+} absorption with age. This would assume that the CaBP concentration is rate-limiting for Ca^{2+} absorption.

AGE-RELATED CHANGES IN INTESTINAL RESPONSIVENESS TO 1,25-DIHYDROXYVITAMIN D

We have begun to examine the effects of 1,25-dihydroxyvitamin D on the Ca^{2+} transport system with age. Knowledge of the action of 1,25-dihydroxyvitamin D with age may be particularly important in terms of finding

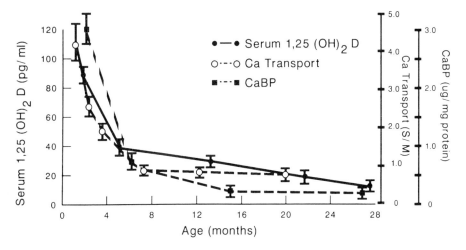

Figure 14.4 Changes in serum 1,25-dihydroxyvitamin D with age. Serum 1,25-dihydroxyvitamin D was quantitated by a competitive binding assay using the calf thymus receptor. Data points for serum 1,25(OH)$_2$D are the mean ± SEM of 6–8 rats. Ca^{2+} transport and intestinal CaBP are plotted for comparison

ways to enhance Ca^{2+} absorption in the elderly. The effect of 1,25-dihydroxyvitamin D on Ca^{2+} absorption was studied in young (3 month) and adult (12 month) rats[17]. Rats were made deficient in 1,25-dihydroxyvitamin D by feeding strontium, which blocks the renal production of 1,25-dihydroxyvitamin D. Rats were then given a single maximal dose of 1,25-dihydroxyvitamin D, and Ca^{2+} transport and intestinal CaBP levels were measured.

1,25-Dihydroxyvitamin D significantly increased Ca^{2+} absorption, as measured by everted intestinal sacs, in both young and adult rats (Table 14.2). Absorption peaked at 6 h in both age groups[17]. However, the increase was much less in the adult and never reached the maximal levels of transport seen in the young. Similar results were seen when Ca^{2+} uptake, rather than Ca^{2+} transport, was measured using everted sacs[8]. In the same experiments, the amount of intestinal CaBP in the segments was quantitated immunologically (Table 14.2). Interestingly, the induction of CaBP by 1,25-dihydroxyvitamin D was actually slightly higher in the adult at 24 h. Twenty-four hours was the time of peak CaBP content in both age groups[17].

CONCLUSION

In summary, there are age-related changes in several components of the intestinal Ca^{2+} transport system. There is a decrease in ATP-dependent Ca^{2+} pumping by the basal lateral membrane, and there is a decrease in the concentration of cytoplasmic CaBP. No age-related changes have been detected in brush-border membrane function, but studies using more sensitive techniques need to be performed.

Table 14.2 Effect of 1,25-dihydroxyvitamin D on calcium absorption and calcium binding protein (data taken from Ref. 17)

Age	Time after dose		
	(0 hours)	(6 hours)	(24 hours)
Calcium absorption (serosal/mucosal)			
Young	1.18 ± 0.04	4.38 ± 0.30	2.05 ± 0.14
Adult	0.71 ± 0.01	1.58 ± 0.14	1.12 ± 0.09
Calcium binding protein (μg)			
Young	n.d.*	20	58
Adult	n.d.*	19	67

Entries are the mean $\pm$ SEM of 4–12 individual animals (Ca^{2+} absorption) or the average determination on tissue pooled from 4–12 animals (CaBP). Young and adult rats were 2–3 and 12–14 months old respectively.
* n.d., not detected

The age-related decline in Ca^{2+} transport is explainable in terms of the decline in serum 1,25-dihydroxyvitamin D levels with age. The intestinal CaBP content parallels the decline of both Ca^{2+} transport and serum 1,25-dihydroxyvitamin D levels. This is consistent with, but does not prove, the idea that this vitamin D-dependent protein mediates the decline in Ca^{2+} absorption.

A second factor in the decline in Ca^{2+} transport may be age-related changes in responsiveness to 1,25-dihydroxyvitamin D. The adult intestine is partially refractory to the action of 1,25-dihydroxyvitamin D in terms of stimulating Ca^{2+} absorption. The defect does not appear to lie in the induction of CaBP. Rather, the defect may be in the enhancement of Ca movement across the brush border and basal lateral membranes. This is currently under investigation. Interestingly, these studies demonstrate that increasing CaBP alone is not sufficient to enhance Ca^{2+} absorption, at least in the adult.

Hopefully, these studies of changes in intestinal Ca^{2+} absorption with age will suggest new ways of enhancing Ca^{2+} absorption, improving Ca^{2+} balance, and decreasing bone loss in the elderly.

Acknowledgements

The author acknowledges the excellent technical assistance of Monica Boltz, William Doubek, and Susan Porter in carrying out these studies. This work was supported by the Veterans Administration.

References

1. Avioli, L. V., McDonald, J. E. and Lee, S. W. (1965). Influence of aging on the intestinal absorption of ^{47}Ca in women and its relation to ^{47}Ca absorption in postmenopausal osteoporosis. *J. Clin. Invest.*, **44**, 1960–7

2. Bullamore, J. R., Gallagher, J. C., Wilkinson, R. and Nordin, B. E. C. (1970). Effect of age on calcium absorption. *Lancet*, **2**, 535–7

3. Alevizaki, C. C., Ikkos, D. G. and Singhelakis, P. (1973). Progressive decrease of true intestinal calcium absorption with age in normal man. *J. Nucl. Med.*, **14**, 760–2

4. Armbrecht, H. J., Zenser, T. V., Bruns, M. E. H. and Davis, B. B. (1979). Effect of age on intestinal calcium absorption and adaptation to dietary calcium. *Am. J. Physiol.*, **236**, E769–E774

5. Armbrecht, H. J., Zenser, T. V., Gross, C. J. and Davis, B. B. (1980). Adaptation to dietary calcium and phosphorus restriction changes with age. *Am. J. Physiol.*, **239**, E322–E327

6. Armbrecht, H. J., Gross, C. J. and Zenser, T. V. (1981). Effect of dietary calcium and phosphorus restriction on calcium and phosphorus balance in young and old rats. *Arch. Biochem. Biophys.*, **210**, 179–85

7. Kalu, D. N., Hardin, R. H., Cockerham, R. and Yu, B. P. (1984). Aging and dietary modulation of rat skeleton and parathyroid hormone. *Endocrinology*, **115**, 1239–47

8. Armbrecht, H. J. (1986). Age-related changes in calcium and phosphorus uptake by rat small intestine. *Biochim. Biophys. Acta*, **882**, 281–6

9. Horst, R. L., DeLuca, H. F. and Jorgenson, N. A. (1978). The effect of age on calcium absorption and accumulation of 1,25-dihydroxyvitamin D in intestinal mucosa of rats. *Metab. Bone Dis. Rel. Res.*, **1**, 29–33

10. DeLuca, H. F. (1979). The vitamin D system in the regulation of calcium and phosphorus metabolism. *Nutr. Rev.*, **37**, 161–93

11. Kowarski, S. and Schachter, D. (1980). Intestinal membrane calcium-binding protein. *J. Biol. Chem.*, **255**, 10834–40

12. Wasserman, R. H., Taylor, A. N. and Fullmer, C. S. (1974). Vitamin D-induced calcium-binding protein and the intestinal absorption of calcium. *Biochem. Soc. Spec. Publ.*, **3**, 55–74

13. Ghijsen, W. E. J. M., De Jong, M. D. and Van Os, C. H. (1982). ATP-dependent calcium transport and its correlation with Ca-ATPase activity in basolateral plasma membranes of rat duodenum. *Biochim. Biophys. Acta*, **689**, 327–36

14. Ghijsen, W. E. J. M. and Van Os, C. H. (1982). 1,25-Dihydroxyvitamin D$_3$ regulates ATP-dependent calcium transport in basolateral plasma membranes of rat enterocytes. *Biochem. Biophys. Acta*, **689**, 170–2

15. Doubek, W. G. and Armbrecht, H. J. (1987). Changes in intestinal glucose transport over the lifespan of the rat. *Mech. Age. Dev.*, **39**, 91–102

16. Reinhardt, T. A., Horst, R. L., Orf, J. W. and Hollis, B. W. (1984). A microassay for 1,25-dihydroxyvitamin D not requiring high performance liquid chromatography: Application to clinical studies. *J. Clin. Endocr. Metab.*, **58**, 91–8

17. Armbrecht, H. J., Zenser, T. V. and Davis, B. B. (1980). Effects of vitamin D metabolites on intestinal calcium absorption and calcium binding protein in young and adult rats. *Endocrinology*, **106**, 469–75

Section 3
Liver Morphology and Physiology

15
Liver morphology with aging

H. DAVID and P. REINKE

INTRODUCTION

No substantial information on aging of the liver is provided in well-established manuals and text-books – the 'old liver' is generally characterized by 'brown atrophy' essentially caused by malnutrition and diseases resulting in cachexia. Absolute and relative weight losses have been emphasized as the most important macroscopic alterations to the liver[1]. Munroe and Young (1978)[2] found the relative weight of human liver to drop from 4% in newborn infants to 2% in aged persons; this was thought to be accompanied by numerical drop of hepatocytes and was suggested to depend, among other things, on race.

Alterations at histological level

Livers of persons aged between 69 and 91 years exhibited only minor histological changes that might be interpreted as signs of aging[3] but would not be specific of aging at all. Hence, no reliable diagnosis of liver aging can be derived from histological findings.

In the rat, age-related alterations are based on endocrine effects on metabolism and morphology of the liver. Aging rats of different strains exhibit spontaneous neoplastic and non-neoplastic lesions of the liver as well as secondary liver changes in parallel to neoplasia of haematopoietic tissue. Findings include fatty degeneration, focal degenerative alterations, eosinophilic, basophilic, and/or bright cell regions, necroses, focal chronic hepatitis and periportal inflammation (non-specific reactive hepatitis), cholangitis, bile duct proliferation, biliary cysts, sinusoid dilatation, chronic passive congestion, hepatocellular atrophy, nodular regeneration, neoplastic nodules/adenomas, carcinomas, haemangiomas/sarcomas, leukaemia, and lymphomas[4].

Age-induced cell death is believed to occur in the form of apoptosis, with damaged hepatocytes being disintegrated to fragments which are then phagocytized by surrounding macrophages, without any inflammatory change developing.

Alterations to hepatocytes

Cell volume

The life span of hepatocytes in the body is relatively long. It accounts for 190 days for the liver cell of rat. They divide only once or twice in a lifetime in the absence of growth stimuli, such as disease-induced loss of hepatocytes or hepatectomy.

Watanabe and Tanaka (1982)[5] recorded from autopsy cases cell enlargement relative to nuclear size, increase in nuclear DNA relative to nuclear size, and growing amounts of binuclear cells in the lobular periphery. Increase of average cell size in persons above 60 years of age was obviously attributable to numerical increase of cells with high ploidy[5,6].

The number of nuclei per unit volume of mouse liver was found to drop by 40% over the period 1–27 months of age, with half of that reduction taking place between 12 and 27 months[7]. Enlargement of cell volume was found to be a result. Hepatocyte volumes in male Fischer-344 rats, aged 1 to 16 months went up during that period by 65% in the centrolobular region and by 35% in the periportal region[8]. However, the volumes at 1 month of age were restored when the animals had reached an age of 30 months.

Meihuizen and Blansjaar (1980)[9] reported that in advanced age cellular and nuclear volumes increased in all three zones of the acinus of liver.

Our own studies into rat liver suggested the hepatocyte volume at birth to be $5776\,\mu m^3$. It increased to about $10\,000\,\mu m^3$ up to 2 months of age and stayed approximately at that level by 6 months, whereafter it was reduced to $7389\,\mu m^3$ by 24–27 months. The hepatocyte volume of female animals differed from that of males, in that it went up continuously to reach a limit of $17\,001\,\mu m^3$ by the end of 27 months. Grouping of liver cells showed some shift during post-natal development towards higher percentage of large cells. While at birth, only 33% of all cells were $> 5000\,\mu m^3$ and only 3.4% were $> 10\,000\,\mu m^3$, 76.7% were $\leqslant 5000\,\mu m^3$ at the age of 4 days, and the limit of $10\,000\,\mu m^3$ had been surpassed by 36.7% at the end of 6 months and by 43% after 18 months. Cell volume variations were larger in older animals due to polyploidization, with both very small and very large hepatocytes being present in higher quantity[10,11].

In relation to the average volumes of hepatocytes of female Wistar rats aged 24 and 27 months ($14\,305.2 \pm 1708.6\,\mu m^3$ or $17\,091.1 \pm 1405.5\,\mu m^3$), the population of mini-hepatocytes amounted to something between 16.7 and 48.9% of the median value, while that of mega-hepatocytes accounted for something between 140.2 and 204.8% of the median value[12] (Figure 15.1).

Increase in cell size and decline in cell count, indicated by the number of nuclei per unit area, are major characteristics of senile atrophy of the liver. Numerical decline has been attributed to an effect of extracellular inhibition factors upon cell division.

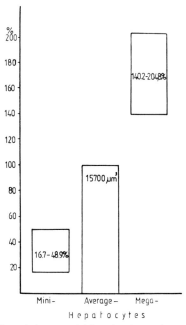

Figure 15.1 Volume relations between mini-hepatocytes and mega-hepatocytes in livers of female rats aged 24 and 27 months.

Various findings are likely to suggest that the share of body weight of a hepatocyte nucleus rises by more than 40% during life. That would mean that complex liver functions in the aged animal are much less perfectly accomplished, even under the assumption that nuclear information remained constant throughout life.

Cell nucleus

The number of large nuclei with higher DNA levels in the human liver was found to rise along with advancing age. Mean nuclear section surface is $22.5\,\mu m^2$. Amounts of large nuclei were found to rise from 1.7% in the first decade to 10.3% in the third, 14.9% in the sixth, and to 22.5% in the eighth[13].

In the rat, the volume of hepatocyte nuclei is $412.7\,\mu m^3$ at birth. It rises to $549.5\,\mu m^3$ by 6 months of age to reach $841.9\,\mu m^3$ towards the end of 12 months, whereafter it drops to $474.8\,\mu m^3$. Values were much higher in female rats in advanced age, that is $622.1\,\mu m^3$ at the end of 12 months and $851.5\,\mu m^3$ at the end of 27 months[10,11].

Nuclear volumes of small cells were usually above average $(551.5 \pm 51.3\,\mu m^3)$ in animals aged 24 months, whereas the volumes of mega-hepatocytes were below the average from 63.7 to 89.0%, which was probably attributable to the development of binuclearity and multinuclearity. In animals aged 27 months, some of the nuclear volumes of mini-hepatocytes

145

(17.7–47.2%) were below average ($851.5 \pm 67.8 \, \mu m^3$), while the volumes of the mega-hepatocyte population were clearly above average (118.7–129.3%)[12].

Two additional classes of larger nuclei were recordable, on top of the small diploid nuclei, from the human liver in the fourth decade of age and even more in the fifth and sixth decades[14]. Mononuclear diploidy was recorded from 50 to 70% of all hepatocytes in young adult rats.

The percentages of binuclear cells rose from 2% in the first 2 weeks of age to 40% in animals aged 30 months or, according to other studies, from 19% in animals aged between 3 and 4 months to 28% in animals aged 29–30 months[15,16].

Changes to proliferative kinetics represented a major factor for senile alterations to the liver[17]. The mode of proliferation was found to change from a fast to slow form in old adult and senile animals. Hepatocytes then lost their divisibility and became incorporated in the pool of the 'non-growth fraction'. The amount of indivisible liver epithelia was found to grow continuously up to advanced age. The 'non-growth fraction' amounts to 0.6% in juvenile animals and grows to 21% in adult animals and accounts for 70% of all hepatocytes in senile rats. Yet, this means that 30% of the hepatocytes remain to be proliferative even at greatest age, a percentage which may be increased again by regenerative stimuli, such as partial hepatectomy or intoxication of the liver[17].

The cells of the 'non-growth fraction' are acino-centrally located in juvenile animals. They may be also in intermediary and peripheral positions in animals aged 2–2.5 years. In old animals, the proliferative activity of regenerating hepatocytes must be higher, if the same regenerative effect is to be accomplished[17].

Variations in the karyogram of the liver are relating to functional changes in the achromatic apparatus and to severe damage to its formation and may grow manifest in many ways, including chromosomal aberration, chromosomal dispersion, formation of double nuclei, pseudo-amitosis, changes to spindle formation, tripolar and multipolar spindle configurations, and monopolar mitosis[14].

Structural changes also may grow manifest through invaginations of the nuclear membrane, build-up of inclusions, such as cytoplasm components and crystals, as well as through vacuoles and heterochromatinization.

The changes to the nucleolus are closely related to genesis and formation of DNA, RNA synthesis as well as to protein synthesis in nucleus and cytoplasm. Studies conducted into livers of humans aged between 69 and 91 years revealed a numerical rise of nucleoli from six to seven and of nucleolar vacuoles to 87% of the nucleoli[3].

In rats aged 1 day, 19% of all nucleoli were of polymorphous structure, while 80.5% were amphinucleoli and 0.5% bipartite nucleoli. The amount of polymorphous nucleoli was reduced to 0.9% after 19 days, with 97.9% being amphinucleoli and 1.2% bipartite nucleoli. The values recordable at an age of 33 months were zero percent of polymorphous nucleoli, 19.7% of amphinucleoli, and 80.3% of the bipartite form[18].

Endoplasmic reticulum, ribosomes, Golgi apparatus

Granular and agranular reticulum as well as free ribosomes and polysomes and their relationship with each other are of particular importance to hepatocyte function. The volume density of these three components is 0.090 at birth. Free ribosomes and granular endoplasmic reticulum are inversely correlated[11,19]. Total endoplasmic reticulum, according to Schmucker, *et al.* (1978)[8], was found to double in the centrolobular cells, between 1 and 10 months of age, and was found to rise to 165% in the portal cells, but after 30 months proved to drop to values similar to animals at 1 month of age. The surface of granular endoplasmic reticulum was clearly reduced in female rats aged 27 months, which could offer an explanation for reduced protein synthesis[7].

Volume density of granular endoplasmic reticulum, according to our own studies, was 0.0470 in hepatocytes of rat liver at birth and dropped to 0.0311 by the age of 3 days. It went up to 0.0545 by 6 months and, again dropped to 0.0498 by 27 months, that is, close to the value at birth[11,19].

Agranular endoplasmic reticulum in the periportal acinus zone was found to be unchanged in advanced age by Schmucker et al. (1978)[8], but in comparison to rats aged 1 month it was increased to 190% in the centrolobular acinus zone in rats aged 30 months. The need for differentiated assessment of age-related changes, depending on sex, was derived from findings according to which granular endoplasmic reticulum in male rats dropped from 0.0545 to 0.0238 (43.7%) from 6 to 18 months of age, but rose from 0.0336 to 0.0445 (132.4%) in females[11]. The higher rates of protein synthesis which were recorded from livers of rats in advanced age probably reflected the existence of a mechanism of compensation for increased protein loss. They demonstrated that livers from old rats were capable of exhibiting highly differentiated responses to protein loss and that protein metabolism did not necessarily decrease in advancing age. For man, however, reduction of protein synthesis rates has been described, in the context of advanced age[20].

The metabolism of pharmaceuticals in the liver of old male rats was considerably lowered, primarily by reduction of microsomal cytochrome P-450 level as well as of NADPH cytochrome P-450 reductase activity. The general validity of these findings, however, was limited by the impossibility of observing them in female rats and mice of either sex[20]. Inducibility of some enzymes was even significantly higher in advanced age. The impact of aging on microsomal polyfunctional oxidase systems of primates was less clearly pronounced than the impact on rodents[21].

Disorganized endoplasmic reticula with few parallel cisterns were recordable from hepatocytes of mice in advanced age. Close relationships were found to exist between mitochondria and cisterns of the endoplasmic reticulum. Fibrous material and opaque granules were recorded from glycogen areas of the endoplasmic reticulum[22]. Decomposition products, some of them in crystalline form, were found to be capable of accumulating in the cisterns of the granular endoplasmic reticulum[23].

The volume densities of ribosomal areas of rat hepatocytes were 0.0381 at birth[11,19] and were between 0.0224 and 0.0145 by the age of 12 months. The minimum value of 0.0113 was recorded at the end of 18 months and was followed by another increase. Similar values were recordable from female rats. The amount of ribosomes, relative to granular endoplasmic reticula, was 44.8%, on the day of birth. Free ribosomes reached levels between 20 and 35% from 7 days to 27 months of age, with 22.1% being recorded at the end of 27 months. Findings obtained from female animals were similar to those of males.

Reduction of free and membrane-bound ribosomes was related to protein synthesis[24,25]. There was no need for hepatocytes of rats aged 3 months to compensate for age-related lesions, such as rise of proteolytic activity or occurrence of changed malfunctional proteins; in other words, their reserve capacity was not required. However, hepatocytes of rats aged 24 months had to compensate for an increased rate of protein degradation or for a quantitative rise in functionally-altered proteins and, therefore, had to use their own reserve capacity in order to be capable of synthesizing higher amounts of albumin and protein. Volume densities of agranular endoplasmic reticulum were 0.0051 in newborn rats and went up to 0.0226 by 21 days, before they declined to something between 0.01 and 0.023. From 6 to 18 months of age (Figure 15.2) they dropped from 0.0186 to 0.0109 (58.6%) in males and from 0.0411 to 0.0370 (90%) in females in which, however, the initial values had been much higher[11]. The levels of agranular endoplasmic reticula relative to the total amount of endoplasmic reticula were 5.7% at birth, 21.4% by 21 days of age, and around 20% by 27 months.

Agranular endoplasmic reticula, according to Pieri et al. (1975)[7], dropped to 75% of the 1-month value after 12 months and to 20% of the 1-month value in animals aged 27 months. However, according to Meihuizen and Blansjaar (1980)[9], levels of agranular endoplasmic reticula rise with age. The reduced surface of agranular endoplasmic reticula might provide an answer to the question why liver capacity for metabolism of drugs is reduced in advanced age.

Volume density of the Golgi apparatus in rat hepatocytes was 0.017 at birth. It dropped to 0.015 by 1 month of age, and values between 0.008 and 0.012 were recorded up to 12 months. The volume was 0.005 at the end of the 27 months. The absolute volume of the Golgi apparatus was 80.1 μm^3 at birth and 31.3 μm^3 at the end of 27 months. Values of female animals in advanced age were much higher, with volumes between 92 μm^3 and 139.2 μm^3 being recorded[11,19]. However, no substantial changes in surface density of Golgi membranes or in relative volume of Golgi areas were recorded as functions of age by Schmucker et al. (1978)[8]. In old hepatocytes, the Golgi apparatus can exhibit degeneration or reduction of components, but there can be multiple occurrence as well.

Mitochondria

Volume density of mitochondria in old rats was found to be 10.48% below that in juvenile animals[26]. Per-cell mitochondrial volumes recorded from female rats by Pieri et al. (1975)[7] were 1.036 μm^3 at 1 month of age, 868 μm^3 after 12 months, and 1.236 μm^3 after 27 months. Decline in mitochondrial

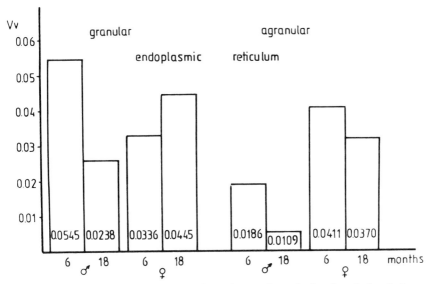

Figure 15.2 Volume densities (V_v) of granular and agranular endoplasmic reticulum in hepatocytes of male and female rats aged 6 and 18 months.

volume density in advancing age was recorded also by Tate and Herbener (1976)[27] and by Herbener (1976)[57]. Volume density dropped concomitant with advancing age; it amounted to 0.283 in animals aged 8 months, 0.257 at 30 months, and 0.181 in animals between 43 and 44 months of age.

From rat liver, we recorded mitochondrial volume densities of 0.165 at birth and 0.236 at the age of 14 days (Figure 15.3). It was subsequently continuously reduced to 0.138 at the end of 12 months. A moderate rise was followed by the lowest recorded value of 0.128 at the end of 27 months[11,29–31]. The absolute mitochondrial volume per cell was 782.8 μm^3 at birth and reached a level of 1418.8 μm^3 towards the end of 6 months of age. It then went down to 1056.1 μm^3 by the end of 12 months and further to 802.9 μm^3 by the end of 27 months (following a rise at 18 months). So, the value at birth was actually restored. In female animals, on the other hand, absolute mitochondrial volume increased to 2464.4 μm^3. Absolute mitochondrial volumes were, generally, lower in mini-hepatocytes of rats in advancing age, that is between 19.2 and 55.3% of the average value in rats aged 24 and 27 months. Yet mitochondrial volumes in mega-hepatocytes were between 131.5 and 178.4% above the mean value[12].

The number of mitochondria in the liver of humans aged over 70 years, according to Sato and Tauchi (1975)[32], was below that recorded from persons under 50 years, while size and overall percentage were increased.

The absolute number of mitochondria to one hepatocyte in male rats was 204 at birth[11,29]. It went up to 708 by the end of 1 month and further to 1441 by the end of 2 months, and to 2199 by the end of 6 months, representing a rise of 1078% from birth. It began to decline from 12 months and was found to remain at 1516 by the end of 27 months.

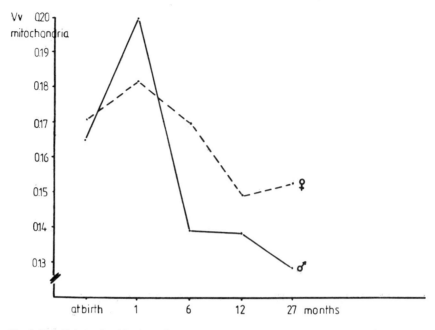

Figure 15.3 Volume densities (V_v) of mitochondria in hepatocytes of male and female rats aged from birth to 27 months.

Mitochondrial areas were $0.81\,\mu m^2$ in female rats aged 6 months and $1.03\,\mu m^2$ in females aged 26 months. Giant mitochondria with areas above $2.5\,\mu m^2$ accounted for 0.17% in juvenile animals and for 5.82% in old animals. Number and length of cristae were reduced in some mitochondria of senile rats, with some of them being shifted to peripheral positions[33]. Smaller mitochondria in livers of senile rats were described by Tauchi (1961)[34].

Mitochondrial sizes were not substantially different in, and between, mice aged 70 days as well as 1 and 2 years[35].

The volume of the average mitochondrion was $3.83\,\mu m^3$ at birth and dropped continuously in the course of development to levels of $1.68\,\mu m^3$ at the age of 7 days and to $0.64\,\mu m^3$ by the end of 6 months, which actually reduced the value to 16.7% of the volume at birth (Figure 15.4). The volume measured at the end of 27 months[11,29] was as small as $0.53\,\mu m^3$.

Reduced mitochondrial numbers were established by Sato and Tauchi (1975)[32] from livers of humans older than 60 years of age. The number of cristae per mitochondrion went up to compensate for this, and so did the size of organelles up to formation of mega-mitochondria. This process possibly corresponded to polyploidization of the cell nucleus.

In mice aged 30 months, mitochondria were enlarged and rounded. The matrix was vacuolized. Cristae were short, and high-density granules were lost[36].

Age-related alterations to mitochondria were found to depend more

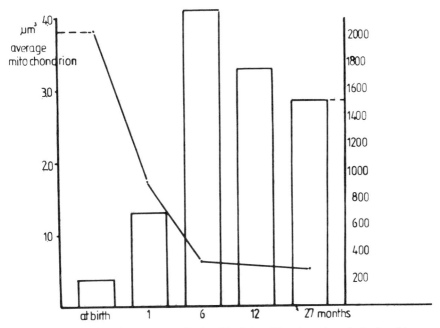

Figure 15.4 Volume (μm^3) of average mitochondria (left scale) and number of mitochondria per hepatocyte (right scale) of rats from birth to 27 months.

strongly on age and function of the individual cells than on age of the whole organ[37].

When examining mitochondrial aging, it should be borne in mind that the turnover rate of mitochondrial molecules is usually between 9 and 11 days. A half-life of 10.3 days was calculated from turnover of proteins, lipids, and cytochrome C, whereas 9.6 days was derived from other findings. So, the conclusion may be drawn that all hepatocytes do possess mitochondrial populations of different ages up to their own death.

Qualitative alterations to mitochondria growth are manifested through more bizarre forms, reduction of cristae, and shifting of cristae to peripheral locations. There has been frequent occurrence of inflated forms, accumulation of substance, paracrystalline inclusions, vacuoles and mega-mitochondria.

Protein levels were reduced in mitochondria of old rats, but protease activities were clearly increased. Impaired performance and higher fragility of mitochondria in old rats were, possibly, attributable to higher mitochondrial neutral protease activity[38].

The matrix protein loss recorded from mitochondria isolated from rats aged 28 months and placed in hypo-osmotic media was higher than loss recorded from animals aged between 7 and 14 months. This seemed to suggest alterations to permeability of the mitochondrial outer membrane[39].

Mitochondrial water levels were found to be considerably reduced with aging[40], which was accompanied by an approximately 100% rise of ion concentration. Water levels thus reduced to about 35% came close to those of bones (20–30%). Hence, limitation to diffusion of substrates to enzyme sites may be expected as a consequence. Such changes would result in reduced energy capacity, and this would offer an explanation for the age-related cellular alterations, such as lipofuscin accumulation due to incomplete decomposition of cross-linked membrane components.

Peroxisomes

The volume density of peroxisomes of rat liver amounted to 0.021 at birth and reached its maximum of 0.027 by 4 months. This was followed by decline to 0.014 up to 12 months and by strong reduction of minimum values at 18 months and later (0.004–0.006).

The absolute volume of peroxisomes to one hepatocyte was $98.9\,\mu m^3$ at birth. It remained continuously above $200\,\mu m^3$ up to 6 months and declined to $127.1\,\mu m^3$ by 12 months and to $36.3\,\mu m^3$ at 24 months. A similar decline was recorded from female animals, with $47.7\,\mu m^3$ at 24 months[11,31,41].

One hepatocyte was found to contain 130.4 peroxisomes at the time of birth. An increase to 868.5 at the end of 6 months was followed by a decrease to 181 by 24 months and a slight increase again to 247.8 by the end of 27 months. The number of peroxisomes was higher in female animals in advanced age.

The volume of one peroxisome dropped from $0.76\,\mu m^3$ at birth to $0.19\,\mu m^3$ at 27 months. In female animals in advanced age, peroxisomes were still smaller, dimensions being $0.13–0.14\,\mu m^3$.

Lysosomes

Higher numbers of enlarged lysosomes with different inclusions were recordable from liver cells of old rats[37]. The cathepsin-D activity was increased, whereas the arylsulphatase-B activity was hardly changed at all[42]. Lysosome volume density grew by 45.5% from juvenile to adult age[26]. The amount of lysosomes was increased particularly in the centrolobular region[9].

Lysosome volume densities in rat liver were 0.0054 at birth, 0.022 at the end of 12 months, and reached a maximum of 0.029 by the end of 27 months, that is five times as high as at birth[11,19,31,43]. This result was in agreement with findings according to which lysosome-related deposits, such as lipofuscin, were found to increase throughout one life span.

Total lysosome volume went up from $25.6\,\mu m^3$ at birth to $94.0\,\mu m^3$ by the end of 27 months. Much higher values were recorded from female animals in advanced age. The number of lysosomes to one cell increased from 31.4 at birth to 198.3 by the end of 27 months. While primary lysosomes were numerically predominant at birth, the number of secondary lysosomes was found to go up in the course of life and accounted for 68.7% by the end of 27 months and was thus substantially higher than the number of primary lysosomes (Figure 15.5).

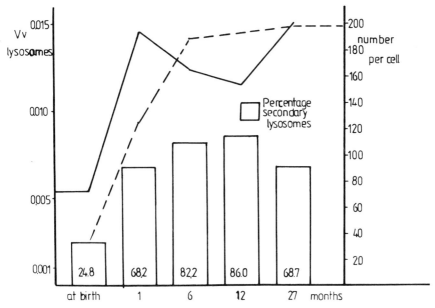

Figure 15.5 Volume densities (V_v) of lysosomes (left scale), number of lysosomes per hepatocyte (right scale), and percentage of secondary lysosomes in hepatocytes of rats from birth to 27 months.

Glycogen, lipids, ground plasma

The glycogen level of hepatocytes in rats exhibited a volume density of 0.0125 at birth. Values between 0.08 and 0.12 were observed at 21 days and were 0.102 at 27 months. Absolute glycogen levels were 589 μm³ at birth, 1293.8 μm³ by 18 months, and were lowered to 640.3 μm³ by 27 months. The maximum for female animals was 1565 μm³ at the end of 24 months, which was followed by decline to 750.3 μm³ by the 27 months[11,44].

Investigations conducted by Onishi *et al.* (1972)[45] on rats aged 70, 250, and 500 days showed total lipid, triglyceride and cholesterol levels to increase during the above periods and phospholipids to remain constant. Our own investigations gave lipid volume densities of 0.007 at birth, 0.116 up to 4 days, and a maximum of 0.179 after 14 days. That was followed by a decline to values between 0.001 and 0.014 during subsequent months. A value of 0.034 was reached after 12 months, and the lipid level of hepatocytes at the end of 27 months was 0.008 (Figure 15.6). Lipid levels in female animals increased with age (Figure 15.7) and were almost eight times as high as at birth, when they had reached a limit of 0.06 by the end of 27 months[11,44].

Absolute levels of unstructured ground plasma in rat hepatocytes went up from 3167 μm³ at birth to 4054 μm³ by 27 months of age, though volume densities did not differ significantly (0.682 at birth and 0.647 at 27 months)[11]. The number of microfilaments and microtubules in ground plasma is thought to rise. Ferritin and haemosiderin deposits were more frequently recordable.

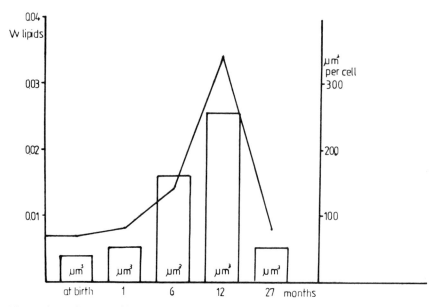

Figure 15.6 Volume densities (V_v) of lipids (left scale) and total volume per hepatocyte (μm^3) of male rats from birth to 27 months.

Plasma membrane

The three different domains of the plasma membrane in the liver cell (sinusoidal, lateral, close to bile canaliculi)[11,46] are characterized, during differentiation and development, not only by differentiated enzyme formation but also by quantitative changes. The sinusoidal surface, absorbing and discharging substances to the blood stream, is crucially affected in this context. The surface area is expanded by factors between 1.8 and 3.7 due to the formation of microvilli. The numbers of microvilli were 1323 at birth and 5471 at 27 months (Figure 15.8). This would, at the same time, enlarge the sinusoidal surface from $688.7\,\mu m^2$ to $1225.9\,\mu m^2$ and that of the entire hepatocyte from $1900\,\mu m^2$ to $2783\,\mu m^2$. The bile canaliculi were also affected by the changes, though to a lesser extent, including formation of microvilli. Values recorded from bile canaliculi were 249 microvilli and a surface of $120.5\,\mu m^2$ at birth and 792 microvilli and a surface of $164.1\,\mu m^2$ at the end of 27 months[10,11,47,48].

Alterations to the composition of the hepatocyte plasma membrane might offer explanations for changes in functional processes, for example, decelerated uptake and discharge of ouabain by isolated hepatocytes[20]. However, no change has so far been recorded in investigations from various membrane-bound enzymes and receptors, when tested for developments along with rising age.

The amount of ^{125}I-labelled dimeric IgA secreted by young adult Fischer-344 rats (aged 3–4 months) was six times higher than that secreted by animals

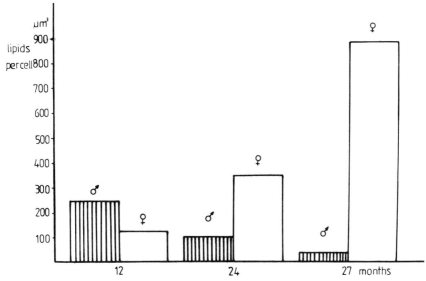

Figure 15.7 Total volume (μm^3) of lipids per hepatocyte in livers of male and female rats aged 12 and 24 months.

aged 12 or 24 months[49]. Total bile acid secretion dropped by between 35 and 40% during the above period, though the number of hepatocytes to one gram of liver was more or less unchanged (130 ± 15 or $146 \pm 20 \times 10^6$) as was the hepatocyte volume (6800 μm^3 or 6500 μm^3). The decline in IgA secretion was probably caused to a large extent by reduction of intracellular translocation processes.

Perisinusoidal functional unit

Data are very scanty on the 'perisinusoidal functional unit' in relation to aging (endothelial, Kupffer, Ito, and pit cells, Disse space, sinusoidal hepatocyte pole)[46,50,51]. Systematic studies are lacking almost entirely. The extrahepatocytic space in rat liver was found to grow from 11.8% in the first months to 16.2% by 6 months and 20.3% by 27 months[7]. The percentage amount of that space, according to Schmucker et al. (1978)[8], did not undergo any significant change between 1 and 30 months, neither in the centrolobular nor in the peripheral acinus region.

Metabolism and quantity of connective tissue components in the liver were considered by Lindner et al. (1977)[52] as being of substantial importance to liver aging. Increase in collagen fibrils, in that context, was primarily attributed to reduced catabolism.

Extremely little information has so far become available on non-hepatocytes in advanced age. The endocytosis function of Kupffer cells is said to be restricted, for example, for heat-denatured and colloidal albumin

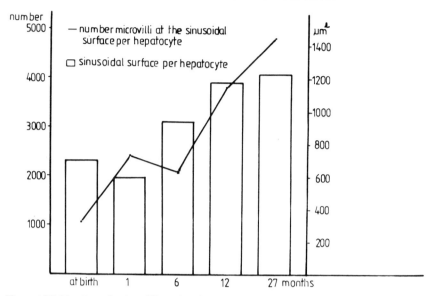

Figure 15.8 Number of microvilli at the sinusoidal surface per hepatocyte (left scale) and sinusoidal surface area (μm^2) (right scale) of rats from birth to 27 months.

and for erythrocyte membranes[53]. Endothelial cells, on the other hand, are believed to retain their capability of ingesting colloidal albumin[54]. The endo-cytosis activity of Kupffer cells in rats aged 30 and 36 months was clearly lower than that recordable from animals aged 3 months[55]. Kupffer cells more strongly bulged into the Disse space, which might explain the reduced clearance[56]. The clearance capacity of the reticulo-endothelial system in man was found to decline to about 15% from 30 to 80 years of age. The hepatic clearance differences for drugs are possibly attributable to decreased intrahepatic blood circulation in advancing age[20].

CONCLUSION

Assessment of age-related alterations to the liver has proved to be quite difficult on account of general and liver-specific problems in the context of ageing. Here are some of the questions to which so far no, or only partial, answers have been found:

(a) Relationships between ages of various species of experimental animals, on the one hand, and those of man, on the other, are still hypothetical, which limits applicability of experimental results.
(b) The definition of 'old' and linkage of this term to age still is disputed among various authors.
(c) Life expectancies may differ considerably within one and the same animal species and between different human races.

(d) Animal species and man differ considerably from each other for numerous parameters of metabolism and liver structure.

(e) Recent investigations have confirmed differences between sexes to which little attention had been given in the past.

(f) Individuals differ from each other by pathographies,with polymorbidity being more frequently recorded from older age groups.

(g) Hepatocytes of different age groups may be present in one and the same liver, and so may organelle populations of different ages in one hepatocyte.

(h) A particular role may be played by quantitative and qualitative changes to structure and function of non-hepatocytes and by the 'perisinusoidal functional unit' at large.

Today, 'liver morphology with ageing' at macroscopic, microscopic, ultrastructural, and molecular levels can be defined only as a combination of findings which are most common in advanced age. They are by no means specific in genesis and may be observed in isolation or in combination under varying pathological conditions. Neither the morphological nor functional alterations are substantially irreversible. Hence, various views and postulations will have to be reconsidered, including rigid specification of age limits for donor livers for transplantation.

The liver appears to offer particularly strong resistance to age-related alterations[54], which seems to be primarily attributable to the following three factors:

1. Blood supply is far beyond demand and arteriosclerosis hardly exists.
2. Proliferative–regenerative processes can be induced up to advanced age.
3. The functional reserve capacity is high.

References

1. Mooney, H., Roberts, R., Cooksley, W. G. E., Halliday, J. W. and Powell, L. W. (1985). Alterations in the liver with ageing. *Clin. Gastroenterol.,* **14,** 757–71
2. Munroe, H. N. and Young, V. R. (1978). Protein metabolism in the elderly. *Postgrad. Med.,* **63,** 143–8
3. Findor, J., Perez, V., Bruch Igartua, E., Giovanetti, M. and Fiaravantti, N. (1973). Structure and ultrastructure of the liver in aged persons. *Acta Hepato-gastroenterol.,* **20,** 200–4
4. Zurcher, C. I., Van Zwieten, M. J., Solleveld, H. A., Van Bezooijen, C. F. A. and Hollander, C. F. (1982). Possible multiple pathological changes in aging rats on studies of influence of organ aging, with emphasis on the liver. In *Liver and Aging* pp. 19–36. Kitani, K. (ed.) (Amsterdam: Elsevier Biomedical Press)
5. Watanabe, T. and Tanaka, Y. (1982). Age-related alterations in the size of human hepatocytes. A study of mononuclear and binucleate cells. *Virchows Arch. (B), Cell Pathol.,* **39,** 9–20
6. Sato, T., Cespedes, R. F., Goyenaga, P. H. and Tauchi, H. (1979). Age changes in the livers of Costa Ricans. *Mech. Age Dev.,* **11,** 171–8
7. Pieri, C., Nagy, I. Zs., Mazzufferi, G. and Guili, C. (1975). The aging of rat liver as revealed by electron microscopic morphometry. I. Basic parameters. *Exp. Gerontol.,* **10,** 291–304
8. Schmucker, D. L., Mooney, J. S. and Jones, A. L. (1978). Stereological analysis of hepatic fine structure in the Fischer 344 rat; influence of sublobular location and animal age. *J. Cell Biol.,* **78,** 319–37

9. Meihuizen, S. P. and Blansjaar, N. (1980). Stereological analysis of liver parenchymal cells from young and old rats. *Mech. Age. Dev.*, **13**, 111–18

10. David, H. (1979). Veränderungen des Volumens und des Oberfläche von Leberzellen männlicher Ratten während der postnatalen Entwicklung. *Acta Biol. Med. Germ.*, **38**, 935–52

11. David, H. (1985). The hepatocyte. Development, differentiation, and ageing. *Exp. Pathol.*, (Suppl. 11), 1–148

12. David, H. (1983). Populations of megahepatocytes and minihepatocytes and their components in liver of old rats. *Exp. Pathol.*, **24**, 77–82

13. Barz, H., Kunze, K. D., Voss, K and Simon, H. (1977). Image processing in pathology. IV. Age dependent changes of morphometric features of liver cell nuclei in biopsies. *Exp. Pathol.*, **14**, 55–64

14. Klinge, O. (1973). Kernveränderungen und Kernteilungsstörungen der Altersleber. *Gerontologia*, **19**, 314–29

15. Van Zwieten, M. J. and Hollander, C. F. (1985). Polyploidy, liver rat. In Jones, T. C., Mohr, U. and Hunt, R. D. (eds.) *Digestive System*. pp. 83–6. (Berlin: Springer-Verlag)

16. Van Zwieten, M. J. and Hollander, C. F. (1985). Intranuclear and intracytoplasmic inclusions, liver, rat. In Jones, T. C., Mohr, U. and Hunt, R. D. (eds.) *Digestive System*. pp. 86–92. (Berlin: Springer-Verlag)

17. Stöcker, E. (1975). Altersabhängige Proliferationskinetik in parenchymatosen Organen von Ratten. *Verh. Dtsch. Ges. Pathol.*, **59**, 78–94

18. Adamstone, F. B. and Taylor, A. B. (1979). Nucleolar reorganization in liver cells of the aging rat. *J. Morphol.*, **61**, 221–2

19. David, H. (1980). Quantitative changes of the endoplasmic reticulum, ribosomes and GERL in the hepatocytes during postnatal development of male rats. *Pathol. Res. Pract.*, **166**, 381–99

20. Kitani, K. (1986). Does the liver age in man? *Hepatology* (Falk), **18/19**, IX–XIX

21. Schmucker, D. L. and Wang, R. K. (1980). Age-related changes in liver drug metabolism: structure vs function. *Proc. Soc. exper. Biol. Med.*, **165**, 178–87

22. Essner, E. (1967). Endoplasmic reticulum and the origin of microbodies in fetal mouse liver. *Lab. Invest.*, **17**, 71–87

23. Basler, J. W. and Agris, P. P. (1976). Accumulation of a semi-crystalline substance in aging human fibroblast cultures. *J. Cell Biol.*, **70**, 314a

24. Van Bezooijen, C. F. A. and Knock, D. L. (1977). Aging changes in bromsulfophthalein uptake, albumin and total protein synthesis in isolated hepatocytes. In Platt, D. (ed.) *Liver and Ageing*. pp. 227–35. (Stuttgart, New York: Schattauer Verlag)

25. Van Bezooijen, C. F. A. (1978). Cellular basis of liver aging studied with isolated hepatocytes. p. 149. (Delft: W. D. Meina, B.V.)

26. Fleischer, M., Meiss, R., Robenek, W. and Themann, H. (1979). Die altersabhängige Wirkung polychlorierter Biphenyle auf die Rattenleber. Eine feinstrukturell-morphometrische Untersuchung. *Int. Arch. Occup. Environ. Health*, **44**, 25–43

27. Tate, E. L. and Herbener, G. H. (1976). A morphometric study of the density of mitochondrial cristae in heart and liver of aging mice. *J. Gerontol.*, **31**, 129–33

28. Henke-Lubarsch (ed.) (1930). *Leber. Handbuch der speziellen pathologischen Anatomie und Histologie*. Vol. 5, Part 1. (Berlin: Springer-Verlag)

29. David, H. (1979). Quantitative and qualitative changes of the mitochondria in hepatocytes during postnatal development of male rats. *Exp. Pathol.*, **17**, 359–73

30. David, H. (1981). Zum Verhalten von Zellorganellen im Entwicklungs- und Alternsprozess von Herz und Leber. *Gegenbaurs Morphol. Jahrbuch*, **127**, 564–73

31. David, H. (1983). Quantitative characterisation of ageing hepatocytes. *Acta Stereol.*, **2**, 408–12

32. Sato, T. and Tauchi, H. (1975). The formation of enlarged and giant mitochondria in the aging process of human hepatic cells. *Acta Pathol. Jap.*, **25**, 403–12

33. Shamoto, M. (1968). Age differences in the ultrastructure of hepatic cells of thyroxine-treated rats. *J. Gerontol.*, **23**, 1–8

34. Tauchi, H. (1961). On the fundamental morphology of the senile changes. *Nagoya J. Med. Sci.*, **24**, 97–132

35. Tauchi, H., Sato, T. and Kobayashi, W. (1984). Effect of age on ultrastructural changes of cortisone treated mouse hepatic cells. *Mech. Age. Dev.*, **3**, 279–90

36. Wilson, P. D. and Franks, L. M. (1975). The effect of age on mitochondrial ultrastructure. *Gerontologia*, **21**, 81–94
37. Tauchi, H. and Sato, T. (1968). Age changes in size and number of mitochondria of human hepatic cells. *J. Gerontol.*, **23**, 454–61
38. Forbeck, M. L. and Martin, A. P. (1976). Mitochondrial membrane-associated functions in aging. *J. Cell Biol.*, **70**, 2(2), 36a
39. Spencer, J. A. and Horton, A. A. (1978). An age-dependent release of matrix proteins from rat liver mitochondria. *Exp. Gerontol.*, **13**, 227–32
40. Zglinicki, Th. (1986). Die Bedeutung der Röntgenmikroanalyse für die experimentelle Medizin und Diagnostik. Dissertation B. Math., Nat. Fak., Humboldt University
41. David, H. (1980). Morphometric analysis of peroxisomes in the liver cells of male rats during postnatal development. *Exp. Pathol.*, **18**, 321–8
42. Knook, D. L. (1977). Lysosomes in the aging process of the rat liver. *Fifth European Symposium on Basic Research in Gerontology*. pp. 595–8
43. David, H. (1982). Morphometrical findings in the liver cell during its postnatal development and connection with quantitative findings in the heart. In Collan, Y. and Romppanen, T. (eds.) *Morphometry in Morphological Diagnosis*. pp. 115–22. (Kuopio: Kuopio University Press)
44. David, H. and Uerlings, I. (1979). Quantitative ultrastrukturelle Befunde über das Verhalten von Lipiden und Glykogen in der Rattenleber während der postnatalen Entwicklung. *Zbl. Allg. Pathol. Pathol. Anat.*, **123**, 85–103
45. Onishi, H., Tsukada, S., Hayashi, Y., Ogawa, N., Yagima, G., Masugi, Y., Aihara, K. and Suzuki, K. (1972). Effects of cytochrome C on liver functions of old rats. *Nature (New Biol.)*, **239**, 84–6
46. David, H. and Reinke, P. (1987). The 'perisinusoidal functional unit' of the liver – importance to pathological processes. *Exp. Pathol.*, **32**, 193–224
47. David, H. (1980). Methodische Probleme und Ergebnisse der Volumen- und Oberflächenbestimmung von Leberzellen von Ratten während der postnatalen Entwicklung. *Gegenbaurs Morphol. Jahrbuch*, **126**, 285–92
48. David, H. (1982). Methodische Probleme der Berechnung der Mikrovilli von Leberzellen. *Acta Histochemica* (Suppl. XXVI), 357–60
49. Schmucker, D. L., Gilbert, R., Jones, A. L., Hradek, G. T. H. and Bazin, H. (1985). Effect of aging on the hepatobiliary transport of dimeric immunoglobulin A in the male Fischer rat. *Gastroenterology*, **88**, 436–43
50. David, H. and Reinke, P. (1988). Die Heterogenität der Leber und das Konzept der 'Perisinusoidal Funktionseinheit'. Abhandl. Akad. Wiss. DDR, Klasse Med. (In press)
51. Reinke, P. and David, H. (1987). Struktur und Funktion der Sinusoidwand der Leber ('Die Perisinusoidale Funktionseinheit'). *Z. Mikr. Anat. Forsch.*, **101**, 91–136
52. Lindner, J., Grasedycck, K., Bittmann, S., Mongold, I., Schutte, B. and Ueberberg, H. (1977). Some morphological and biochemical results on liver ageing, especially regarding connective tissue. In Platt, D. (ed.) *Liver and Ageing*. pp. 23–38. (Stuttgart, New York: Schattauer Verlag)
53. Knook, D. L., Praaning van Dalen, D. P. and Brouwer, A. (1982). The clearance function of Kupffer and endothelial liver cells in relation to drugs and aging. In K. Kitani, (ed.) *Liver and Aging*. pp. 269–81. (Amsterdam: Elsevier Biomedical Press)
54. Popper, H. (1986). Aging and the liver. In Popper H. and Schaffner, F. (eds.) *Progress in Liver Disease*. Vol. 8, pp. 659–83. (Orlando: Grune & Stratton)
55. Brouwer, A. and Knook, D. L. (1983). The reticuloendothelial system and aging. *Mech. Age. Dev.*, **21**, 205–28
56. Dubuisson, L., Bedin, C. and Balaband, C. (1986). Cell to cell interactions in rat liver sinusoidal cells: age related ultrastructural changes. *Falk Symp.*, **43**, 161
57. Herbener, G. H. (1976). A morphometric study of age dependent changes in mitochondrial populations of mouse liver and heart. *J. Gerontol.*, **31**, 8–12

16
Influence of age on biliary lipid metabolism in man

B. ANGELIN and K. EINARSSON

Cholesterol gallstones occur frequently in the Western world. An increased prevalence of gallstone disease with increasing age is a well-established clinical observation[1], as is the preponderance of females (Figure 16.1). However, the mechanisms behind these clinical relationships have not been characterized until recently. In this presentation, we want to summarize data from our studies describing risk factors for cholesterol gallstone development, and discuss some possible mechanisms for gallstone development with advancing age.

When considering risk factors for cholesterol gallstone disease, it is pertinent to first briefly recapitulate some aspects of the normal biliary lipid metabolism (for review, see ref. 2). The major lipid fractions in human bile are bile acids, phospholipids, and cholesterol, their relative molar percentages being 70–75%, 20–25% and 4–8%, respectively. In addition, bile contains proteins and bile pigments, among other substances. The secreted hepatic bile is concentrated 3- to 5-fold in the gallbladder. In human bile, the quantitatively most important bile acids are cholic acid (30–40%), chenodeoxycholic acid (30–40%) and deoxycholic acid (20–30%). Together with small amounts of ursodeoxycholic and lithocholic acid, these bile acids are excreted in the bile conjugated with glycine or taurine. They are very efficiently (95–98%) reabsorbed from the intestine, mainly by an active process in the distal ileum. Reabsorbed bile acids are transported in the portal vein and efficiently extracted by the liver. The formation of bile acids in the liver is assumed to be regulated homeostatically by the inflow of bile acids via the portal vein. The rate-determining enzyme has been demonstrated to be cholesterol 7α-hydroxylase, which catalyzes the first reaction in the degradation of cholesterol to bile acids. Under steady-state conditions, the synthesis rate of bile acids (equalling the faecal excretion) is 0.5 to 1.5 mmol (200–600 mg)/day. Normally, the formation of cholic acid is 1.5 to 2 times that of chenodeoxycholic acid. Owing to the efficient enterohepatic circulation, the bile pool circulates 5 to 10 times/day.

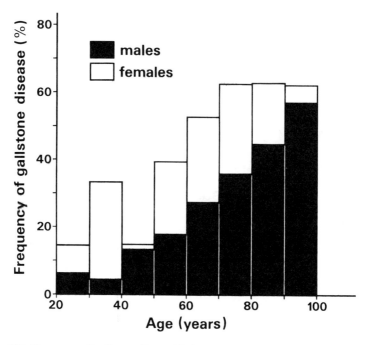

Figure 16.1 Frequency of gallstone disease (cholecystectomy or cholelithiasis) in various age groups. Data from a Swedish autopsy study[1]

Lecithin is the main phospholipid in human bile, generally containing a saturated fatty acid at position 1 and an unsaturated fatty acid at position 2. The secretion and probably the synthesis of biliary lecithin is stimulated by the flux of bile acids through the liver, although the mechanisms are not known.

Biliary cholesterol is secreted in non-esterified form from the liver (Figure 16.2)[3]. This cholesterol may be derived from both extrahepatic (diet and lipoproteins) and intrahepatic (synthesis and stored, esterified cholesterol) sources. The daily intake of cholesterol is generally about 0.5 to 1.5 mmol (200–600 mg), and between 30 and 60% of this cholesterol is absorbed, together with a similar proportion of the cholesterol secreted in the bile. In chylomicrons, absorbed cholesterol reaches the plasma via the lymphatic duct, and in the form of partially degraded chylomicron remnants this cholesterol is taken up by the liver by receptor-mediated endocytosis. The body synthesis of cholesterol is quantitatively more important than the amount derived from the diet, about half of cholesterol production assumed to occur in the liver. By an intricate regulation of the activity of the rate-determining enzyme (3-hydroxy-3-methylglutaryl coenzyme A reductase), the hepatic cholesterol synthesis is regulated by the inflow of cholesterol and possibly also by the inflow of bile acids to the liver. About 30–50% of the daily cholesterol turnover (synthesis + absorption) is catabolized to bile acids in humans. Compared to several other species, this low fractional conversion

INTESTINE

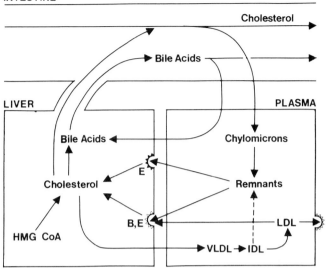

Figure 16.2 Cholesterol metabolism in man. Reprinted from Angelin[3] with permission

in man increases the amount of cholesterol available for biliary secretion and may explain the high cholesterol content of human bile relative to other species.

Cholesterol is completely insoluble in aqueous media, and has to be solubilized in bile, either in the form of mixed micelles with bile acids and lecithin, or in the form of vesicles containing cholesterol and lecithin. The solubility of cholesterol is determined by the relative composition of gallbladder bile, by the total lipid concentration, and by the pattern of individual bile acids. Carey and Small have defined limits of cholesterol solubility using artificial model bile systems and predicted that when the amount of cholesterol is in excess of what can theoretically be kept in solution, bile becomes supersaturated with cholesterol[4]. The degree of supersaturation is generally expressed as a percentage of the cholesterol-holding capacity. Two types of supersaturated solution have been defined: in metastable solutions, bile is mildly supersaturated and cholesterol can be kept in solutions several hours before precipitation occurs, whereas in labile bile, cholesterol precipitates rapidly.

According to current view, the presence of mixed micelles is probably the most important mechanism for holding cholesterol in solution in gallbladder bile. The relative concentrations of the respective lipids is determined to a major degree by the hepatic secretion rates of the three biliary lipids. The hepatic secretion of bile acids is dependent on the enterohepatic circulation. One factor of importance here is the pool size of bile acids, which is related to the balance between input and output and to the recycling frequency of the bile acid pool. The cycling frequency is in turn dependent on the storage capacity and the contraction of the gallbladder, on the intestinal transit time and on the intestinal and hepatic uptake of bile acids. As mentioned above, the hepatic secretion of lecithin is tightly linked to that of bile acids. The secretion of cholesterol into bile is also related to bile acid secretion, but not at all as closely. Theoretically, several possibilities exist which may result in the secretion of supersaturated bile: a reduction of bile acid secretion and a small bile acid pool, a reduction of lecithin secretion, and an increase of cholesterol secretion or combination of these situations.

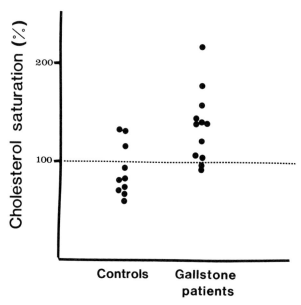

Figure 16.3 Cholesterol saturation of gallbladder bile in gallstone-free subjects and patients with cholesterol gallstones[6]. Reprinted from Einarsson and Angelin[2] with permission

Finally, it should be very clearly stressed that although supersaturation of bile is an obligatory metabolic condition for the development of cholesterol gallstones, also other factors are required for the actual crystallization process to occur[5]. Thus, although bile is almost invariably supersaturated in patients with cholesterol gallstones, such bile is also present in a considerable proportion of individuals without gallstone disease (Figure 16.3). However, the presence of saturated bile in populations has been shown to be linked to an increased risk for subsequent development of cholesterol gallstone disease. Thus, clinical situations such as obesity, hypertriglyceridaemia, oestrogen therapy, and clofibrate treatment are associated with an increased prevalence of supersaturated bile. In all these situations, the major factor responsible for the increased cholesterol saturation appears to be an absolute increase in the secretion rate of cholesterol from the liver[2].

In order to characterize the possible effect of age on biliary lipid composition, we determined the biliary lipid composition in a large series of gallstone-free, healthy Scandinavians of varying age[7]. As seen in Figure 16.4,

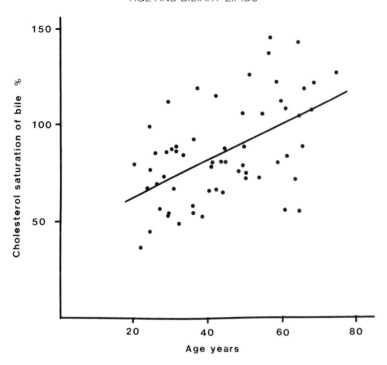

Figure 16.4 Relation between age and cholesterol saturation of bile. All subjects (29 females and 31 males) were gallstone-free, normolipidaemic and less than 120% ideal body weight. Reprinted from Einarsson *et al.*[7] with permission

almost 30% of these healthy subjects had supersaturated bile. There were no differences between the sexes with regard to biliary lipid or bile acid composition, or to cholesterol saturation. However, there was a clear increase in cholesterol saturation of bile with increasing age for both sexes. This may well explain the increased prevalence of gallstone disease known to occur with age. Thus, in a given population a progressive increase in saturation would result in an increased number of individuals exposed to the risk of cholesterol crystal precipitation. It is very clear that other factors, such as nucleating agents, or lack of anti-nucleating substances, are essential in determining whether or not an individual actually will develop gallstone disease, however (cf. ref. 5).

To investigate the possible mechanisms for this relation between age and biliary cholesterol saturation, we performed studies on the rates of secretion of biliary lipids in a subset of the patients (Figure 16.5). It was evident that cholesterol secretion increased progressively with increasing age in both sexes, whereas there was no relationship to age of bile acid or phospholipid secretion[7]. Furthermore, the degree of saturation of bile was positively correlated with the secretion rate of cholesterol in these individuals[7]. In agreement with these findings, we have recently found that in patients with overt gallstone disease, the secretion rate of cholesterol is enhanced compared to

cholesterol secretion
μmol/h

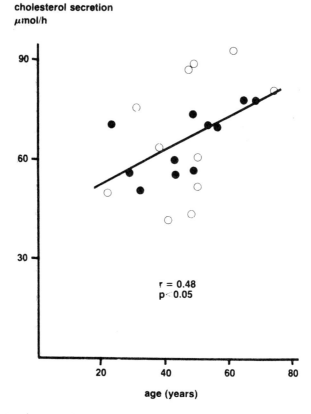

Figure 16.5 Relation between age and hepatic secretion of cholesterol in 22 healthy individuals. ○ , Females; ●, males. Reprinted from Einarsson et al.[7] with permission

normal controls, whereas the rate of bile acid secretion is normal[8]. Thus, biliary 'hypersecretion' of cholesterol is obviously of major importance for the generation of supersaturated bile, at least in the Scandinavian population.

As an explanation to the increased cholesterol secretion, we considered the possibility that a reduced fraction of hepatic cholesterol was converted to bile acids (cf. Figure 16.2). By measuring bile acid production in a series of normal volunteers of varying age, we were indeed able to demonstrate an inverse relationship between age and bile acid synthesis in both sexes (Figure 16.6). Furthermore, we observed a negative correlation between bile acid production and biliary cholesterol saturation, and between bile acid synthesis and cholesterol secretion[7]. It is of interest to consider the mean difference in cholesterol conversion into bile acids between a 20- and a 60-year-old subject: assuming that cholesterol production is unchanged, an additional 30 μmoles (12 mg) of cholesterol would be available for secretion each hour in the older subject[7]. This compares very favourably with the observed mean difference in cholesterol secretion, 20 μmoles (8 mg) per hour.

Finally, it is relevant to consider the possible importance of these age-

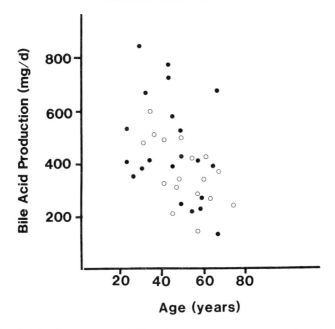

Figure 16.6 Relation between age and bile acid production rate (measured using Lindstedt's isotope dilution technique) in 38 healthy individuals. ○, Females; ●, males. Reprinted from Angelin *et al.*[9] with permission

dependent changes in biliary lipid metabolism for the overall regulation of hepatic lipoprotein metabolism (Figure 16.2). In animals, the expression of hepatic receptors for low-density lipoproteins (apolipoprotein B,E receptors) can be modulated by experimental interference with bile acid production[3,10]. Whether this occurs in man is not known. However, the concentration of low-density lipoproteins in humans is known to increase with age, as well as during suppression of bile acid synthesis owing to chenodeoxycholic acid therapy[3]. Preliminary studies indicate that the catabolism of low-density lipoproteins is in fact retarded in older subjects, suggesting a reduced hepatic receptor expression[9]. Further studies on the possibilities to influence the age-dependent changes in lipoprotein and biliary lipid metabolism by pharmacologic interference with bile acid metabolism will be of great interest.

Acknowledgements

The authors' work is supported by the Swedish Medical Research Council (03X-4793 and 03X-7137) and by the King Gustaf V and Queen Victoria Foundation. We thank Ms Lena Ericsson for skilful editorial assistance.

References

1. Lindström, C.G. (1977). Frequency of gallstone disease in a well-defined Swedish population. A prospective necropsy study in Malmö. *Scand. J. Gastroenterol.*, **12**, 341–6
2. Einarsson, K. and Angelin, B. (1986). Hyperlipoproteinemia, hypolipidemic treatment, and gallstone disease. In Grundy, S.M. (ed.) *Bile Acids and Atherosclerosis.* pp. 67–97 (New York: Raven Press)
3. Angelin, B. (1984). Regulation of hepatic lipoprotein receptor expression. In Calandra, S., Carulli, N. and Salvioli, G. (eds.) *Liver and Lipid Metabolism.* pp. 187–201 (Amsterdam: Elsevier)
4. Carey, M.C. and Small, D.M. (1978). Physical chemistry of cholesterol solubility in bile: Relationship to gallstone formation and dissolution in man. *J. Clin. Invest.*, **61**, 998–1026
5. Holzbach, R.T. (1986). Recent progress in understanding cholesterol crystal nucleation as a precursor to human gallstone formation. *Hepatology*, **6**, 1403–6
6. Ahlberg, J., Angelin, B. and Einarsson, K. (1981). Hepatic 3-hydroxy-3-methylglutaryl coenzyme A reductase activity and biliary lipid composition in man: Relation to cholesterol gallstone disease and effects of cholic acid and chenodeoxycholic acid treatment. *J. Lipid Res.*, **22**, 410–22
7. Einarsson, K., Nilsell, K., Leijd, B. and Angelin, B. (1985). Influence of age on secretion of cholesterol and synthesis of bile acids by the liver. *N. Engl. J. Med.*, **313**, 277–82
8. Nilsell, K., Angelin, B., Liljeqvist, L. and Einarsson, K. (1985). Biliary lipid output and bile acid kinetics in cholesterol gallstone disease. Evidence for an increased hepatic secretion of cholesterol in Swedish patients. *Gastroenterology*, **89**, 287–93
9. Angelin, B., Berglund, L., Einarsson, K., Ericsson, S. and Eriksson, M. (1987). Disturbances of bile acid metabolism and abnormalities of lipoprotein turnover. In Paumgartner, G., Stiehl, A. and Gerok, W. (eds.) *Bile Acids and the Liver.* pp. 277–80 (Lancaster: MTP Press)
10. Angelin, B. and Einarsson, K. (1986). Bile acids and lipoprotein metabolism. In Grundy, S.M. (ed.) *Bile Acids and Atherosclerosis.* pp. 41–66 (New York: Raven Press)

17
Bile acids in aging

K. KITANI

Bile acids are one of the important components of bile lipids and their excretion determines bile flow itself (bile-salt-dependent bile). The majority of bile acids excreted into the duodenum undergo an extensive enterohepatic circulation after efficient intestinal absorption and subsequent hepato-biliary transport.

A variety of pathologic conditions (e.g. cholesterol gallstone, cholestatic liver diseases, bile duct obstruction, intestinal malabsorption, etc.) are known to be associated with various abnormalities in each process, such as bile acid synthesis, uptake, excretion, catabolism and reabsorption. There are a vast number of clinical and experimental studies of the physiological as well as pathophysiological aspects of bile acid metabolism and kinetics. In contrast, very little is known on the relationship between bile acids and the age of subjects either in men or experimental animals. This chapter will look at this unexplored field from both the clinical and experimental points of view. Since the most important aspect of bile acids and aging, namely bile acids in relation to cholesterol, was covered by another author, this paper will be limited to other clinical aspects of bile acids and the aging liver and mostly to experiments performed in the author's own laboratory.

CLINICAL ASPECTS
Bile salt excretion

The increase of cholesterol gallstone with age is a well established fact in most areas of the world, although the incidence and the age-related increase rate vary considerably among different ethnic groups[1-3]. The rise of cholesterol gallstone frequency with age has been correlated with changes in the biliary excretion of relative concentrations of biliary lipids and several studies agree that the bile lithogenicity index significantly increases with age[4-8].

After Einarsson and his co-workers found a decrease in the cholic acid pool size and an increase in cholesterol excretion in elderly Swedes they suggested that this could be the result of the decrease in the conversion of cholesterol of extrahepatic pool to cholic acid with age[6]. They further suggested that the latter may result from a decrease in the LDL receptors of hepatocyte surface membranes. A decrease in bile salt pool size in the elderly reported by Einarsson *et al.*[6], however, is not supported by other investigations[5]. Leiss *et al.*[7] and Roda *et al.*[8] reported a significant increase in the deoxycholate fraction in biles of the elderly. They hypothesized that an increase in cholesterol concentration in the bile of the elderly may be due to the increased excretion of deoxycholate. This could occur if the 7α-dehydroxylation of primary bile acids is enhanced in the elderly. In agreement with the above arguments, Van der Werf *et al.* had previously found evidence that the 7α-dehydroxylation of bile acids is enhanced in the elderly[9]. Recently, Hellemans and co-workers in Belgium reported the results of a bile acid breath test in the elderly[10]. They found that a considerable number of elderly people, even if they looked healthy or were judged by a physician to be healthy

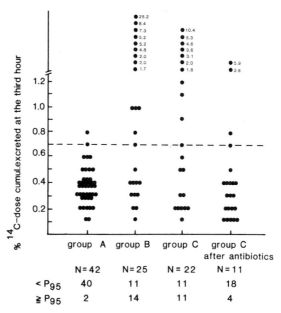

Figure 17.1 The cumulative percentage dose excretion of $^{14}CO_2$ in the expired air at 3 h after the ingestion of [^{14}C]glycocholic acid in four different groups: Group A, young subjects (19–24 years old); group B, healthy elderly subjects (65–89 years old); group C, ill elderly subjects (65–92 years old).
Reproduced with the permission of the publisher and authors: Hellemans, J. *et al.* (1984). *Age and Ageing*, **13**, 138–43

had abnormally high ^{14}C-glycocholic acid breath test values (Figure 17.1). This test is based on the principle that the rate of appearance of the $^{14}CO_2$ molecule in the expired air represents the rate of deconjugation in the intestine of orally administered cholic acid conjugated with ^{14}C-labelled glycine. The results suggest an enhanced deconjugation of conjugated bile acids which is believed to take place by means of intestinal bacterial flora enzymes. Thus, the abnormally increased productions of $^{14}CO_2$ in the bile acid breath test indicates that in many apparently healthy elderly subjects, there exists a latent but excessive growth of intestinal flora. In accordance with this finding, high breath test values in a majority of patients returned to the normal range after an administration of antibiotics (Figure 17.1)[10]. Although no definite conclusion can be drawn as to what is responsible for this phenomenon (i.e. age *per se* or age-associated gastrointestinal disorders), it appears that many elderly subjects, even if they look healthy, have an excessive growth of intestinal bacterial flora. The association of colon cancer with an increased intestinal deoxycholate concentration has been previously reported[11,12]. It is now believed that deoxycholate is a cancer promotor[13,14]. Thus, enhanced intestinal production of this bile salt would present a potential risk for colonic cancer in the elderly.

Experimental aspects

Table 17.1 shows our findings for bile flow and total bile salt excretion rate in rats of various ages[19]. In contrast to our expectation that these parameters

Table 17.1 Bile flow and total bile salt excretion rate of various rat groups of different ages (all values are expressed as mean ± S.D.).
Reproduced with the permission of the publisher: Kitani, K. *et al.* (1981) *Mech. Age. Dev.*, **7**, 381–93

Rat group	Baseline bile flow rate (μl/min/g liver)	Baseline bile salt excretion rate (nmol/min/g liver)
BN♀3m (n=17)	2.25 ± 0.35	73.7 ± 25.4
BN♀12 m (n=8)	1.85 ± 0.76*	107.0 ± 7.5*
BN♀24 m (n=8)	1.98 ± 0.31	71.6 ± 19.1
BN♀30 m (n=8)	1.80 ± 0.17*	72.5 ± 23.8
WAG♀3 m (n=9)	2.63 ± 0.25	75.8 ± 14.6
WAG♀12 m (n=6)	1.79 ± 0.19*	66.4 ± 11.3
WAG♀24 m (n=15)	2.00 ± 0.25*	68.7 ± 22.9
WAG♀30 m (n=11)	2.72 ± 0.31	76.3 ± 22.3
WAG♂3 m (n=18)	2.62 ± 0.46	64.7 ± 15.9
WAG♂12 m (n=14)	2.24 ± 0.24*	53.7 ± 13.3
WAG♂24 m (n=8)	2.07 ± 0.24*	47.0 ± 14.4*
WAG♂30 m (n=6)	2.38 ± 0.22	62.1 ± 14.0

* Significantly different from values of 3-month-old rats ($p < 0.05$)

would decline with age, most of the data we obtained from rats of different strains indicated that neither the bile flow nor bile salt excretion rate per gram of liver declined with age[15–17]. The only exception to this rule is a mild decline in both parameters in female Fischer-344 rats[17]. Furthermore, as is shown in Figure 17.2, we found some old animals with exceptionally high values comparable to the youngest rats.

Uchida, in Osaka, Japan, analysed bile salts of rats of various ages and concluded that the excretion of chenodeoxy- (and β-muri) cholic acid in the bile decreases with age[18,19]. He hypothesized that there are two different cholesterol compartments for bile acid metabolism, one for cholic acid and the other for chenodeoxycholate acid and related bile acids such as β-muricholic acid. He suggested that the conversion of cholesterol to chenodeoxy-(and β-muri) cholic acid may preferentially decline with age. According to his hypothesis, the cholesterol compartment to be converted to chenodeoxy-(and β-muri) cholic acid is of largely extra-hepatic origin and is taken up by the liver[19]. In other words, he suggested an age-dependent decline in hepatic receptor function for exogenous cholesterol may be the cause of the decrease

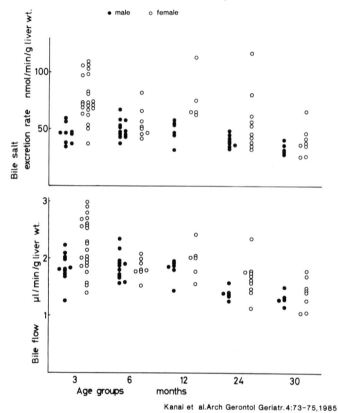

Kanai et al.Arch Gerontol Geriatr.4:73–75,1985

Figure 17.2 The bile flow and total bile salt excretion rate in aging Fischer-344 rats. For both parameters, there is a tendency to decrease with age. Note, however, that there are several old animals which exhibited an unusually high flow (and excretion values).
Reproduced with the permission of the publishers: Kanai, S. *et al.* (1985). *Arch. Gerontol. Geriatr.*, **4**, 73–85

in chenodeoxycholate excretion. It is interesting to see some similarity between the hypotheses of Einarsson for man[6] and Uchida for rats, but Uchida suggested a decline in the conversion to chenodeoxycholate[19] while Einarsson[6] suggested that decline was in the conversion to cholic acid. Uchida also showed the orally administered ^{14}C-cholesterol was converted to chenodeoxy- (and β-muri) cholic acid in smaller amounts in old rats than in young rats which is compatible with his hypothesis.

In collaboration with his laboratory, we recently examined concentrations of various bile acids in young and old F-344 rats of both sexes. In male rats, we could confirm his earlier observation that the relative proportion of cholic acid increases and that of chenodeoxy- (and β-muri) cholic acid declines with age. However, in females we could not reproduce their results (Figure 17.3). This emphasizes the caution that bile acid metabolism in rats in relation to age should be carefully interpreted in view of the notorious sex-related difference in liver functions in aging rats[20-22].

The key enzyme for the conversion of cholesterol to bile acids is 7α-hydroxylase, and other important enzymes for subsequent metabolism such as 12α- and 6β-hydroxylases are all P-450 dependent enzymes. P-450 function changes with age are known to be very much sex-dependent in rats[20-22]. In male rats, the P-450 concentration and many mono-oxygenase activities dependent on this system decline drastically with age, while in female rats,

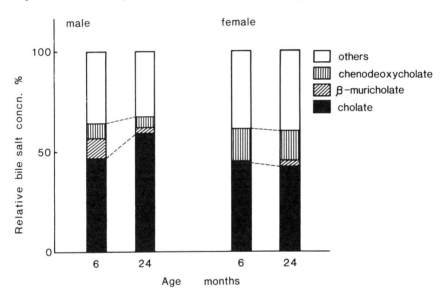

Figure 17.3 Relative concentrations of bile acids in biles of male and female F-344 rats of different ages.

little alteration occurs during aging. We have demonstrated that this is largely owing to an alteration in the P-450 isozyme population in male rat liver during aging as is shown in Figure 17.4[22]. The decline in the proportion of 6β-muricholic acid in old males may be at least partially explained by the possible differences between male and female rats in the age effect on the enzyme activity. Thus, we need to be very careful about generalizing the results on bile salt metabolism change with age in rat studies. Earlier studies of this enzyme activity change with age by Story and Kritchevsky suggested that changes are also very much strain-specific[23]. This may explain some discrepancies between the observation by Uchida[18,19] and that of our's.

Bile salts are also known to undergo an efficient entero-hepatic circulation which, of course, requires an efficient hepatic uptake and biliary excretion of bile salts. Hepatic uptake mechanisms for bile salts have been extensively studied by many investigators. It is known that the uptake of conjugated and trihydroxy bile salts is a relatively Na^+-dependent and saturable process but that unconjugated and dihydroxy bile salt uptake is mediated mainly by Na^+-independent and non-saturable process[24-26], although both mechanisms are operative in the uptake of most bile salts. Saturation kinetics have been demonstrated for many bile salts, both in hepatic uptake and biliary excretory systems, but little information is available with regard to the hepato-biliary transport of bile acids in relation to age. Only a single study suggested that for taurocholic acid aging may affect the biliary excretion process more than the uptake mechanism[27].

We have demonstrated previously that sulfobromophthalein (BSP) biliary transport maxima (T_{max}) values tend to decrease in all rat strains examined [15-17]. In addition, our recent data suggest that the T_{max} of conjugated BSP with glutathione also declines with age[28], which suggests that transport mechanism *per se* may decline with age. Furthermore, another of our studies revealed that the biliary excretion of i.v. injected ouabain, a neutral cardiac glycoside which is efficiently excreted into the bile without any biotransformation, also declines with age in both male and female rats[29]. We also found that the ouabain uptake rate of isolated hepatocytes declines in an almost linear fashion with age[30], which largely accounts for the delayed biliary recovery of i.v.-injected ouabain in old rats previously observed by us[29].

These studies prompted us to examine possible alterations in the hepatic uptake and biliary excretion of bile salts in aging rats. We found that the V_{max} value of hepatic uptake velocity for ouabain (nmol/mg/min) by isolated hepatocytes significantly decreases with age (2.98 ± 1.05, $n=4$, vs. 1.03 ± 0.39, $n=3$, $P < 0.05$), while K_m value (μM) changed little with age (31.08 ± 9.31 vs. 23.47 ± 10.92). Figure 17.4 is a summary of our bile salt T_{max} study in aging male Wistar rats. The T_{max} value for taurocholic acid expressed per gram of liver was significantly lower in old rats. It was found previously that the T_{max} for tauroursodeoxycholate is more than two-fold higher than that of taurocholate among young rats of both sexes[31,32]. Thus, the age effect, if any, may be more clearly demonstrated for tauroursodeoxycholic acid. The right panel in Figure 17.5 shows a summary of tauroursodeoxycholic acid T_{max} studies. Again, T_{max} changes were significant. From these studies, it can be tentatively concluded that for bile salts, too, the hepato-biliary transport function declines with age in rats as has been demonstrated for BSP and ouabain. Since carriers for these substances are believed to differ, these data may suggest that the carrier units for cholephilic substances universally decrease in number with age. Alternatively, as we suggested recently, the ouabain uptake data (and probably bile salt uptake, too) may be generally explained by a qualitative alteration of membrane proteins, namely a decrease in the lateral mobility of membrane located proteins which was demonstrated by a technique called fluorescence recovery after photo-bleaching (FRAP)[33-36].

As is shown in Figure 17.6, we found a linear decline in the lateral diffusion constant of membrane proteins in both male and female rats[34] and more

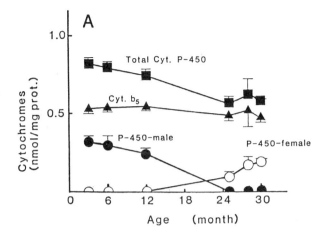

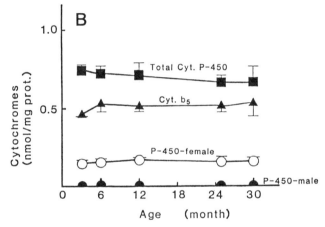

Figure 17.4 Age-related changes in the contents of cytochrome (Cyt) P-450 and Cyt B_5 in liver microsomes of male (A) and female (B) rats. Analysis of variance indicates significant changes in the contents of the cytochromes with respect to ages, sexes and age × sexes ($P < 0.05$) except in the content of Cyt b_5 between ages. Vertical bars show S.D. ($n \geqslant 6$, except 12-month-old female rats in which $n = 4$).
Reproduced with the permission of the authors and the publisher: Kamataki, T. *et al.* (1985). *J. Pharmacol. Exp. Ther.*, **233**, 222–8.

recently in mice of both sexes (Zs.-Nagy *et al.* unpublished data), although the slope value varied depending on sex and species. If the lateral protein movements in hepatocyte surface membranes generally decline with age, it can cause a general decline in the uptake velocities for many compounds that are carrier mediated in membranes. A similar change is also conceivable for canalicular membrane proteins, although there is no proof available for this possibility at the moment. Furthermore, it is as yet not elucidated whether such a change is present in old human livers. Moreover, considering the very efficient hepato-biliary transport systems for bile salts, the physiological

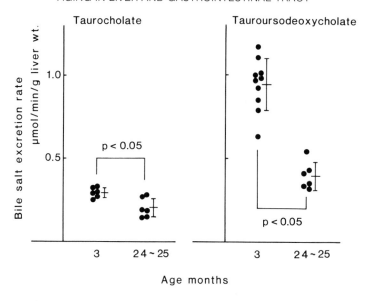

Figure 17.5 The transport maxima values for taurocholic acid and tauroursodeoxycholic acid in young and old male Wistar rats.

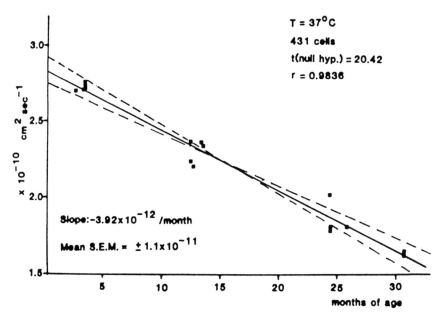

Figure 17.6 Age-related alterations in the lateral mobility (diffusion constant) of surface proteins of hepatocytes in rats of various ages.
Reproduced with the permission of the publisher: Zs.-Nagy, I. *et al.* (1986). *Arch. Gerontol. Geriatr.*, **5**, 131–57

alterations in transport functions with age shown in these studies do not appear to induce any age-related clinical abnormalities for bile salt kinetics in healthy conditions. However, these may be potential risk factors for elderly subjects with liver diseases (for example jaundice), assuming that these alterations are present in humans. Lowered transport functions for bile salts and probably for other substances like bilirubin may worsen the jaundice and also retard the recovery of hepatobiliary diseases in the elderly.

SUMMARY

(1) A possible increase in bacterial growth in the intestine of the elderly, may enhance deconjugation of bile salts and 7α-dehydroxylation resulting in an enhanced production, absorption and excretion of the more noxious secondary bile salts such as deoxycholate. This may be related to the higher incidence of cholesterol gallstone diseases in the elderly and also may increase risk of colon cancer.

(2) In rats, the basal bile flow and bile salt excretion rate barely declines with age.

(3) However, the hepatic uptake and especially biliary transport maximum decline with age regardless of rat sex and strain.

(4) These alterations observed in aging animals may have little clinical significance for the healthy elderly humans but may be a potential risk for the aged with liver diseases.

References

1. Lieber, M. M. (1952). The incidence of gall stones and their correlation with other diseases. *Ann. Surg.*, **135**, 394–405
2. Torvik, A. and Hoivik, B. (1960). Gallstones in an autopsy series. Incidence, complications and correlations with carcinoma of the gallbladder. *Acta Chir. Scand.*, **120**, 168–74
3. Marinovic, I., Guerra, C. and Larach, G. (1972). Incidencia de litiasis biliar en material de autopsiasis y análisis de composición de los cálculos. *Re. Med. Chil.*, **100**, 1320–7
4. Sampler, R. E., Bannett, P. H., Comess, L. J. *et al.* (1970). Gallbladder disease in Pima Indians: demonstration of high prevalence and early onset by cholecystography. *N. Engl. J. Med.*, **283**, 1358–64
5. Valdidideso, V., Palma, R., Wunkhaus, R., Antezana, C., Severin, C. and Contreras, A. (1978). Effect of aging on biliary lipid composition and bile acid metabolism in normal Chilean women. *Gastroenterology*, **74**, 871–4
6. Einarsson, K., Nilsell, K., Leijd, B. and Angelin, B. (1985). Influence of age on secretion of cholesterol and synthesis of bile acids by the liver. *N. Engl. J. Med.*, **313**, 277–282
7. Leiss, O., Becker, M. and von Bergman, K. (1987). Effect of age and individual endogenous bile acids on biliary lipid secretions in humans. In Paumgartner, G., Stiehl, A. and Gerok, W. (eds.) *Bile Acids and the Liver*, pp. 217–224. (Lancaster, Boston, The Hague, Dordrecht: MTP Press)
8. Roda, E., Bazzoli, F., Mazzella, G., Villanova, N., Simoni, P., Festi, D., Petronelli, A., Ronchi, M. and Barbara, L. (1987). Effect of age and sex on bile acid metabolism and biliary lipid secretion in normal subjects and gallstone patients. In Paumgartner, G., Stiehl, A. and Gerok, W. (eds.) *Bile Acids and the Liver*, pp. 225–227. (Lancaster, Boston, The Hague, Dordrecht: MTP Press)
9. Van der Werf, S. D. J., Huijbregts, A. W. M., Lanners, H. L. M., van Berge Henegouwen, G. P. and van Tongeren, J. H. M. (1981). Age dependent difference in human bile acid metabolism and 7α-dehydroxylation. *Eur. J. Clin. Invest.*, **11**, 425–31
10. Hellemans, J., Joosten, E., Ghoos, Y., Carchon, H., Vantrappen, G., Pelemans, W. and

Rutgerts, P. (1984). Positive $^{14}CO_2$ bile acid breath test in elderly people. *Age Ageing*, **13**, 138–43

11. Hill, M. J., Crowther, J. S., Draser, B. S., Hawksworth, G., Aries, V. and Williams, R. E. O. (1971). Bacteria and aetiology of cancer of large bowel. *Lancet*, **1**, 95–100

12. Cook, J. W., Kennaway, E. L. and Kennaway, N. M. (1940). Production of tumors in mice by deoxycholic acid. *Nature*, **145**, 627

13. Narisawa, T., Magadia, N. E., Weisberger, J. H. and Wynder, E. L. (1974). Effect of acids on colon carcinogenesis after intrarectal instillation of N'-methyl-N-nitro-N-nitrosoguanidine in rats. *J. Natl. Cancer Inst.*, **53**, 1093–7

14. Narisawa, T. (1983). Bile acid metabolism and colonic carcinogenesis. *Rinshokagaku*, **19**, 188–192. (In Japanese)

15. Kitani, K., Kanai, S. and Miura, R. (1978). Hepatic metabolism of sulfobromophthalein (BSP) and indocyanine green (ICG) in aging rats. In Kitani, K. (ed.) *Liver and Aging – 1978*, pp. 145–56. (Amsterdam: Elsevier/North-Holland)

16. Kitani, K., Zurcher, C. and van Bezooijen, C. F. A. (1981). The effect of aging on the hepatic metabolism of sulfobromophthalein in BN/Bi female and Wag/Rij male and female rats. *Mech. Age. Develop.*, **7**, 381–93

17. Kanai, S., Kitani, K., Fujita, S. and Kitagawa, H. (1985). The hepatic handling of sulfobromophthalein in aging Fischer-344 rats: *in vivo* and *in vitro* studies. *Arch. Gerontol. Geriatr.*, **4**, 73–85

18. Uchida, K., Matsubara, T., Ishikawa, Y. and Ito, N. (1982). Age-related changes in cholesterol-bile acid metabolism and hepatic mixed function oxidase activities in rats. In Kitani, K. (ed.) *Liver and Aging – 1982, Liver and Drugs* pp. 192–211. (Amsterdam: Elsevier/North-Holland Biomedical Press)

19. Uchida, K. and Takeuchi, N. (1986). Changes in cholesterol and bile acid metabolism during aging. In Yonago, H. (ed.) *Proc. 15th Symposium on Pharmacological Activity and Mechanism*. pp. 41–6. (In Japanese)

20. Fujita, S., Uesugi, T., Kitagawa, H., Suzuki, T. and Kitani, K. (1982) Hepatic microsomal monooxygenase and azoreductase activities in aging Fischer-344 rats. Importance of sex difference for aging study. In Kitani, K. (ed.) *Liver and Aging – 1982, Liver and Drugs*, pp. 55–71. (Amsterdam: Elsevier/North-Holland Biomedical Press)

21. Kitani, K. (1986). Hepatic drug metabolism in the elderly. *Hepatology*, **6**, 316–19

22. Kamataki, T., Maeda, K., Shimada, M., Kitani, K., Nagai, T. and Kato, R. (1985). Age-related alteration in the activities of drug-metabolizing enzymes and contents of sex-specific forms of cytochrome P-450 in liver microsomes from male and female rats. *J. Pharmacol. Exp. Ther.*, **233**, 222–8

23. Story, J. A. and Kritchevsky, D. (1978). Age-related changes in cholesterol. In Kitani, K. (ed.) *Liver and Aging – 1978*, pp. 193–203. (Amsterdam: Elsevier/North-Holland)

24. Schwarz, L. R., Burr, R., Schwenk, M., Pfaff, E. and Greim, H. (1975). Uptake of taurocholic acid into isolated rat-liver cells. *Eur. J. Biochem.*, **55**, 617–23

25. Van Dyke, R., Jeffery, W., Stephens, E. and Scharschmidt, B. F. (1982). Bile acids transport in cultured rat hepatocytes. *Am. J. Physiol.*, **243**, G484–G492

26. Anwer, M. S., Kroker, R. and Hegner, D. (1976). Cholic acid uptake into isolated rat hepatocytes. *Hoppe-Seyler's Z. Physiol. Chem.*, **357**, S-1477–1486

27. Kroker, R., Hegner, D. and Anwer, M. S. (1980). Altered hepatobiliary transport of taurocholic acid in aged rats. *Mech. Age. Dev.*, **12**, 367–73

28. Kanai, S., Kitani, K., Sato, Y. and Nokubo, M. (1988) Biliary transport maximum of conjugated sulfobromophthalein in aging F-344 rats. *Arch. Gerontol. Geriatr.* (Submitted)

29. Sato, Y., Kanai, S. and Kitani, K. (1987). Biliary excretion of ouabain in aging male and female F-344 rats. *Arch. Gerontol. Geriatr.*, **6**, 141–52

30. Ohta, M., Kanai, S., Sato, Y. and Kitani, K. (1988). Age-dependent decrease in the hepatic uptake and biliary excretion of ouabain in rats. *Biochem. Pharmacol.*, **37**, 935–42

31. Kitani, K. and Kanai, S. (1981). Biliary transport maximum of tauroursodeoxycholate is twice as high as that of taurocholate in the rat. *Life Sci.*, **29**, 269–75

32. Kitani, K., Kanai, S., Ohta, M. and Sato, Y. (1986). Differing transport maxima values for taurine conjugated bile salts in rats and hamsters. *Am. J. Physiol.*, **251**, G852–G858

33. Zs-Nagy, I., Ohta, M., Kitani, K. and Imahori, K. (1984). An automated method for measuring lateral mobility of proteins in the plasma membrane of cells. *Mikroskopie*, **41**, 12–25

34. Zs.-Nagy, I., Kitani, K., Ohta, M. and Imahori, K. (1986). Age-dependent decrease in lateral diffusion constant of proteins in the plasma membrane of hepatocytes as revealed by fluorescence recovery after photobleaching in tissue smears. *Arch. Gerontol. Geriatr.*, **5,** 131–57

35. Zs.-Nagy, I., Kitani, K., Ohta, M., Zs.-Nagy, V. and Imahori, K. (1986). Age-estimations of rats based on the average lateral diffusion constant of hepatocyte membrane proteins as revealed by fluorescence recovery after photobleaching. *Exp. Gerontol.*, **21,** 555–63

36. Kitani, K., Zs.-Nagy, I., Kanai, S., Sato, Y. and Ohta, M. (1988). Correlation between the biliary excretion of ouabain and lateral mobility of hepatocyte plasma membrane proteins in the rat. The effect of age and spironolactone pretreatment. *Hepatology*, **8,** 125–31

18
Age related perturbations of vesicular transport and ligand processing in hepatocytes

A. L. JONES, C. K. DANIELS, S. J. BURWEN and D. L. SCHMUCKER

HISTORICAL PERSPECTIVE

The liver plays a prominent role in maintaining the homeostasis of the organism. To fulfill this function, the liver parenchymal cell relies almost exclusively on receptor-mediated endocytosis and vesicular transport to bind, internalize and process a wide variety of macromolecules. Aging of an organism is generally characterized by a diminished ability to maintain homeostasis and adapt or respond to environmental stresses. At the beginning of our research on intracellular vesicular movement of macromolecules within liver parenchymal cells, essentially nothing was known about the effects of aging on these important transport processes. It was our feeling that potential age-related perturbations in the hepatic processing of macromolecules might provide a tool for dissecting and understanding these transport pathways.

Two main pathways of ligand processing have been identified in hepatocytes[1] (Figure 18.1). The first pathway, referred to as the transcellular pathway, utilizes shuttle vesicles to transport receptor-bound protein from the sinusoidal membrane to the bile canalicular membrane for exocytosis. Since these vesicles are segregated from the lysosomal elements of the hepatocyte, their contents are usually delivered into the bile intact. Immunoglobulin A (IgA) is typical of ligands transported by this pathway[2]. The second pathway, known as the lysosomal or degradative pathway, involves the integration of endocytic vesicles with multivesicular bodies and lysosomes. This pathway is utilized by ligands destined for degradation, such as low-density lipoproteins, lipoprotein remnants and desialylated glycoproteins[3,4]. In general, the specific receptors for ligands that utilize this pathway are recycled.

For our studies on the effect of aging on vesicular transport and processing of macromolecules by hepatocytes, we chose three representative ligands,

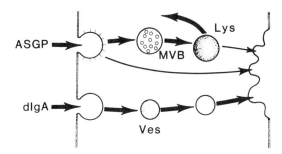

Figure 18.1 This highly schematic diagram depicts the principal features of the lysosomal (degradative) or transcellular pathways for macromolecular transport across hepatocytes and into the bile canaliculi. The arrows reflect the movement of [125]I. See text for details. ASGP, asialoglycoprotein; MVB, multivesicular bodies; Lys, lysosomes; dIgA, dimeric IgA; Ves, vesicle

utilizing the different intracellular transport pathways: Immunoglobulin A (IgA), asialoorosomucoid (ASOR), and epidermal growth factor (EGF).

Fisher *et al.* had previously shown that IgA binds rapidly to a non-recyclable receptor, called secretory component, on the sinusoidal surface of the rat hepatocyte[5]. IgA enters the bile still bound to a portion of its receptor. Renston *et al.* demonstrated that the transport of IgA from sinusoid to bile involves endocytic vesicles that do not enter the lysosomal pathway, resulting in the biliary secretion of intact IgA[2].

In contrast to IgA, ASOR is transported almost exclusively by the lysosomal pathway. Hubbard and Stukenbrok showed that receptor-bound ASOR is internalized into endocytic vesicles that fuse to form endosomes[3]. The endosomes comprise a pre-lysosomal compartment, that is, they become acidified and give rise to multivesicular bodies, which eventually fuse with primary lysosomes to form secondary lysosomes. The exposure of endocytic vesicle contents to lysosomal acid hydrolases results in their degradation. In rodents, only about 3% of injected ASOR is secreted into bile intact; the remainder enters the bile as degradation products. In the primate, however, approximately 8% of injected ASOR is secreted intact. In addition, ASOR taken up by the liver forms a lobular concentration gradient.

EGF was shown to utilize both the transcellular and lysosomal transport pathways[6]. St Hilaire *et al.* demonstrated that the liver clears the majority of EGF from the blood via a single pass, and that it, too, forms a lobular concentration gradient[7]. They also observed that, although most of the EGF secreted into bile is in degraded form, approximately 20% of the biliary EGF is immunoprecipitable with anti-EGF antibody. Burwen *et al.* demonstrated that the two transport pathways were indeed separate. Following an intra-portal injection of a single bolus of EGF, the biliary secretion of immu-noprecipitable EGF peaked at 20 min, whereas the peak secretion of degradation products occurred 40 min after injection. Furthermore, the immunoprecipitable EGF in bile was capable of specifically binding to cul-tured hepatocytes. In addition, inhibition of the lysosomal pathway with chloroquine dramatically decreased the biliary secretion of degradation products, but had essentially no effect of the secretion of intact EGF into bile[6].

Regardless of the pathway utilized, microtubules, which are a major component of the liver cell cytoskeleton, are essential for the vectorial movement of intracellular vesicles. Colchicine, an inhibitor of microtubule function, had a marked effect on the transcellular transport of all three macromolecules used in these studies. In colchicine-treated hepatocytes, IgA was endocytosed, but not transported to the pericanalicular areas of the cells[8]. Biliary secretion of IgA by *in situ* rat liver was also dramatically reduced in the presence of colchicine. Similarly, colchicine also reduced the biliary secretion of EGF, and affected both intact and degraded forms to the same extent (Burwen and Barker, unpublished observations). In cultured hepatocytes, the degradation of endocytosed ASOR was inhibited in the presence of colcemid (an analog of colchicine), since ASOR was prevented from reaching the lysosomes. Furthermore, this inhibition was proportional to the concentration of colcemid[9].

In summary, all three macromolecules selected for these studies utilize receptor-mediated endocytosis and intracellular vesicles, and rely on functionally dynamic microtubules, for their transport by hepatocytes. But ASOR and EGF form lobular concentration gradients. In contrast, IgA does not form a lobular concentration gradient. ASOR has a receptor that recycles. The EGF receptor is degraded in the lysosomes along with its ligand. And the IgA receptor, or at least a portion of it, is secreted into bile still attached to its ligand.

METHODS

The methods used in these studies are all published procedures, and are described in detail in the cited references. In brief, we:

1. Radiolabel EGF with ^{125}I using the chloramine T method, and IgA and ASOR using the monochloride method[10].
2. Use Fischer-344 male rats between the ages of 3 and 27 months.
3. Cannulate the common bile duct *in situ*, inject ligand into the portal or femoral vein, collect bile over timed intervals, and analyse the bile for secreted ligand.
4. Process the liver for light and electron microscopic autoradiography to localize ligand within hepatocytes.
5. Isolate highly purified rat liver plasma membranes for quantitative ligand binding studies.

RESULTS

IgA studies

Biliary secretion and intracellular distribution of IgA were compared in young vs. old rats. ^{125}I-IgA was injected into the portal veins of 3-, 12- and 24-month-old Fischer male rats, and bile was collected for 90 min over 10-min intervals. During the peak of secretory activity, at approximately 40 min after injection, the biliary secretion of IgA in the 3-month-old rats was 5 times greater than that of the 12-month-old rats, and 6 times greater than that of the 24-month-old rats[11] (Figure 18.2). At the termination of the experiments, the intact livers from both young and old rats retained the same amount of radioactivity. Since the liver weight of the older rats was 30% greater, the amount of IgA per cell was much higher in the livers of young rats (Table 18.1). These data, taken together with the 6-fold higher rate of biliary IgA secretion by the younger rats, indicate that the livers of older rats do not clear IgA from the plasma as effectively as young rat livers.

The intracellular distribution of IgA was shown by light and electron microscopic autoradiography. Autoradiographic grains, representing IgA, were located in the pericanalicular regions of the hepatocyte in young rats, whereas in old rats, grains were primarily associated with hepatocyte plasma membranes, indicating a decreased ability, on the part of old hepatocytes, to transport endocytosed IgA (Figures 18.3 and 18.4).

To see whether age-related changes in IgA receptors could account for the observed age-dependent decrease in IgA transport and biliary secretion, IgA receptors from livers of young and old rats were compared. Isolated liver plasma membrane preparations were used for quantitative binding studies (Table 18.2). For all age groups, the binding of IgA to plasma membranes demonstrated a single class of specific receptors[12]. As calculated from Scatchard plots, IgA binding decreased almost 4-fold, from 2.61×10^{12} to 0.72×10^{12} sites per mg membrane protein, between the 3-month-old and 27-month-old rats (Figure 18.5)

Therefore, the age-dependent decrease in the liver's ability to take up IgA from the plasma is certainly consistent with this observed decrease in liver plasma membrane IgA binding activity. However, the 4-fold loss of binding activity alone cannot account for the 6-fold loss in biliary secretion of IgA. In summary, the livers from aging rats have markedly decreased ability in both uptake of IgA from the plasma and transport of IgA to the pericanalicular region of the hepatocyte.

ASOR studies

Studies with ASOR were conducted in a very similar manner to those for IgA. ^{125}I-ASOR was injected into rat femoral veins, and bile was collected and analysed for secretion of both intact and degraded ASOR. In addition, quantitative binding studies were performed with isolated plasma membranes. And finally, light microscopic autoradiography was used to assess the effect of aging on the distribution of ASOR within the liver lobule.

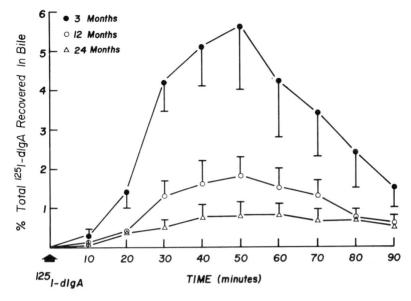

Figure 18.2 Effect of animal age on the hepato-biliary secretion of ^{125}I-labelled rat dimeric immunoglobulin A (dIgA) after administration via the femoral vein. The radiolabelled ligand was injected at time 0, and the amount recovered in the bile was measured at 10-min intervals over the subsequent 90 min. The values are expressed as the percentage of administered ^{125}I/g bile/g liver/10 min. Each point represents the mean of 3–5 animals ± SD.
[From Schmucker, D. L. *et al.* (1985). *Gastroenterology*, **88**, 436–43]

Table 18.1 Effect of animal age on liver weight and hepatic content of ^{125}I-labelled dimeric immunoglobulin in the rat (all values represent the mean ± S.D. of 3–6 animals)

	Animal age (months)		
	3–4	12	24–25
Liver weight (g)	8.1 ± 2	10.9 ± 1.7	11.3 ± 1.7
Hepatic content of dIgA*	3.3 ± 0.4	2.5 ± 0.9	2.3 ± 0.7
^{125}I-dIgA/g liver			
^{125}I-dIgA/liver	28 ± 3	27 ± 10	26 ± 4

*Values expressed as percent of administered dose per gram liver or per liver. dIgA = dimeric IgA.
[From Schmucker, D. L. *et al.* (1985). *Gastroenterology*, **88**, 436–43]

In contrast to the findings with IgA, there was no difference in the biliary secretion of ASOR in young vs. old animals. Analysis of the bile indicated that the secretory rate and amount of intact and degraded ASOR was the same in all age groups. However, quantitative binding studies with isolated liver plasma membranes did show a 40–50% decrease in specific binding activity for ASOR in old rats. The point is that, even with remarkably reduced

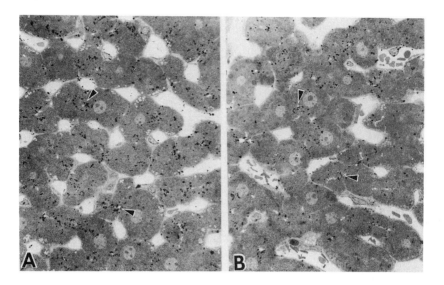

Figure 18.3 Light-microscopic autoradiographs of liver tissue from young adult (A) and senescent (B) rats injected with ^{125}I-labelled dimeric IgA via the femoral vein. The animals were sacrificed and the tissue was prepared 35 min after the administration of the ligand, i.e., immediately preceding peak biliary secretion of IgA. The number of autoradiographic grains concentrated within the pericanalicular cytoplasm in the 3-month-old rats is greater than that observed in the old animals. (Arrowheads show bile canaliculi.) × 600.

[From Schmucker, D. L. *et al.*, (1985). *Gastroenterology*, **88**, 436–43]

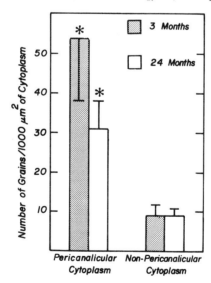

Figure 18.4 Quantitative analysis of autoradiographic grain distribution, representing ^{125}I-labelled dimeric IgA, either in the pericanalicular or non-pericanalicular cytoplasm of rat hepatocytes, as a function of animal age. The pericanalicular cytoplasm comprised 10% of the hepatocellular cytoplasm in the micrographs analyzed, the remainder was designated as non-pericanalicular cytoplasm. The pericanalicular cytoplasm of 'young' hepatocytes contained approximately twice the number of autoradiographic grains as did the same subcellular zone in 'old' liver cells. There was no apparent age-related difference in the number of grains associated with the non-pericanalicular zone, consistent with the observation that there were fewer grains per 'old' liver cell. Each bar represents the mean (± S.D.) of 4 animals and the asterisk denotes a statistically significant difference ($p < 0.05$).

[From Schmucker, D. L. *et al.*, (1985). *Gastroenterology*, **88**, 436–43]

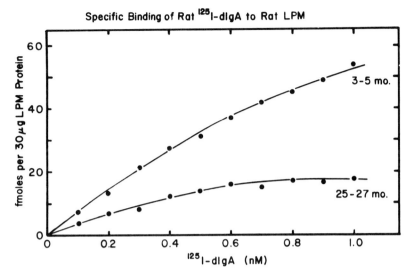

Figure 18.5 Effect of animal age on specific binding of ^{125}I-dIgA to isolated liver plasma membrane (LPM). Specifically-bound ^{125}I-dIgA; the difference between totally bound and the amount bound in the presence of a 2000-fold molar excess of unlabelled ligand is plotted vs. increasing concentrations (0.1 to 1.0 nM) of labelled rat dIgA for two age groups of rats from a typical experiment.

[From Daniels, C. K. et al., (1985). *J. Immunology*, **134**, 3855–8]

Table 18.2 Effects of animal age on the isolation and properties of LPM*

	Animal age (months)		
	3–6	12–14	24–27
Liver weight (g)	8.3 ± 0.2	9.7 ± 0.4	10.3 ± 0.5
Protein yield**	1.0 ± 0.1	1.1 ± 0.1	0.98 ± 0.2
5′ − Nucleotidase activity†			
Homogenate	41.1	–	48.6
Liver plasma membrane (LPM)	1136	–	1070
Relative enrichment††	28	–	22

* Values are mean ± S.E.M. for 3–7 samples, where each sample represents an LPM preparation from 2 or 4 livers. Individual values are the mean of two samples
** Milligrams of LPM protein per gram wet weight of liver
† Nanomoles of product formed per minute per mg protein
†† Defined as the ratio of the specific activity in the LPM to specific activity in the homogenate
[From Daniels, C. K. et al., (1985). *J. Immunology*, **134**, 3855–8]

ability for the old liver plasma membranes to bind ASOR, the livers were still capable of secreting ASOR to the same extent as the young livers (Figure 18.6).

The means by which the old livers could compensate for their loss in ASOR binding capabilities and maintain their secretory output was revealed by light

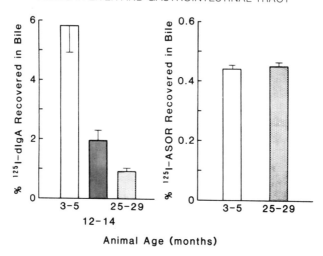

Figure 18.6 Histogram comparing the transport of dIgA and asialoorosomucoid (ASOR) into the bile as a function of age

autoradiographic studies on the age-dependent lobular distribution of ASOR. In young rat livers, ASOR was taken up primarily by zone 1 cells, and the lobular concentration gradient formed extended across 30–50% of the liver lobule. However, in old rat livers, the lobular concentration gradient was diminished; that is, the uptake of ASOR extended into zone 3 cells, across most of the lobule. Therefore, even though, on a per cell basis, old livers have a diminished capacity to take up ASOR, it is offset by the reserve capacity of cells further down the lobular gradient. In other words, by recruiting cells further down the lobule, the liver as a whole can compensate for the diminished binding capacity of its individual cells.

EGF studies

Preliminary studies on the biliary secretion of EGF by young and old rats showed that, in all age groups, both intact and degraded EGF were secreted. However, the total quantity of EGF transported to bile decreased markedly in 18-month-old rats as compared to young rats. Biliary secretions of both intact and degraded EGF were decreased to the same extent. In addition, the peak of secretion of degradation products was delayed, occurring at 50 min instead of 40 min. These data were very similar to data on the biliary secretion of EGF in the presence of the microtubule inhibitor, colchicine.

Preliminary quantitative binding studies with liver plasma membranes isolated from both young and old rats demonstrated that there was an age-dependent decrease in EGF binding activity by approximately 50%. However, the amount of the decrease in binding activity was not sufficient to account for the amount of decrease in biliary secretion of EGF.

WORKING HYPOTHESIS

We have identified three important factors that contribute to age-related changes in vesicular transport, processing and biliary secretion of macromolecules by hepatocytes: receptor binding, recruitment of cells from portal to central areas of the liver lobule, and microtubules.

Two indirect lines of evidence suggest that microtubule function declines as a function of age: (1) Endocytosed IgA does not get transported to the pericanalicular region of hepatocytes in old livers; (2) the delayed and diminished biliary transport of both IgA and EGF in the presence of colchicine closely resembles the age-related decline in biliary transport of these two ligands.

Specific receptor-binding activity for all three macromolecules declines significantly as a function of age. In the case of ASOR transport, the old liver is able to compensate by recruitment of additional cells down the lobule for transport duty. Since IgA does not form a lobular concentration gradient, there is no reserve capacity in the liver to compensate for the age-related decline in receptor binding activity. EGF, however, normally forms a lobular concentration gradient like ASOR, so it is surprising that the reserve transport capacity of cells further down the lobule cannot make up for the age-dependent decline in its biliary secretion. Differences in the availability of receptors for EGF and ASOR may account for the differences in their transport by old livers.

ASOR receptor is normally recycled, and EGF receptor is normally degraded in lysosomes. Both IgA and EGF receptor replenishment require *de novo* synthesis, whereas ASOR receptor does not. A loss of microtubule function with age might selectively adversely affect the rate of receptor replenishment, without having a similar detrimental effect on the rate of receptor recycling. If this is true, then hepatocytes even further down the lobule (zone 3) could lack the necessary receptors to compensate for diminished EGF uptake by zone 1 cells.

There is currently no data available to support the speculations presented in this working hypothesis. Further research is clearly required to elucidate the mechanisms by which aging affects vesicular transport processes.

Acknowledgements

The authors wish to acknowledge the excellent technical assistance of Sandra Huling, Rose Wang and Anna Feren. The data presented in this manuscript were from work done and supported by the United States Veterans Administration and by NIH grants P50 AM18520, RO1 DK38436, RO1 AM25878 and R23 AG04897.

References

1. Jones, A. L. and Burwen, S. J. (1985). Hepatic receptors and their ligands: problems of intracellular sorting and vectorial movement. *Semin. Liver Dis.*, **5**, 136–46
2. Renston, R. H., Jones, A. L., Christiansen, W. D., Hradek, G. T. and Underdown, B. J. (1980). Evidence for a vesicular transport mechanism in hepatocytes for biliary secretion of immunoglobulin A. *Science*, **208**, 1276–8
3. Hubbard, A. L. and Stukenbrok, H. (1979). An electron microscope autoradiographic study of the carbohydrate recognition systems in rat liver. II. Intracellular fates of the ^{125}I-ligands. *J. Cell Biol.*, **83**, 65–81
4. Jones, A. L., Hradek, G. T., Hornick, C., Renaud, G., Windler, E. E. T. and Havel, R. J. (1984). Uptake and processing of remnants of chylomicrons and very low density lipoproteins by rat liver. *J. Lipid Res.*, **25**, 1151–8
5. Fisher, M. M., Nagy, B., Bazin H. *et al.* (1979). Biliary transport of IgA: role of secretory component. *Proc. Natl. Acad. Sci. USA*, **76**, 2008–12
6. Burwen, S. J., Barker, M. E., Goldman, I. S., Hradek, G. T., Raper, S. E. and Jones, A. L. (1984). Transport of epidermal growth factor by rat liver: evidence for a nonlysosomal pathway. *J. Cell Biol.*, **99**, 1259–65
7. St Hilaire, R. J., Hradek, G. T. and Jones, A. L. (1983). Hepatic sequestration and biliary secretion of epidermal growth factor (EGF): evidence for a high capacity uptake system. *Proc. Natl. Acad. Sci. USA*, **80**, 3797–801
8. Goldman, I. S., Jones, A. L., Hradek, G. T. and Huling, S. (1983). Hepatocyte handling of immunoglobulin A in the rat: the role of microtubules. *Gastroenterology*, **85**, 130–40
9. Caron, J. M., Jones, A. L. and Kirschner, M. W. (1985). Autoregulation of tubulin synthesis in hepatocytes and fibroblasts. *J. Cell Biol.*, **101**, 1763–72
10. Helmkamp, R. W., Goodland, R. L., Bale, W. F. *et al.* (1960). High specific activity iodination of γ-globulins with iodine-131 monochloride. *Cancer Res.*, **20**, 1495–1500
11. Schmucker, D. L., Gilbert, R., Hradek, G. T., Jones, A. L. and Bazin, H. (1985). Effect of aging on the hepatobiliary transport of dimeric immunoglobulin A in the male Fischer rat. *Gastroenterology*, **88**, 436–43
12. Daniels, C. K., Schmucker, D. L. and Jones, A. L. (1985). Age-dependent loss of dimeric immunoglobulin A receptors in the liver of the Fischer 344 rat. *J. Immunol.*, **134**, 3855–8

19
Hepatocyte co-culture: a model system in liver age research?

A. GUILLOUZO, B. CLEMENT, D. RATANASAVANH, C. CHESNE, J.-M. BEGUE and C. GUGUEN-GUILLOUZO

The aging of the liver is indicated by morphologic alterations, disturbances in adaptation and regulation, and changes in biochemical or metabolic features. Since the liver is under the influence of other organs this makes it difficult to distinguish key events in the aging process from other hepatic manifestations occurring in the aged[1]. An approach to overcome this major problem could be to use isolated hepatocytes from donors of different ages for investigating cellular and molecular aspects of the aging process in the liver.

Parenchymal cells from various species including man can be easily obtained by the two-step collagenase method[2]. Freshly isolated cells express most of the functions they possess just before their isolation. Therefore, they enter the culture medium with a prior history or memory of signals to which they were responding *in vivo*. In addition suspected hepatocytes have no intercellular contacts, exhibit some functional alterations particularly at the plasma membrane level and do not survive for more than a few hours. All these features might represent limitations in the use of isolated hepatocytes as a model system to analyse the key events related to aging.

For prolonged survival *in vitro* hepatocytes need to attach to a support. When placed in conventional culture conditions, these cells may survive for 1–3 weeks. However, they undergo rapid phenotypic changes[3]. As example, the cytochrome P-450 level is markedly decreased[4,5] and transcription of specific liver genes is very low after 24 h[6,7]. Addition of soluble factors such as hormones and growth factors, and the use of extracellular matrix components as supports may improve specific functions and enhance cell survival. However, whatever the culture conditions used, adult hepatocytes do not remain functionally stable beyond a few days[3,8].

This limitation was recently overcome in our laboratory. We reported that hepatocytes from various species including man, could remain differentiated in primary culture for several weeks by addition of another liver cell type isolated from rat liver[9-11]. This review discusses the potential applications and interest of this co-culture system in liver age research.

THE HEPATOCYTE CO-CULTURE SYSTEM

A few hours after the hepatocytes have attached to the support, rat liver epithelial cells are added. These attach to free surfaces, rapidly divide and establish close contacts with parenchymal cells[9] (Figure 19.1). Confluency may be obtained within 24 h when the two cell populations are plated in an appropriate density and such cultures may be maintained for several weeks, even in a serum-free medium.

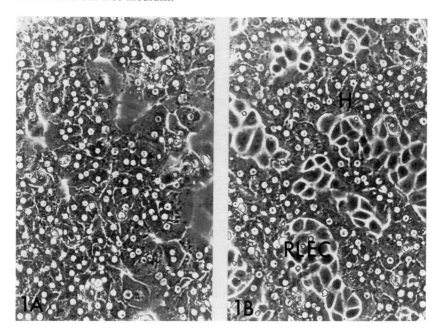

Figure 19.1 Phase-contrast micrographs of cultured adult human hepatocytes: 3-day pure culture (A) and co-culture (B). When added to hepatocyte (H) cultures, rat-liver epithelial cells (RLEC) occupy all the free surfaces. Note the more globular shape of co-cultured hepatocytes. (× 270)

Rat liver epithelial cells probably derive from the undifferentiated cells which line the canal of Hering; they are isolated by trypsinisation of young rat livers, cloned and subcultivated[12]. These cells interact with hepatocytes only before they undergo spontaneous transformation, i.e. during about 30 passages. The intimate contacts between the two cell types are discontinuous and do not involve intercellular junctions. This was recently confirmed by microinjection of Lucifer yellow in either hepatocytes or epithelial cells. The dye did not diffuse from one cell type to another[13].

Since rat liver epithelial cells may interact with hepatocytes from various species including man, at different ages, this makes the co-culture system suitable for studying liver development and aging in various species.

A number of specific functions have been found to be well preserved. However, the stability of the system is dependent upon the presence of corticosteroids into the medium. When the hormone is absent or at a too low

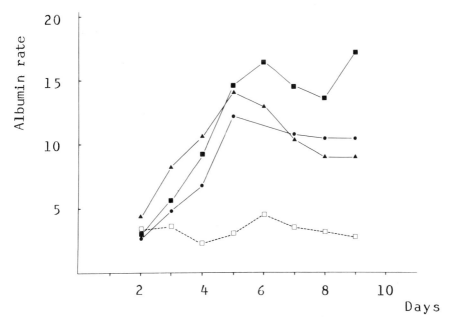

Figure 19.2 Albumin secretion by rat hepatocytes co-cultured with rat liver epithelial cells in the absence (□ ---- □) or presence of various concentrations of hydrocortisone (■ − − ■, 1.4×10^6 M; ▲ − ▲, 7×10^{-6} M; ● − ●, 7×10^{-7} M). The nutrient medium is expressed in micrograms per millilitre of medium per day. Each point represents the mean of triplicate cultures. (From ref. 14)

concentration, a decline in the expression of specific functions is observed (Figure 19.2) and hepatocytes die[14]. The production of various plasma proteins has been demonstrated i.e. albumin[9,10], hemopexin[15], haptoglobin[15], α_2-macroglobulin[15] and α_1-acid glycoprotein[16]. By using the immunoperoxidase technique, it was demonstrated that all the hepatocytes whether in contact or not with rat liver cells, produce albumin[9,10]. Moreover, it was found that Golgi complexes were preferentially located near bile canaliculi indicating that parenchymal cells were polarized as in the *in vivo* situation[10].

Other studies have been carried out in order to evaluate the capacity of co-cultured hepatocytes to transcribe specific genes. Both indirect and direct evidence was provided that these cells continue to transcribe specific genes[7]. Neosynthesized albumin and transferrin mRNAs were demonstrated by run-off experiments. It is not excluded that maintenance of high levels of specific mRNAs in co-culture is favoured by a stabilizing effect of hydrocortisone.

Indeed it has been reported that mRNAs are stabilized in pure rat hepatocyte culture maintained in a hormonally-defined medium[17].

DRUG METABOLISM CAPACITY

Since the cytochrome P-450-dependent mono-oxygenase system plays a major role in drug metabolism we have first measured the total cytochrome P-450 content by a spectral assay. While it declines rapidly in pure rat hepatocyte culture and more slowly in pure human hepatocyte culture, it remains relatively stable in hepatocyte co-cultures from both species[18,19]. Moreover, two isozymes which are components belonging to the two major cytochrome P-450 families in human liver and have a different lobular distribution were studied *in vitro*. As *in vivo*, the 4-mephenytoin hydroxylase isozyme was found in all hepatocytes and the nifedipine oxidase isozyme only in a fraction of cells[20]. These observations indicate that there is no cell selection during the isolation process and that the functional heterogeneity is retained in culture. Cytochrome P-450 responds to inducers; it is markedly increased after treatment with sodium phenobarbital and erythromycin estolate[19]. After a daily treatment for 3 days, 2.1- and 1.8-fold increases in cytochrome P-450 concentration were found in 9-day human hepatocyte co-cultures in the presence of phenobarbital and erythromycin estolate, respectively.

Metabolism of several drugs has been investigated in human hepatocyte co-cultures. In all studies, most of the main metabolites formed *in vivo* were identified *in vitro*, even after several days[21,22]. Thus the two main metabolites of ketotifen formed in humans, namely reduced ketotifen and a glucuronide, were still demonstrated after 3 weeks of co-culture while the glucurono-conjugated compound was no longer demonstrated in 6-day pure culture[21]. Biotransformation of pindolol and fluperlapine was found to be well preserved. Fluperlapine which has the highest first pass *in vivo* was also metabolized faster *in vitro*[22].

These results provide argument indicating that the co-culture system is suitable for studying drug-metabolism interactions and cytotoxicity without the influence of some factors related to the donor or cell preparation. This is particularly important for suspended and short-term cultured human hepatocytes of which functional activities can be greatly influenced by various environmental factors related to the donor (premedication, nutritional status) or by the conditions of cell isolation (duration of the time separating liver resection from the beginning of the dissociation process)[23]. The obtention of hepatocyte cultures from young and old donors should allow determination of whether the drug-metabolizing enzyme capacity is impaired and whether the toxicity of some drugs is more severe in the aged.

FORMATION OF AN EXTRACELLULAR MATRIX

A number of studies have shown that hepatocytes become able to manufacture matrix components, including collagens, fibronectin and glycosaminoglycans but these components remain soluble in the medium[24–26]. After a few days, accumulation of extracellular material can be easily demonstrated in rat hepatocyte co-cultures by the presence of reticulin fibres around and over hepatocyte colonies, using the silver impregnation method[9]

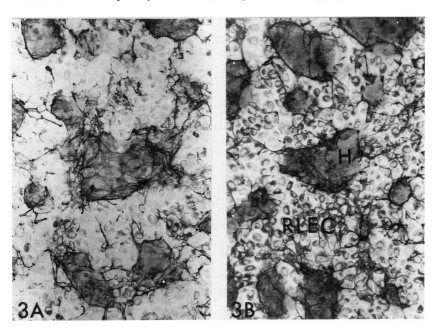

Figure 19.3 Extracellular matrix component accumulation in rat hepatocyte (H) co-cultures. A, reticulin staining; B, immunoperoxidase staining of type III pro-collagen. Note the intracellular staining for type III pro-collagen in rat-liver epithelial cells (RLEC). Day 4 of co-culture. (× 110)

(Figure 19.3A). Among the components already identified in this material are types I, III and IV collagen, fibronectin and laminin[10,27] (Figure 19.3B). The same components were also found in human hepatocyte co-cultures but they accumulate more slowly and remain in lower amounts. In order to evaluate the participation of hepatocytes in this process, we have separated the two cell types by collagenase treatment and the levels of both types I and IV collagen mRNAs were determined in rat hepatocytes after 3 and 7 days of co-culture. Compared to the levels found in freshly isolated cells, mRNAs for both collagens were markedly increased in culture[28].

CO-CULTURE OF CRYOPRESERVED HEPATOCYTES

Availability of human liver samples is limited and irregular but large numbers of cells can often be obtained from a single perfusion. In addition, inter-individual variations in their functional capacity may extensively vary owing to the influence of various factors as stressed above. Therefore it is desirable to store cells in excess in order to run parallel experiments on several cell populations or to reproduce some studies at different times. The only conceivable method for long-term storage of hepatocytes is cryopreservation.

Most of the freezing protocols described until now have been tested on rat hepatocytes and do not result in the restoration of full activity after thawing[29-31]. Recently, we have reconsidered both freezing protocols and culture conditions of frozen cells. When frozen in a nutrient medium added with dimethylsulfoxide, and stored in liquid nitrogen, 50–60% of rat hepatocytes are still able to attach to a support and be cultured, as compared to unfrozen cells. Only when put in co-culture were they capable to restore the capacity to secrete plasma proteins and to metabolize paracetamol at levels close to those found in co-cultures of unfrozen cells[32]. Similar results have been obtained with human hepatocytes. This gives further argument supporting the interest of the co-culture system for the study of differentiated hepatocytes *in vitro*.

CONCLUSIONS

When in co-culture both young and old hepatocytes from various species may be maintained functionally differentiated for several days or weeks. This culture system should become a suitable tool to investigate the key events related to the aging process.

Acknowledgments

We are indebted to Mrs A. Vannier for typing the original manuscript.

REFERENCES

1. Popper, H. (1986). Aging and the liver. In Popper, H. and Schaffner, F. (eds.) *Progress in Liver diseases*. Vol. VIII, pp. 659–83. (Orlando: Grune and Stratton)
2. Guguen-Guillouzo, C. and Guillouzo, A. (1986). Methods for preparation of adult and fetal hepatocytes. In Guillouzo, A. and Guguen-Guillouzo, C. (eds.) *Isolated and Cultured Hepatocytes*. pp. 1–12. (Paris: Les Editions INSERM; and London: John Libbey)
3. Guguen-Guillouzo, C. and Guillouzo, A. (1983). Modulation of functional activities in cultured rat hepatocytes. *Mol. Cell. Biochem.*, **53/54**, 35–56
4. Guzelian, P. S., Bissell, D. M. and Meyer, U. A. (1977). Drug metabolism in adult rat hepatocytes in primary monolayer culture. *Gastroenterology*, **72**, 1232–9
5. Fahl, W. E., Michalopoulos, G., Sattler, G. L., Jefcoate, C. R. and Pitot, H. C. (1979). Characteristics of microsomal enzyme controls in primary cultures of rat hepatocytes. *Arch. Biochem. Biophys.*, **192**, 61–72

6. Clayton, D. F. and Darnell, J. E. (1983). Changes in liver-specific compared to common gene transcription during primary culture of mouse hepatocytes. *Mol. Cell Biol.*, **3**, 1552–61

7. Fraslin, J. M., Kneip, B., Vaulont, S., Glaise, D., Munnich, A. and Guguen-Guillouzo, C. (1985). Dependence of hepatocyte specific gene expression on cell–cell interactions in primary culture. *EMBO J.*, **4**, 2487–91

8. Bissell, D. M. and Guzelian, P. (1980). Phenotypic stability of adult rat hepatocytes in primary monolayer culture. *Ann. NY Acad. Sci.*, **349**, 85–98

9. Guguen-Guillouzo, C., Clément, B., Baffet, G., Beaumont, C., Morel-Chany, E., Glaise, D. and Guillouzo, A. (1983). Maintenance and reversibility of active albumin secretion by adult rat hepatocytes co-cultured with another liver epithelial cell type. *Exp. Cell Res.*, **143**, 47–54

10. Clément, B., Guguen-Guillouzo, C., Campion, J. P., Glaise, D., Bourel, M. and Guillouzo, A. (1984). Long-term co-cultures of adult human hepatocytes with rat liver epithelial cells: modulation of albumin secretion and accumulation of extracellular material. *Hepatology*, **4**, 373–80

11. Guguen-Guillouzo, C. (1986). Role of homotypic and heterotypic cell interactions in expression of specific functions by cultured hepatocytes. In Guillouzo, A. and Guguen-Guillouzo, C. (eds.) *Isolated and Cultured Hepatocytes.* pp. 259–84. (Paris: Les Editions INSERM; and London: John Libbey)

12. Morel-Chany, E., Guillouzo C., Trincal, G. and Szajnert, M. F. (1978). 'Spontaneous' neoplastic transformation *in vitro* of epithelial cell strains of rat liver: cytology, growth and enzymatic activities. *Eur. J. Cancer*, **14**, 1341–52

13. Mesnil, M., Fraslin, J. M. Piccoli, C., Yamasaki, H. and Guguen-Guillouzo, C. (1987). Cell contact but not junctional communication with biliary epithelial cells is required for hepatocytes to maintain differentiated functions. *Exp. Cell Res.*, **173**, 524–33

14. Baffet, G., Clément, B., Glaise, D., Guillouzo, A. and Guguen-Guillouzo, C. (1982). Hydrocortisone modulates the production of extracellular material and albumin in long-term co-culture of adult rat hepatocytes with other liver epithelial cells. *Biochem. Biophys. Res. Commun.*, **109**, 507–12

15. Guillouzo, A., Delers, F., Clément, B., Bernard, M. and Engler, R. (1984). Long-term production of acute phase proteins by adult rat hepatocytes co-cultured with another liver cell type in serum-free medium. *Biochem. Biophys. Res. Commun.*, **120**, 311–17

16. Le Breton, J. P., Daveau, M., Hiron, M., Fontaine, M., Biou, M., Gilbert, D. and Guguen-Guillouzo, C. (1986). Long-term biosynthesis of complement C3 and α-1 acid glycoprotein by adult rat hepatocytes in a co-culture system with an epithelial liver cell type. *Biochem. J.*, **235**, 421–7

17. Jefferson, D. M., Clayton, D. F., Darnell, J. E. Jr and Rein, L. M. (1984). Post-transcriptional modulation of gene expression by media conditions in cultured rat hepatocytes. *Mol. Cell Biol.*, **4**, 1929–34

18. Bégué, J. M., Guguen-Guillouzo, C., Pasdeloup, N. and Guillouzo, A. (1984). Prolonged maintenance of active cytochrome P-450 in adult rat hepatocytes co-cultured with another liver cell type. *Hepatology*, **4**, 839–42

19. Guillouzo, A., Beaune, P., Gascoin, M. N., Bégué, J. M., Campion, J. P., Guengerich, F. P. and Guguen-Guillouzo, C. (1985). Maintenance of cytochrome P-450 in cultural adult human hepatocytes. *Biochem. Pharmacol.*, **34**, 2991–5

20. Ratanasavanh, D., Beaune, P., Baffet, G., Rissel, M., Kremers, P., Guengerich, F. P. and Guillouzo, A. (1986). Immunocytochemical evidence for the maintenance of cytochrome P-450 isozymes, NADPH cytochrome *c* reductase and epoxide hydrolase in pure and mixed primary cultures of adult human hepatocytes. *J. Histochem. Cytochem.*, **34**, 527–33

21. Bégué, J. M., Le Bigot, J. F., Guguen-Guillouzo, C., Kiechel, J. R. and Guillouzo, A. (1983). Cultured human adult hepatocytes: a new model for drug metabolism studies. *Biochem. Pharmacol.*, **32**, 1643–6

22. Guillouzo, A., Bégué, J. M., Maurer, G. and Koch, P. (1988). Identification of metabolic pathways of pindolol and fluperlapine in adult human hepatocyte cultures. *Xenobiotica.* (In press)

23. Guillouzo, A., Ratanasavanh, D., Bégué, J. M. and Guguen-Guillouzo, C. (1987). Utilisation des hépatocytes isolés pour l'évaluation de l'hépatotoxicité des médicaments. In *Développement et évaluation du médicament*, **157**, 163–74. (Paris: Les Editions INSERM)

24. Diegelmann, R. F., Cohen, I. K. and Guzelian, P. S. (1980). Rapid degradation of newly synthetized collagen by primary cultures of adult rat hepatocytes. *Biochem. Biophys. Res. Commun.*, **97**, 819–26

25. Voss, B., Allam, S., Rauterberg, J., Ulrich, K., Gieselmann, V. and Von Figura, K. (1979). Primary cultures of rat hepatocytes synthesize fibronectin. *Biochem. Biophys. Res. Commun.*, **90**, 1348–54

26. Gressner, A. M. and Grouls, P. (1982). Stimulated synthesis of glycosaminoglycans in suspension cultures of hepatocytes from subacutely injured livers. *Digestion.* **23**, 259–64

27. Clément, B., Rescan, P. Y., Baffet, G., Loréal, O., Lehry, D., Campion, J. P. and Guillouzo, A. (1988). Hepatocytes may produce laminin in fibrotic liver and in primary culture. *Hepatology.* (In press)

28. Clément, B., Laurent, M., Guguen-Guillouzo, C., Lebeau, G. and Guillouzo, A. (1988). Types I and IV procollagen gene expression in cultured rat hepatocytes. *Coll. Rel. Res.* (In press)

29. Fuller, B. J., Grout, B. W. and Woods, R. J. (1982). Biochemical and ultrastructural examination of cryopreserved hepatocytes in rat. *Cryobiology*, **19**, 493–502

30. Novicki, D. L., Irons, G. P., Strom, S. C., Jirtle, R. and Michalopoulos, G. (1982). Cryopreservation of isolated rat hepatocytes. *In Vitro*, **18**, 393–9

31. Jackson, B. A., Davies, J. E. and Chipman, J. K. (1985). Cytochrome P-450 activity following cryopreservation and monolayer culture. *Biochem. Pharmacol.*, **34**, 3389–91

20
Albumin synthesis in aging

C. F. A. VAN BEZOOIJEN and G. J. M. J. HORBACH

INTRODUCTION

The lifespan of organisms is generally considered to be partially under genetic control. Changes in the genetic apparatus and/or in the flow of genetic information to proteins, therefore, could be one of the mechanisms involved in the aging process. Aging and protein synthesis have been studied extensively; however, most studies performed on this topic can be considered as generalizations, since they do not take into account that aging may exert a differential influence on the synthesis of individual proteins. For a full understanding of the influence of aging on protein synthesis, it is of importance to study the synthesis of individual proteins with age. This chapter will deal with the influence of age on the synthesis and elimination of one individual protein, i.e. rat serum albumin.

The study started by measuring the albumin synthesis of hepatocytes isolated from rats of different ages. To determine whether possible changes in albumin synthesis with age reflect overall changes in the protein synthesis of the hepatocytes or a change in the capacity to synthesize an individual liver-specific protein, the protein synthesizing capacity was also measured. The following questions were posed:

- Are possible changes in albumin synthesis *in vitro* with age correlated with possible age-related changes in albumin elimination *in vivo*?

- Are possible changes in albumin synthesis regulated at the level of the albumin mRNA, and/or by changes in the translational capacity of this mRNA?

- Are possible age-related changes in albumin mRNA levels attributable to changes in the rate of transcription of the albumin gene and/or to a changed turnover rate with age?

- Are there qualitative changes in albumin mRNA with age?

RESULTS

Albumin synthesis by hepatocytes isolated from rats of different ages

Hepatocytes freshly isolated from 3-, 12-, 24-, 31- and 36-month-old rats were used to measure their capacity for albumin synthesis. Methods and optimal incubation conditions have been previously published[1-3]. Table 20.1 shows a significant decrease in the amount of albumin synthesized per 10^6 hepatocytes isolated from female WAG/Rij rats between 3 and 24 months of

Table 20.1 Albumin synthesis by hepatocytes isolated from female WAG/Rij rats of different ages*

Age (months)	Protein content of paren-chymal cells (mg/10^6 cells)	Albumin synthesis	
		$\mu g/h \cdot 10^6$ cells	$\mu g/h \cdot mg$ cellular protein
3	1.47 ± 0.10 (11)	5.77 ± 0.79 (12)	3.94 ± 0.60
12	1.80 ± 0.10 (4)**	3.73 ± 0.34 (8)**	2.06 ± 0.20**
24	2.03 ± 0.09 (3)**	2.29 ± 0.30 (7)**·†	1.13 ± 0.15**·†
31	–	6.36 ± 0.78 (3)†·††	–
36	2.01 ± 0.11 (5)**	9.8 ± 1.7 (7)**·†·††	4.88 ± 0.89†·††

* Mean ± S.E.; number of different cell preparations in parentheses
** Value differs significantly ($p < 0.05$) from the 3-month value
† Value differs significantly ($p < 0.05$) from the 12-month value
†† Value differs significantly ($p < 0.05$) from the 24-month value

age. Contrasting with this, a sharp increase was found after 24 months up to 36 months. When the albumin-synthesizing capacity was expressed on a protein basis, approximately the same pattern of age-related changes was observed, with the exception that hepatocytes isolated from 36-month-old rats did not significantly synthesize more albumin than cells isolated from 3-month-old ones. This latter phenomenon was due to an increase in protein content of the cells with age.

Protein synthesis by hepatocytes isolated from rats of different ages

The influence of age on the capacity to synthesize protein was determined with hepatocytes isolated from 3-, 12-, 24-, 31- and 36-month-old rats. Methods and optimal incubation conditions have been previously published[4,5]. The cells used for measuring the protein synthesis were obtained from the same cell isolation as those used for measuring the albumin synthesis. A significant decrease was observed between 3 and 12 months (Table 20.2). Thereafter, no change was observed up to 24 months of age. A considerable increase in protein synthesis was measured after 24 months of age up to the age of 36 months. The value obtained for the protein synthesizing capacity of 36-month-old rats did not differ significantly from that obtained for 3-month-old rats (Table 20.2).

Table 20.2 Total protein synthesis by liver parenchymal cells from female WAG/Rij rats of different ages*

Age (months)	Protein content of paren-chymal cells (mg/10⁶ cells)	Incorporation of leucine	
		nmol/h·10⁶ cells	nmol/h·mg cellular protein
3	1.47 ± 0.10 (11)	14.4 ± 1.4 (10)	8.70 ± 1.10
12	1.80 ± 0.10 (4)**	9.8 ± 1.4 (6)**	5.53 ± 0.91**
24	2.03 ± 0.09 (3)**	8.4 ± 1.2 (5)**	4.14 ± 0.62**
31	–	12.9 ± 2.8 (4)	–
36	2.01 ± 0.11 (5)**	14.7 ± 1.2 (7)† ·††	7.32 ± 0.70††

*Mean ± S.E.; number of different cell preparations in parentheses
** Value differs significantly ($p < 0.05$) from the 3-month value
† Value differs significantly ($p < 0.05$) from the 12-month value
†† Value differs significantly ($p < 0.05$) from the 24-month value

The ratio of albumin versus total protein synthesis by isolated hepatocytes with age

One of the reasons for choosing the protein-synthesizing capacity as a functional characteristic of isolated hepatocytes was to find out whether changes in albumin-synthesizing capacity with age are representative for changes in all proteins. To some extent, the age-related pattern of albumin synthesis by hepatocytes was comparable with that observed for total protein synthesis (Tables 20.1 and 20.2)—a decrease early in life and an increase in old age. However, hepatocytes isolated from 36-month-old rats synthesized significantly more albumin than did cells from 3-month-old ones. With respect to protein synthesis, cells isolated from 3- and 36-month-old rats did not

Table 20.3 The relationship between the ratio of albumin versus total protein synthesis and the age of the rats from which the hepatocytes were isolated

Age (months)	Ratio albumin versus total protein synthesis*
3	0.40 ± 0.70 (11)
12	0.38 ± 0.06 (7)
24	0.27 ± 0.05 (6)
31	0.49 ± 0.12 (4)
36	0.67 ± 0.13 (7)††

*The data are expressed as: (μg/albumin/h·10⁶ cells)/(nmol leucine/h·10⁶ cells). Mean ± S.E. number of different cell preparations in parentheses
†† Value differs significantly ($p < 0.05$) from 24-month value

differ. As a consequence, the ratio between albumin and protein synthesis did not change during the first 24 months and increased significantly between 24 and 36 months (Table 20.3). An increase only in albumin synthesis is possible, since albumin synthesis represents only 7–10% of total protein synthesis[6,7].

Age-related changes in albumin elimination

In order to determine whether the increase in albumin synthesis observed with hepatocytes isolated from the older rats might be explained as a compensatory effect for a loss of albumin in these rats, the elimination of albumin *in vivo* was measured with age. Methods have been previously published[8]. From individual plasma radioactivity curves (obtained after injection of albumin isolated from 3-month-old rats into rats which are longitudinally studied at different ages), the elimination half-life ($t_\frac{1}{2}$, the apparent volume of distribution (Vd_{app}) and the systemic clearance (Cl_s) were calculated. Age-related

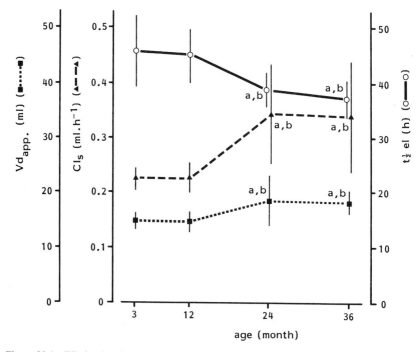

Figure 20.1 Elimination half-life, apparent volume of distribution and systemic clearance of albumin in female WAG/Rij rats determined longitudinally. The number of rats used at 3, 12, 24 and 36 months were 30, 29, 27, 6, respectively. (a) Value differs significantly ($p < 0.05$) from 3-month value. (b) Value differs significantly ($p < 0.05$) from 12-month value. Values expressed as means ± S.D.

changes in these three characteristics are shown in Figure 20.1 The elimination $t_\frac{1}{2}$ decreased between 12 and 24 months and remained constant thereafter. The Vd_{app} increased between 12 and 24 months. After 24 months no significant change in Vd_{app} was observed. The albumin clearance increased between 12 and 24 months of age. All rats showed this increase. After 24 months no significant change in the clearance was found.

When albumin was isolated from rats of the same age as the recipients, about the same figures were obtained except for the elimination $t_\frac{1}{2}$, Vd_{app} and Cl_s of the 36-month-old rats. Their elimination $t_\frac{1}{2}$ did not differ from the 3-

and 12-month value, whereas their Vd_{app} and the Cl_s were higher than that of 24-month-old rats, indicating that the albumin molecule might be changed in 36-month-old rats.

Three main processes are responsible for the albumin elimination: urinary albumin excretion, gastrointestinal protein loss and fluid-phase endocytosis. The increase in albumin elimination is mainly owing to increased fluid-phase endocytosis. The urinary albumin excretion only accounted for 2.4% of the total albumin elimination in the old rats. Gastrointestinal protein loss, probably an estimation of albumin elimination, remained constant with age[8–10].

MOLECULAR REGULATION OF THE ALBUMIN SYNTHESIS WITH AGE

Another objective of the study was to investigate the molecular basis of the age-related increase in albumin synthesis, specifically, whether this change was caused by a change in the level of messenger RNA and/or by a change in the translational capacity of this messenger RNA. Total post-nuclear RNA and polyribosomes, both membrane-bound and free, were prepared from liver homogenates. For technical details see Horbach et al.[11].

No change in the RNA content of the several fractions prepared from liver homogenate was observed[11]. The albumin mRNA content was determined in the various RNA fractions by a molecular hybridization technique using a labelled albumin cDNA probe[11]. The amount of albumin mRNA sequences per mg RNA is greater at 24 and 36 months of age than at 3 and 12 months of age in the post-nuclear RNA fraction. This higher content of albumin mRNA is attributed to the increased albumin mRNA content in the membrane-bound polyribosomal fractions and especially in the poly(A)$^-$-RNA fraction (Table 20.4). The albumin mRNA content per whole liver increased between 12 and 36 months of age (see Table 20.5). Apart from the increase in albumin mRNA concentration at between 12 and 24 months of age, an increase in total liver albumin mRNA content at between 24 and 36 months is observed, owing to an increase in liver weight. It is notable that at 24 and 36 months of age, more albumin mRNA is present in the poly(A)$^-$-RNA than in the poly(A)$^+$-RNA, indicating the absence or shortening of the poly(A)-tail of albumin mRNAs with age.

In order to study the translational capacity of the albumin mRNA, liver polyribosomes (both free and membrane-bound) were isolated from rats of different ages.

No change with age was found in the protein synthetic activity of either free or membrane-bound polyribosomes. The albumin synthesis by free polyribosomes remained unchanged with age[11] whereas the albumin synthetic activity per μg RNA of membrane-bound polyribosomes was higher at 24 and 36 months of age when compared with younger animals (Figure 20.2).

Although the results of the increased albumin synthesis at 24 and 36 months are consistent with the findings of the increased albumin mRNA levels, albumin synthesis is not proportionally increased with the elevated albumin

Table 20.4 Age-related changes in the relative amount of albumin mRNA in several RNA-fractions prepared from liver homogenates of female WAG/Rij rats

	Relative albumin mRNA content as percentage of total RNA* Age (months)			
	3	12	24	36
Total post-nuclear RNA	0.15 ±0.01	0.17 ±0.02	0.31 ±0.02**·†	0.31±0.02**·†
Poly(A)⁺-RNA	3.4 ±0.4	4.0 ±1.3	4.2 ±0.4	4.1 ±0.5
'Poly(A)⁻'-RNA	0.06 ±0.01	0.07 ±0.02	0.20 ±0.02**·†	0.23 ±0.04**·†
Membrane-bound polyribosomes	0.22 ±0.08	0.23 ±0.07	0.44 ±0.10**·†	0.46 ±0.12**·†
Free polyribosomes	0.002±0.000	0.002±0.000	0.002±0.000	0.002±0.000

* Values are expressed as means ± S.D. for a minimum of 3 experiments with 2 livers per experiment
** Value differs significantly ($p < 0.05$) from 3-month value
† Value differs significantly ($p < 0.05$) from 12-month value

Table 20.5 Influence of age on the albumin mRNA content in several RNA-fractions prepared from liver homogenates of female WAG/Rij rats

	Albumin mRNA content per whole liver (µg)* Age (months)			
	3	12	24	36
Total post-nuclear RNA	44.5±4.2	47.8±2.1	96 ±10**·†	137 ±11**·†·††
Poly(A)⁺-RNA	16.8±3.9	28 ±11	24.8±5.5	38 ±13**
'Poly(A)⁻'-RNA	16.1±1.9	20.0±4.0	61.3±4.3**·†	96 ±12**·†·††
Membrane-bound polyribosomes	42 ±15	38.4±9.0	70 ±14**·†	109 ±20**·†·††
Free polyribosomes	0.11±0.01	0.11±0.01	0.13±0.03	0.15 ±0.03

* Values are expressed as means ± S.D. for a minimum of 3 experiments with 2 livers per experiment
** Value differs significantly ($p < 0.05$) from 3-month value
† Value differs significantly ($p < 0.05$) from 12-month value
†† Value differs significantly ($p < 0.05$) from 24-month value

mRNA level (50% (Figure 20.2) vs. 100% (Table 20.4). This suggests that some, if not all, albumin mRNAs present in the liver in older rats are biologically less active than those found in young animals. It can be concluded that the age-related increase in the amount of albumin synthesis is caused by a two-fold increase in the amount of albumin mRNA combined with a 25% decrease in the translational activity of this mRNA.

Molecular basis of the age-related increase in albumin mRNA levels

In the previous section it was shown that the molecular basis for the age-related increase in albumin synthesis is at the level of the albumin mRNA.

204

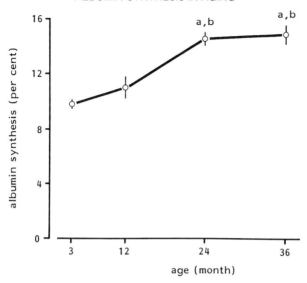

Figure 20.2 Synthesis of albumin-like material by membrane-bound polyribosomes of female WAG/Rij rats of different ages. Cell-free albumin synthesis was investigated in age-matched cell sap. The albumin synthesis is expressed as a percentage of total protein synthesis. Values are expressed as means ± S.D. for a minimum of 3 experiments with two livers per experiment. (a) Value differs significantly ($p < 0.05$) from 3-month value. (b) Value differs significantly ($p < 0.05$) from 12-month value.

Changes in the steady-state levels of mRNA could be due to either of two processes: (1) changes in mRNA synthesis and (2) changes in mRNA turnover. No change with age was observed in the total transcriptional activity of isolated nuclei[11–13]. The rate of transcription of the albumin gene was assessed by hybridizing the newly synthesized RNA molecules with filter-bound albumin specific cDNA[12]. Aging did not influence the transcriptional rate of the albumin gene. The amount of albumin-specific RNA sequences in rat liver nuclei also showed no age-related changes[11–13]. These data yield evidence that the increase in albumin mRNA content in rats with age is not controlled by transcriptional processes, but might be caused by a decreased turnover of this mRNA. Since the data on the influence of age on the albumin mRNA content in several RNA fractions (Table 20.5), indicate that a decrease in the length of the poly(A)-tail of the albumin mRNA may play an important role in the physiological control mechanism of albumin synthesis, additional studies were performed with regard to the length of the poly(A)-tails in total cytoplasmic RNA. An age-related shift in the overall distribution of the poly(A)-tails was observed (Figure 20.3). The relative amount of poly(A)-tails longer than 161A-residues is decreased between the ages of 12 and 24 months, whereas the amount of poly(A)-tail shorter than 115A-residues is increased between these two ages.

The physiological significance of the age-related decrease in the poly(A)-tail length, especially of albumin mRNA is unclear. The shortening of the

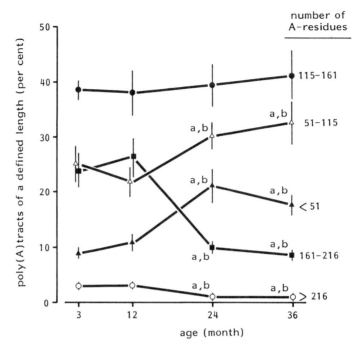

Figure 20.3 The influence of age on the size-distribution of poly(A)-tracts of rat liver mRNA. Values are expressed as means ± S.D. for 5 experiments. (a) Value differs significantly ($p < 0.05$) from 3-month value. (b) Value differs significantly ($p < 0.05$) from 12-month value.

poly(A)-tail of albumin RNA coincides with a diminished translational activity of this mRNA in polyribosomes. Whether there is a direct correlation between these two observations remains to be established.

DISCUSSION

The albumin synthesis by hepatocytes isolated from female WAG/Rij rats of different ages decreased between 3 and 24 months of age. Thereafter, an increase was observed (Table 20.1). For a comparison between the albumin synthesis of isolated hepatocytes with that of membrane-bound poly-ribosomes, calculations should be performed. By multiplying the total amount of albumin mRNA in membrane-bound polyribosomes per whole liver (Table 20.5) with the translatability of this mRNA (100% in 3- and 12-month-old rats and 75% in 24- and 36-month-old ones) 'albumin synthesis' per liver could be estimated. This albumin synthesis increased after 12 months. At 36 months of age the albumin synthesis is twice as high as that of 3- and 12-month-old rats. So there is a discrepancy between the data obtained with isolated hepatocytes and those obtained with polyribosomes. Several expla-nations are possible. Among them are the intracellular organization of the hepatocyte, the amount of polysomes per hepatocyte and the number of hepatocytes per liver. Contradictory data were also found with respect to protein synthesis. Again a biphasic pattern was observed with the isolated hepatocytes – a decrease during the first year of life and an increase during the third year of life. Protein synthesis by free and membrane-bound poly-ribosomes, however, remained constant with age. Nevertheless, the ratio of albumin synthesis versus protein synthesis increased in old age in both experimental systems.

The observed increase in albumin synthesis in old age with the isolated hepatocytes as well as with the membrane-bound polyribosomes is in agree-ment with the increase in *in vivo* synthesis of albumin observed by Beauchene *et al.*[14], by Salatka *et al.*[15] and by Ove *et al.*[16]. Studies by Chen *et al.*[17] showed that also in isolated rat liver microsomes, albumin synthesis increased with age. This increase in albumin synthesis in old age can be explained by a compensation of the liver for the increased albumin elimination in late age (Figure 20.1). The observed increase in albumin elimination in this longitudinal study is in agreement with the previously observed increase in albumin elimination in a cross-sectional study[8]. This increased elimination was mainly owing to an increased fluid-phase endocytosis.

The increase in albumin synthesis was regulated by an increase in the albumin mRNA content of the liver (Tables 20.4 and 20.5), whereas its translation capacity decreased by 25%.

The increase in the amount of albumin mRNA was not owing to an increased albumin gene transcription rate but probably to a decreased turn-over of this mRNA. The albumin mRNA revealed a shortening of the poly(A)-tails which can be probably attributed to an increase in stability. Poly(A)-tails in the cytoplasm are continually subjected to the action of nucleases which results in a shortening of the tail over time. Therefore, the observed shortening of the poly(A)-tail of albumin mRNA could be due to its prolonged presence in the cytoplasm.

The results obtained in this study demonstrate that an individual protein is not regulated via a general pattern but in its own individual way. In addition, a number of age-related changes (both at the molecular and the organ level) are observed that influence the metabolism of rat serum albumin. Despite these changes (which affect both albumin synthesis rates and albumin elimination rates), the aging female WAG/Rij rat is still capable of main-taining an unchanged plasma albumin level[8] and possesses sufficient flex-ibility, as far as albumin is concerned, to maintain homeostasis with age.

References

1. Van Bezooijen, C. F. A., Grell, T. and Knook, D. L. (1976). Albumin synthesis by liver parenchymal cells isolated from young, adult and old rats. *Biochem. Biophys. Res. Commun.*, **21**, 513
2. Van Bezooijen, C. F. A., Grell, T. and Knook, D. L. (1977). Age-related changes in albumin synthesis of isolated liver parenchymal cells. In Schmidt, U. J., Brüschke, G., Lang, E., Viidik, A., Platt, D., Frolkis, V. V. and Schulz, F. H. (eds.) *Fifth European Symposium on Basic Research in Gerontology*. p. 584. (Erlangen: Verlag Dr Med. D. Staube)
3. Van Bezooijen, C. F. A. and Knook, D. L. (1977). Aging changes in bromsulfophthalein

uptake, albumin and total protein synthesis in isolated hepatocytes. In Platt, D. (ed.) *Liver and Aging*. pp. 227–41. (Stuttgart, New York: Schattauer Verlag)

4. Van Bezooijen, C. F. A., Grell, T. and Knook, D. L. (1977). The effect of age on protein synthesis by isolated liver parenchymal cells. *Mech. Age. Dev.*, **6**, 293

5. Van Bezooijen, C. F. A., Sakkee, A. N. and Knook, D. L. (1981). Sex and strain dependency of age-related changes in protein synthesis of isolated hepatocytes. *Mech. Age. Dev.*, **17**, 11

6. Peters, T. and Peters, J. C. (1972). The biosynthesis of rat serum albumin. Intracellular transport of albumin and rates of albumin and liver protein synthesis *in vivo* under various physiological conditions. *J. Biol. Chem.*, **247**, 3858

7. Edwards, K., Schreiber, G., Dryburgh, H., Urban, J., Fleischer, S. and Inglis, A. S. (1976). Synthesis of albumin via a precursor protein in cell suspensions from rat liver. *Eur. J. Biochem.*, **63**, 303

8. Horbach, G. J. M. J., Yap, S. H. and Van Bezooijen, C. F. A. (1983). Age-related changes in albumin elimination in female WAG/Rij rats. *Biochem. J.*, **216**, 309

9. Horbach, G. J. M. J., Van Leeuwen, R. E. W., Yap, S. H. and Van Bezooijen, C. F. A. (1986). Changes in fluid-phase endocytosis in the rat with age and their relation to total albumin elimination. *Mech. Age. Dev.*, **33**, 305

10. Horbach, G. J. M. J., Van Leeuwen, R. E. W., Yap, S. H. and Van Bezooijen, C. F. A. (1984). Age-related changes in fluid-phase endocytosis in female WAG/Rij rats. In Van Bezooijen, C. F. A. (ed.) *Pharmacological, Morphological and Physiological Aspects of Liver Aging*. p. 19. (Rijswijk: EURAGE)

11. Horbach, G. J. M. J., Princen, H. M. G., Van der Kroef, M., Van Bezooijen, C. F. A. and Yap, S. H. (1984). Changes in the sequence content of albumin mRNA and its translational activity in the rat liver with age. *Biochim. Biophys. Acta*, **783**, 60

12. Horbach, G. J. M. J. Albumin Metabolism and Aging, thesis, 1986. (Maastricht)

13. Horbach, G. J. M. J., Van der Boom, H., Van Bezooijen, C. F. A. and Yap, S. H. (1986). Molecular aspects of age-related changes in albumin synthesis in rats. In Van Bezooijen, C. F. A., Miglio, F. and Knook, D. L. (eds.). *Liver, Drugs and Aging*, p. 121. (Rijswijk: EURAGE)

14. Beauchene, R. E., Roeder, L. M. and Barrows, C. H. (1970). The inter-relationships of age, tissue protein synthesis, and proteinuria. *J. Gerontol.*, **25**, 359

15. Salatka, K., Kresge, D., Harris, L. Jr., Edelstein, D. and Ove, P. (1971). Rat serum protein changes with age. *Exp. Gerontol.*, **6**, 25

16. Ove, P., Obenrader, M. and Lansing, A. I. (1972). Synthesis and degradation of liver proteins in young and old rats. *Biochim. Biophys. Acta*, **277**, 211

17. Chen. J. C., Ove, P. and Lansing, A. I. (1973). *In vitro* synthesis of microsomal protein and albumin in young and old rats. *Biochim. Biophys. Acta*, **312**, 598

21
Aging of sinusoidal liver cells

A. BROUWER, A. M. DE LEEUW, R. J. BARELDS and D. L. KNOOK

INTRODUCTION

The liver consists of various cell types, each of which has its own functional, morphological and biochemical characteristics. The parenchymal cells are the most abundant liver cell type, constituting about 60% of the total number of cells present and occupying about 85% of the liver volume[1]. The non-parenchymal (or sinusoidal) liver cells are composed of three main cell types, viz. Kupffer, endothelial and fat-storing cells, which, together, account for about 35% of all liver cells, but occupy only 6–7% of the liver volume[1]. Despite this, they are now of primary importance for maintenance of the structure, organization and function of the liver lobule[2,3]. During the last decade, our understanding of sinusoidal cells has increased greatly as a result of the development of techniques for the isolation, purification and cultivation of each of the sinusoidal cell types[2,4–8]. The localization of the sinusoidal cells within the liver and their ultrastructural appearance are illustrated in Figures 21.1–21.4.

Kupffer cells are tissue macrophages, which protect against micro-organisms and clear foreign and endogenous particles and macromolecules from the circulation[2,9,10]. The cells are primarily responsible for the removal of bacteria, bacterial endotoxins, colloidal substances and cellular debris from the blood. In addition, they have the capacity to synthesize and excrete several signal molecules (monokines), which may exert profound effects on the functions of other cells present in the liver and elsewhere in the body. These monokines include pyrogens, immuno-modulators, prostaglandins and other inflammatory mediators, and factors that modulate protein synthesis or proliferation of parenchymal and fat-storing cells in the liver. The ultra-structure of Kupffer cells is very similar to that of other macrophages. They possess a ruffled membrane and their cytoplasm contains numerous lysosomal vacuoles (Figure 21.2).

Endothelial cells, which cover the liver sinusoids, are of a special type[2]. Unlike vascular endothelium, they form a fenestrated lining, without an underlying basement membrane, which facilitates direct contact between

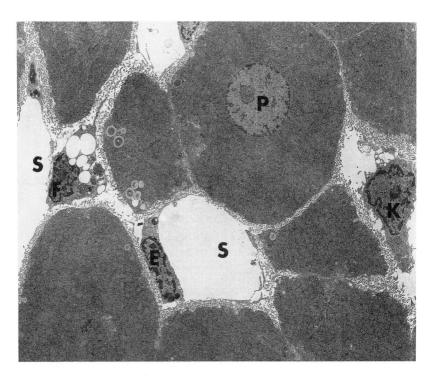

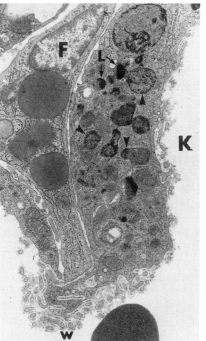

Figure 21.1 Transmission electron micrograph (TEM) of the liver of a 3-month-old female BN/BiRij rat. S, sinusoid; P, parenchymal cell; K, Kupffer cell; E, endothelial cell; F, fat-storing cell. (×2450)

Figure 21.2 TEM of Kupffer cell (K) from a 33-month-old rat, with lipid-like electron dense material (L) and ferritin (arrowheads) inside lysosomal structures. F, fat-storing cell; w: worm-like structures. (×8300)

Figure 21.3 TEM of an endothelial cell (E) from a 30-month-old rat, with lysosomal ferritin accumulation (arrows). Arrowheads indicate fenestrations. (× 8300)

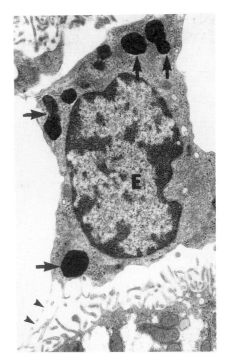

Figure 21.4 TEM of a fat-storing cell (F) from a 24-month-old rat. L, lipid droplets; S, sinusoid; arrows indicate dilated rough endoplasmic reticulum; arrowheads indicate endothelial lining. (× 6650)

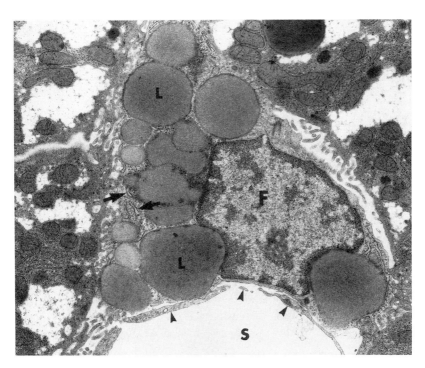

solutes and small particles present in the plasma and the parenchymal and fat-storing cells that are situated beneath the endothelial lining (Figure 20.3). The endothelial cells of the liver have a remarkable capacity to take up and catabolize macromolecules, including glycosaminoglycans, (glyco)proteins and lipoproteins[11,12]. In addition, they, also, can be induced to produce mediators, such as prostacyclin and other vasoactive substances.

Fat-storing cells are located in the space of Disse, between recesses of parenchymal cells (Figure 21.4). Their main function probably is the storage of vitamin A[13]. Despite their relatively small number (they occupy less than 2% of the liver volume[1]), the cells generally contain the majority of all vitamin A in the mammalian body[13]. Fat-storing cells also contain high concentrations of binding proteins and enzymes necessary for the metabolism of vitamin A[14]. The involvement of fat-storing cells in the production of connective tissue components is controversial, although there is strong circumstantial evidence that these fibroblast-like cells have the capacity to synthesize several types of collagen and may contribute to the excess deposition of collagen and glycosaminoglycans during fibrosis of the liver[15].

In this brief review, the influence of aging on the morphology, biochemistry and function of each type of sinusoidal cell is discussed. One study on the age-related changes in the relative numbers of sinusoidal cells[16] shows that

Table 21.1 Relative numbers of endothelial, Kupffer and fat-storing cells in female BN/BiRij rats of different ages*

Age (months)**	Endothelial cells	Kupffer cells	Fat-storing cells
3 (3)	49	20	31
6 (2)	44	23	33
12 (3)	43	21	36
24 (3)	44	24	33
33 (2)	49	23	28

* Data presented as a percentage of the total number of sinusoidal cells
** Number of animals in which cells were counted per age group in parentheses; 150–200 nucleated cells were determined per animal

the relative number of Kupffer, endothelial and fat-storing cells in rat liver is constant throughout the entire life span (Table 21.1). Thus it seems likely, that the numbers of sinusoidal cells per unit liver volume do not change during aging. However, since, in rats, liver weight does increase with age (roughly in parallel with body weight) the total number of sinusoidal cells in liver increases[16]. In contrast, liver weight in humans decreases towards the end of the life span.

SINUSOIDAL LIVER CELLS AND AGING

Morphologic and ultrastructural changes in sinusoidal cells during aging

Kupffer cells

The morphological and ultrastructural changes observed in Kupffer cells during aging do not appear to be dramatic. An increase in haemosiderin pigment and auto-fluorescent material is observed[17] by light microscopy and ultrastructural studies[16] have shown that there is increased accumulation of electron-dense. lipid-like material and of ferritin into membrane-bound vacuoles, probably lysosomes (Figures 21.2 and 21.5).

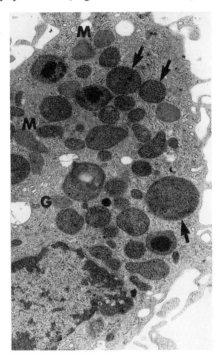

Figure 21.5 TEM of a Kupffer cell from a 36-month-old rat after 24 h in culture. Note the abundance of lysosomal ferritin deposition (arrows). G, Golgi system; M, mitochondria. (× 12 800)

Endothelial cells

Organelles present in the endothelial processes which cover the sinusoids and in the perinuclear cytoplasm, such as the Golgi system, mitochondria and the tubular system show a fairly constant appearance at all ages. However, from after 6 months the vacuoles of the lysosomal system became filled with particulate electron-dense material which closely resembled ferritin (Figure 21.3). Similar particles were observed lying free in the cytoplasm. The ferritin nature of the particles was confirmed by X-ray elemental analysis which revealed the presence of large amounts of iron[16].

Fat-storing cells

Fat-storing cells have shown clear age-related changes in their ultrastructural morphology. Cells in livers of 3-month-old rats contained relatively small numbers of lipid droplets and considerable parts of the cytoplasm were occupied by cell organelles such as a Golgi system, swollen cisternae of the rough endoplasmic reticulum and mitochondria. With advancing age of the animal, fat-storing cells became increasingly filled with lipid droplets (Figure 21.4) and relatively less cytoplasmic space remains for other cell organelles. Concomitantly, the volume of the fat-storing cells increases. Since these lipid droplets[13] in fat-storing cells are known to contain about 80% of all liver vitamin A, it is likely that the increase in their lipid content is related to increased storage of vitamin A during aging.

Biochemical changes during aging

Characterization of the enzyme content of sinusoidal cells during aging

The first studies on the effects of aging sinusoidal liver cells were performed with unseparated sinusoidal cell preparations, containing both endothelial ($\pm 65\%$) and Kupffer cells ($\pm 25\%$)[18,19]. For lysosomal enzymes, some activities were unchanged, while others showed minor increases or decreases[18]. Studies with purified Kupffer, endothelial and parenchymal cells have shown that different aging changes occur in the three liver cell types and for different enzymes (Table 21.2). In Kupffer and endothelial cells, there were no major changes in the activities of most of the key lysosomal enzymes tested[20] (Table 21.2), nor of the multiple forms of acid phosphatase[21]. For cathepsin D, which is a proteolytic enzyme responsible for the degradation of endocytosed proteins (see also below), our data have been variable: in the first series of experiments the activity of this enzyme was about two-fold higher in Kupffer cells from older rats (Table 21.2), while no changes were observed in a second series (Table 21.3) which included two different assays for cathepsin D activity. We conclude that no changes in the different forms of this enzyme are apparent in Kupffer and endothelial cells (Table 21.3).

Cytochemical and biochemical studies have shown a decrease in the activity of glucose-6-phosphatase and Mg-ATPase and in glucagon-stimulated adenyl-cyclase activity of endothelial cells[19]. Alkaline phosphatase activity was increased in endothelial cells from older rats. No changes in the activities of these and other enzymes, including cytochome c reductase, 5'-nucleotidase, γ-glutamyl transferase and gluthatione-S-transferase, were observed in Kupffer cells[19].

Age-related changes in the biochemical properties of fat-storing cells have

Table 21.2 Age-dependent change of lysosomal enzyme activities in parenchymal, Kupffer and endothelial cells isolated from livers of female BN/BiRij rats

Enzyme	Age (months)	Parenchymal cells	Kupffer cells	Endothelial cells
Acid phosphatase	3	36.3 ± 2.1	115.3 ± 14.6	165.3 ± 21.6
	24	45.9 ± 2.0*	186.1 ± 16.7*	192.4 ± 17.0
	32	37.1 ± 3.0	172.9 ± 13.0*	171.1 ± 10.8
Acid Lipase	3	12.4 ± 2.0	53.1 ± 5.3	27.1 ± 1.5
	24	27.1 ± 3.4*	82.8 ± 9.1	35.0 ± 2.2*
	32	16.7 ± 2.4	82.3 ± 8.7	36.8 ± 6.8
Acid DNAse	3	13.9 ± 3.6	235.6 ± 43.4	376.9 ± 40.8
	24	36.6 ± 8.2	374.6 ± 52.1	482.2 ± 117.0
	32	24.3 ± 5.0	286.9 ± 42.6	322.0 ± 22.8
Cathepsin D	3	0.52 ± 0.03	17.0 ± 2.6	6.4 ± 0.4
	24	1.18 ± 0.12*	42.6 ± 4.5*	6.8 ± 1.1
	32	1.01 ± 0.08*	35.8 ± 6.4*	8.1 ± 0.9
Aminopeptidase B	3	7.7 ± 1.0	11.3 ± 1.7	9.2 ± 1.2
	24	8.3 ± 0.3	11.5 ± 0.8	12.4 ± 1.7
	32	6.2 ± 0.3	12.4 ± 0.8	13.5 ± 0.3
β-Galactosidase	3	2.5 ± 0.1	20.7 ± 2.3	24.1 ± 1.2
	24	2.8 ± 0.1	36.0 ± 2.7	27.8 ± 2.6
	32	2.5 ± 0.2	29.3 ± 3.7	26.5 ± 2.8
β-Glucuronidase	3	6.4 ± 0.4	28.0 ± 3.3.	19.6 ± 1.2
	24	5.8 ± 0.1	23.5 ± 1.8	18.7 ± 1.8
	32	4.7 ± 0.3*	20.1 ± 2.1	17.9 ± 1.3
β-N-acetylglucosaminidase	3	88.8 ± 3.3	151.6 ± 8.3	299.7 ± 33.0
	24	50.8 ± 2.2*	171.0 ± 14.0	234.7 ± 28.6
	32	46.6 ± 3.6*	143.8 ± 12.6	226.3 ± 24.0
Arylsulphatase B	3	9.7 ± 0.7	48.1 ± 10.4	149.4 ± 18.0
	24	11.0 ± 0.3	45.0 ± 0.9	143.3 ± 18.2
	32	9.9 ± 0.4	41.0 ± 5.5	163.1 ± 14.9

Enzyme activities are expressed as nanomoles of 4-methylumbelliferone (acid phosphatase, acid lipase, β-galactosidase, β-acetylglucosaminidase), nucleotide equivalents (acid DNAse), tryptophan (cathepsin D), β-naphthylamine (aminopeptidase B), phenolphthalein (β-glucuronidase) or nitrocatechol (arylsulphatase B) released per minute per mg of protein at 37°C. Date are means ± S.E.M. of 4 separate experiments
* $P < 0.05$ versus values at 3 months
Activities of lysosomal enzymes were determined as described previously[5]

not been studied in detail. Under normal nutritional conditions there was a steady increase in vitamin A content with advancing age and which parallels the increase in total liver vitamin A[22]. Recent observations published elsewhere in this volume[23] suggested that the concentrations of vitamin A binding proteins and retinyl palmitate hydrolase in fat-storing cells do not change with age.

Table 21.3 Distribution of cathepsin D activities based on the liberation of tyrosine (Tyr) or tryptophan (Trp) from haemoglobin, in parenchymal, endothelial and Kupffer cells from young and old rats. (Cathepsin D activities were determined as described previously[5,20])

Age (months)	Cell type	Tyr* (nmoles)	Trp* (nmoles)	Tyr**/Trp
3	parenchymal cells	6.90 ± 0.91	0.29 ± 0.04	23.8 ± 2.3
	endothelial cells	53.43 ± 3.60	3.06 ± 0.25	17.5 ± 0.6
	Kupffer cells	230.02 ± 6.64	14.16 ± 0.49	16.3 ± 0.2
33–34	parenchymal cells	11.45 ± 0.84	0.89 ± 0.06	13.1 ± 1.8
	endothelial cells	59.25 ± 3.03	2.97 ± 0.15	20.0 ± 0.4
	Kupffer cells	220.57 ± 42.79	10.84 ± 2.22	20.4 ± 0.8

The values represent the mean ± S.E.M. of three separate experiments
(Cathepsin D activities were determined as described previously[5,20])
* The activities are expressed as nmoles tyrosine (Tyr) or tryptophan (Trp) released per minute per mg protein
** The ratio nmoles Tyr/Trp is 2.4 for intact haemoglobin

Functional changes during aging

Morphology of endocytosis

One of the major functions of Kupffer and endothelial cells is the uptake of materials from the circulation. The uptake of latex, horseradish peroxidase (HRP) and endotoxin was studied qualitatively by electron microscopy using cultured cells obtained from old rats. No major differences in the mechanisms of uptake and the subcellular organelles involved in the processing of the ligands were observed in cells from old rats. For HRP, a similar localization in bristle-coated micro-pinocytotic vesicles, tubular structures and larger lysosomal vacuoles was observed in Kupffer and endothelial cells, both in young and old rats[8] (Figure 21.6).

Age-related changes in the capacity of rat liver Kupffer and endothelial cells to take up colloidal albumin

Rats of different ages were injected with a saturating dose of colloidal albumin (CA), which ensures that the endocytic capacity of the reticulo-endothelial cells is the rate-limiting factor determining the cellular uptake of CA[24,25]. The amount of CA that still present in the circulation in all animals after 6 min was more than 75% of the injected dose (Table 21.4). The low clearance rate of CA from the plasma in this time period made it difficult to assess age-related changes from clearance curves. The uptake of CA by the liver and spleen is shown in Table 21.4. For the whole liver, the uptake of CA amounted to about 8% of the injected dose, without significant age-related changes. The amount of CA endocytosed per gram liver wet weight, which represents the maximum rate of uptake of CA per unit liver tissue, also did not change significantly with age[25].

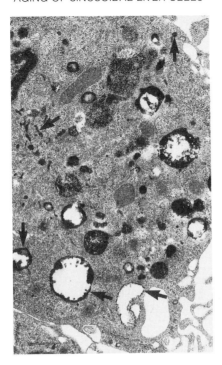

Figure 21.6 TEM of cultured Kupffer cells from a 36-month-old rat after 30 min incubation with horseradish peroxidase (HRP) (125 mg/ml). Reaction product indicating the presence of HRP is observed in various types of endocytic and lysosomal structures (arrows). ($\times$ 12 600)

The uptake of CA by Kupffer and endothelial liver cells *in vivo* was determined by isolation and purification of these cells from animals injected with a saturating dose of CA. The cells were isolated at low temperature to avoid degradation and loss of label during the isolation procedure[12]. The uptake of CA by the two cell types is presented in Table 21.4. The maximum endocytic capacity, expressed as ng CA per minute per 10^6 cells, is similar in both cell types. Since endothelial cells are about twice as abundant as Kupffer cells in the rat liver, these results indicate that the contribution of the endothelial cells to the clearance of CA exceeds that of Kupffer cells. For Kupffer cells, there was a significantly higher uptake in cells from 6-month-old rats when compared with those aged 3 or 36 months. For endothelial cells no age-related changes were observed.

Kinetic analyses of the uptake of CA by Kupffer cells were performed on purified cells in maintenance culture[25]. The cells were incubated with concentrations of CA ranging from 15–4000 μg CA per ml. The age-related changes were analysed by Michaelis–Menten kinetics. Table 21.5 shows that there is a significant age-related decrease in the apparent V_{max}, the maximum rate of uptake of CA, by Kupffer cells per mg protein. Because the protein content of cells increases with age from 92 mg in 3-month-old to 110 mg per 10^6 cells for 30–36 month-old rats[25], the percentage decrease in endocytosis

217

Table 21.4 Plasma and organ distribution and cellular uptake of intravenously injected colloidal albumin (CA)

	Age		
	3-month-old	*6-month-old*	*36-month-old*
Organ distribution (% of dose)			
Liver	8.54 ± 1.0	7.37 ± 0.89	8.88 ± 1.25
Spleen	0.92 ± 0.09	0.80 ± 0.05	0.56 ± 0.06
Plasma	81.4 ± 5.6	85.0 ± 2.7	76.6 ± 1.8
Organ uptake (μg/CA/g)			
Liver	66.2 ± 9.3	57.1 ± 6.9	68.8 ± 9.6
Spleen	104.6 ± 4.4	103.2 ± 8.2	61.5 ± 4.4
Uptake (ng/10^6 cells/min) by			
Kupffer cells	$32.4 \pm 5.3*$	80.1 ± 10.5	$48.4 \pm 6.7*$
Endothelial cells	53.5 ± 8.7	43.3 ± 4.8	44.7 ± 7.7

Rats were injected with 2.5 mg CA per 100 g body weight and sacrificed after about 6 min incubation time. Plasma clearance, organ distribution and cellular uptake were determined as described elsewhere[25]. Values are given as mean $\pm$ S.E.M. In each age group, 5 animals were used
* Differs significantly from 6-month-old rats ($p < 0.05$)

Table 21.5 Kinetics of endocytosis of colloidal albumin (CA) by cultured Kupffer cells from female BNBi/Rij rats of various ages

Age (months)	n	Maximum rate of uptake (V_{max})	K_m
3	5	9.33 ± 1.36	0.124 ± 0.016
12	4	6.04 ± 0.71	0.089 ± 0.004
30	3	$4.99 \pm 0.81**$	0.103 ± 0.025
36	4	$4.28 \pm 0.41* \cdot †$	0.091 ± 0.013

Maintenance cultures of Kupffer cells were incubated with various concentrations colloidal albumin as described (15–4000 μg/ml) elsewhere[25]. The values were calculated, applying Michaelis-Menten kinetics, by linear regression from Lineweaver–Burke plots of the rate of uptake vs. the concentrations of CA. The maximum rate of uptake is expressed as μg taken up per mg cellular protein per 30 min. The K_m is expressed as mg CA[125]I per ml. Values are the mean $\pm$ S.E.M.
* Differs significantly ($p < 0.02$) from 3-month value (Student's t-test)
** Difference with 3-month value: $0.05 < p < 0.10$
† Difference with 12-month value: $0.05 < p < 0.10$

with increasing age is less when V_{max} is expressed per 10^6 cells than per mg protein. The K_m, which indicates the affinity of Kupffer cells for the substrate is unaffected by the age of the donor rat.

Lysosomal degradation of ingested CA by cultured Kupffer cells

After uptake of CA by Kupffer cells in culture, the degradation of CA was monitored. Cells from 24-month-old rats showed a slightly higher rate of appearance of trichloroacetic acid-soluble radioactivity than those from 6-

Table 21.6 Degradation and excretion of ingested colloidal albumin (CA) by cultured Kupffer cells from young and old rats†

Post-incubation	Degradation		Excretion	
	3 months	24 months	3 months	24 months
0 min	10.3 ± 1.3	11.0 ± 1.2	—	—
15 min	27.9 ± 2.7	33.1 ± 1.6	$25.6 \pm 2.0*$	$31.3 \pm 2.0*$
30 min	42.2 ± 3.4	44.1 ± 1.6	38.9 ± 3.1	43.6 ± 2.8
60 min	55.7 ± 3.3	58.2 ± 2.3	55.4 ± 3.3	58.7 ± 3.3
24 h	94.6 ± 1.9 (4)	91.2 ± 1.1 (3)	91.7 ± 1.6 (4)	91.9 ± 1.9 (3)

Cultured Kupffer cells were incubated with 320 mg CA per ml medium for 45 min[25], chilled and extracellular CA was removed by thorough rinsing. The cells were then post-incubated at 37°C for various time intervals and the medium and cells were harvested separately. Degradation was assessed on the basis of trichloroacetic acid-soluble radioactivity.
*$0.05 < p < 0.10$
† Values are expressed as the percentage of the amount of CA present in the cells at 0 min and given as the means $\pm$ S.E.M. ($n = 5$, unless stated otherwise (in parentheses))

month-old rats, but only during the first 15 min of incubation (Table 21.6). This slightly increased rate of degradation might be related to an increase in lysosomal cathepsin D in Kupffer cells from old rats. These results suggest that the lysosomal processing of endocytosed ligands by Kupffer cells is not affected during aging.

Endotoxin clearance in rats of different ages

Kupffer cells are primarily responsible for the removal of bacterial endotoxin from the circulation[11]. After intravenous injection of endotoxin, the plasma disappearance curves of young and old rats were similar in shape[26,27]. The results on the elimination half-life of endotoxin removal are summarized in Table 21.7. Generally, the chromogenic limulus amoebocyte lysate (LAL) assay gave a significantly shorter half-life than the decay of radiolabel but, a significant increase in half-life was observed in older rats by both techniques.

Table 21.7   Plasma half-life of *in-vivo* injected endotoxin in female BN/BiRij rats

Age (months)	Half-life (hours) by radioactive determination	Half-life (hours) by LAL test
3	5.70 ± 0.44	2.00 ± 0.14
6	4.93 ± 0.33	2.28 ± 0.13
24	7.28 ± 0.33*	3.28 ± 0.21*
36	8.13 ± 1.23**	3.29 ± 0.64

Animals were injected with 2 mg of ^{51}Cr-labeled *E. coli* O26 B6 endotoxin per 100 g body weight. Means ± S.E.M., $n = 5$. The elimination half-lives were calculated from the plasma disappearance curves obtained from radioactivity determinations (c.p.m.) and determination of endotoxin by the chromogenic limulus amoebocyte lysate (LAL) assay.
Comparisons by the Mann–Whitney U-test:
   * Significantly different from 3- and 6-month-old rats ($p < 0.05$)
  ** Significantly different from 6-month-old rats ($p < 0.05$)

Survival and tissue damage after endotoxin administration

Death occurred more frequently after injection of endotoxin in old rats over a broad range of concentrations (Table 21.8). Administration of 1, 2 or 4 mg

Table 21.8   Survival of female BN/BiRij rats of different ages after administration of *E. coli* endotoxin

Endotoxin dose (mg/100 g)	Survival* (survivors/total) 3–6 months	Survival* (survivors/total) 24–36 months
1	4/5	0/5
2	10/10	1/10
4	9/10	0/10
10	0/3	–

* Survival was assessed at 24 h

per 100 g body weight killed almost all animals 24 months and older, whereas almost all young adults survived. When 10 mg per 100 g was given all young adult rats died. The process of dying was clearly different in older animals[26,27]. Endotoxin-induced tissue damage detected histopathologically and biochemically appeared to be somewhat more severe in old rats, especially in liver, kidney and lung[26,28].

DISCUSSION

The major morphological and ultrastructural alterations with age of sinusoidal liver cells appeared to be restricted to the lysosomal system, in Kupffer and endothelial cells, and to lipid droplets in fat-storing cells. No changes were observed in the relative numbers of the sinusoidal cell types.

Biochemically, minor changes in the cellular content of lysosomal enzymes were found in Kupffer and endothelial cells, but no consistent pattern was evident. The significance of decreased glucose-6-phosphatase and Mg-ATPase activities in endothelial cells remains to be established. The apparent impairment of endothelial cells from old rats to respond to glucagon stimulation is of particular interest, in view of major metabolic effects of endotoxins in old rats (see below). The functional endocytotic capacity of Kupffer cells decreases with aging, in contrast to endothelial cells. At a high, saturating dose of CA, the clearance of CA by the whole liver was unchanged with age indicating that even with a maximum challenge, the reticuloendothelial (RE) system clearance function is essentially preserved even in advanced age. The endocytic capacity of Kupffer cells does decrease significantly between 6 and 36 months of age, while no changes were observed for endothelial cells, but decreased Kupffer cell function is insufficient to cause a reduction in total liver uptake. This is not unexpected, since Kupffer cells are responsible for only about 30% of the total clearance of CA by the liver. The age-related decline in endocytosis of CA by Kupffer cells was also observed with maintenance cultures *in vitro*, although with a slightly different pattern. A progressive decrease was observed at between 3 and 36 months of age, resulting in a maximum reduction of 40%. The results of both the *in vivo* and the *in vitro* experiments suggest strongly that the endocytic capacity of Kupffer cells decreases during aging.

Our data on hepatic clearance of CA are in apparent contradiction with the thesis that an age-related decline in the clearance capacity of the RE system is present in man[29-31] and rodents[32-34] (see also ref. 24). However, experimental studies in man were performed only with low doses of (different) colloids and probably are indicative of an age-related change in liver blood flow rather than in clearance capacity[24].

Earlier studies in rodents did not include truly senescent animals[32-34] and contradictory results on the patterns of change with age were observed in young and mature animals[24,32-34]. These discrepancies probably result from the use of different species and strains of rodents, different types and concentrations of test colloids and other causes not directly related to age-effects in RE system clearance capacity. Therefore, we have determined the clearance capacity by direct measurement of colloid uptake in the liver under saturating conditions and also determined the uptake in specific liver cell populations. The results show that the capacity of the whole liver to take up colloidal albumin is not significantly affected even at a very old age. However, an age-related decrease in endocytic capacity was observed for Kupffer cells. Since most RE system test substances are, like colloidal albumin, not exclusively cleared by Kupffer cells[11], this decrease can easily remain undetected. However, there are a number of potentially harmful agents, such as bacterial endotoxins, that can be removed from the circulation only by Kupffer cells[11].

Old rats were dramatically more sensitive to endotoxin-induced death than young adult rats. This was evident by 24 months of age but more so at 36 months. This probably is not simply the result of a decreased threshold dose for toxic effects since it appears that the mechanisms responsible for death are different in the older age group. Our observations are in support of a complex response to endotoxin in older animals involving disturbances in liver and kidney function, temperature regulation and probably energy metabolism. It appears unlikely that the increased susceptibility to endotoxin is caused solely by a reduction in the capacity to clear endotoxin from the bloodstream because the increase in half-life is only about 50–60%, whereas lethal doses are at least 4-fold less in older rats. More probably, older animals are more sensitive to the induction by endotoxin of one or more mediators produced by macrophages. Indeed, in various models for endotoxin-induced lethality, an essential role for macrophage secretory products such as interleukin-1, prostaglandins and leukotrienes has been postulated.

In conclusion, some important biochemical and functional parameters of sinusoidal liver cells are significantly altered in aging but, overall no major dysfunction of these cells is seen under normal conditions. However, when the organism is subjected to a challenge, such as evoked by injection of bacterial endotoxins, the response of older individuals may be dramatically affected. Since both Kupffer and endothelial cells play important roles in the protection against endotoxins and in the regulation of the organism's response, this might point to a decreased capacity of sinusoidal cells to maintain homeostasis.

References

1. Blouin, A., Bolender, R. P. and Weibel, E. R. (1977). Distribution of organelles and membranes between hepatocytes and nonhepatocytes in the rat liver parenchyma. *J. Cell Biol.*, **52**, 261–72
2. Wisse, E. and Knook, D. L. (1979). The investigation of sinusoidal cells: A new approach to the study of liver function. In Popper, H. and Schaffner, F. (eds.) *Progress in Liver Diseases.* Vol. VI, pp. 153–71. (New York: Grune and Stratton)
3. Kirn, A., Knook, D. L. and Wisse, E. (eds.) (1986). *Cells of the Hepatic Sinusoid.* Vol. 1. (Rijswijk, The Netherlands: The Kupffer Cell Foundation)
4. Brouwer, A., De Leeuw, A. M., Praaning-van Dalen, D. P. and Knook, D. L. (1982). Isolation and culture of sinusoidal liver cells: Summary of a round table discussion. In Knook, D. L. and Wisse E. (eds.) *Sinusoidal Liver Cells.* pp. 509–16. (Amsterdam: Elsevier Biomedical Press)
5. Knook, D. L. and Sleyster, E. Ch. (1980). Isolated parenchymal, Kupffer and endothelial cells characterized by their lysosomal enzyme content. *Biochem. Biophys. Res. Commun.*, **96**, 250–7
6. Knook, D. L., Seffelaar, A. M. and De Leeuw, A. M. (1982). Fat-storing cells of the rat liver; their isolation and purification. *Exp. Cell Res.*, **139**, 468–71
7. De Leeuw, A., Barelds, R. J., De Zanger, R. and Knook, D. L. (1982). Primary cultures of endothelial cells of the liver. A model for ultrastructural and functional studies. *Cell Tissue Res.*, **223**, 201–15
8. De Leeuw, A. M., Brouwer, A., Barelds, R. J. and Knook, D. L. (1983). Maintenance cultures of Kupffer cells isolated from rats of various ages: ultrastructure, enzyme cytochemistry and endocytosis. *Hepatology*, **3**, 497–506
9. Benacerraf, B. (1964). Functions of the Kupffer cells. In Rouiller, E. (ed.) *The Liver.* Vol. II. pp. 37–62. (New York: Academic Press)
10. Altura, B. M. (1980). Reticuloendothelial cells and host defence. In Altura, B. M. (ed.) *Adv. Microcirc.*, Vol. 9. pp. 252–94 (Basel: Karger)
11. Praaning-van Dalen, D. P., Brouwer, A. and Knook, D. L. (1981). Clearance capacity of rat liver Kupffer, endothelial and parenchymal cells. *Gastroenterology*, **81**, 1036–44
12. Praaning-van Dalen, D. P. and Knook, D. L. (1982). Quantitative determination of *in vivo* endocytosis by rat liver Kupffer and endothelial cells facilitated by an improved cell isolation method. *FEBS Lett.*, **241**, 229–32

13. Hendriks, H. F. J., Verhoofstad, W. A. M. M., Brouwer, A., De Leeuw, A. M. and Knook, D. L. (1985). Perisinusoidal fat-storing cells are the main vitamin A storage sites in rat liver. *Exp. Cell Res.*, **160**, 138–49

14. Blaner, W. S., Hendriks, H. F. J., Brouwer, A., De Leeuw, A. M., Knook,, D. L. and Goodman, D. S. (1985). Retinoids, retinoid-binding proteins, and retinyl palmitate hydrolase distributions in different types of liver cells. *J. Lipid Res.*, **26**, 1241–51

15. Brouwer, A., Wisse, E. and Knook, D. L. (1988). Sinusoidal endothelial cells and perisinusoidal fat-storing cells. In Arias, I. M., Jakoby, W. B., Popper, H., Schachter, D. and Schafritz, D. A. (eds.) *The Liver: Biology and Pathobiology.* (2nd edn). pp. 665–82 (New York: Raven Press)

16. De Leeuw, A. M. and Knook, D. L. (1983). The ultrastructure of sinusoidal liver cells in the intact rat liver at various ages. In Van Bezooijen, C. F. A. (ed.) *Pharmacological, Morphological and Physiological Aspects of Liver Aging.* pp. 91–6. (Rijswijk: EURAGE)

17. Burek, J. D. (1980). *Pathology of Aging Rats.* (West Palm Beach, Florida: CRC Press)

18. Knook, D. L. and Sleyster, E. Ch. (1976). Lysosomal enzyme activities in parenchymal and nonparenchymal liver cells isolated from young, adult and old rats. *Mech. Age. Dev.*, **5**, 389–97

19. Wilson, P. D., Watson, R. and Knook, D. L. (1982). Effects of age on rat liver enzymes. A study using isolated hepatocytes, endothelial and Kupffer cells. *Gerontology*, **28**, 32–43

20. Knook, D. L. and Sleyster, E. Ch. (1978). Lysosomes in Kupffer cells isolated from young and old rats. In Kitani, K. (ed.) *Liver and Aging.* pp. 241–50. (Amsterdam: Elsevier Biomedical Press).

21. Sleyster, E. C. and Knook, D. L. (1980). Aging and multiple forms of acid phosphatase in isolated rat liver cells. *Mech. Age. Dev.*, **14**, 443–52

22. De Leeuw, A. M., Earnest, D. L., Brouwer, A., Hendriks, H. F. J. and Knook, D. L. (1986). Ultrastructure and function of sinusoidal liver cells during aging: correlation with vitamin A status? In Van Bezooijen, C. F. A., Miglio, F. and Knook, D. L. (eds.) *Liver, Drugs and Aging.* pp. 65–70. (Rijswijk: EURAGE)

23. Hendriks, H. F. J., Blaner, W. S., Brouwer, A., Goodman, D. S. and Knook, D. L. (1988). Age-related changes in retinoid status and some parameters of retinoid metabolism. In *Falk Symposium* No. 47, (This volume), p. 349–58. (Lancaster: MTP Press)

24. Brouwer, A. and Knook, D. L. (1983). The reticuloendothelial system and aging: a review. *Mech. Age. Dev.*, **21**, 205–28

25. Brouwer, A., Barelds, R. J. and Knook, D. L. (1985). Age-related changes in the endocytic capacity of rat liver Kupffer and endothelial cells. *Hepatology*, **3**, 362–6

26. Horan, M. A. (1986). *Endotoxin as a Naturally Occurring Immunomodulator.* (Utrecht: State University of Utrecht)

27. Brouwer, A., Horan, M. A., Barelds, R. J., Knook, D. L. and Hollander, C. F. (1986). Age-related changes in the clearance and toxicity of intravenously injected *E. coli* endotoxin. In Van Bezooijen, C. F. A., Miglio, F. and Knook, D. L. (eds.) *Liver, Drugs and Aging.* pp. 77–82. (Rijswijk: EURAGE)

28. Brouwer, A., Horan, M. A., Barelds, R. J. and Knook, D. L. (1986). Cellular aging of the reticuloendothelial system. *Arch. Gerontol. Geriatr.*, **5**, 317–24

29. Antonini, F. M., Cappelli, G., Citi, S. and Serio, M. (1964). Alcune osservazioni sui rapporti fra invecchiamento e potere granulopessico del sistema reticolo-endoteliale. (Studio condotto nell'uomo mediante[198] Au.) *G. Gerontol.*, **12**, 741–50

30. Mundschenk, H., Hromec, A. and Fischer, J. (1971). Phagocytic activity of the liver as a measure of hepatic circulation – A comparative study using [198] Au and ^{99m}Tc-sulfur colloid. *J. Nucl. Med.*, **12**, 711–18

31. Wagner, H. N., Migita, T. and Solomon, N. (1966). Effect of age on reticuloendothelial function in man. *J. Gerontol.*, **21**, 57–62

32. Bilder, G. E. (1975). Studies on immune competence in the rat: Changes with age, sex and strain. *J. Gerontol.*, **30**, 641–6

33. Jaroslow, B. N. and Larrick, J. W. (1973). Clearance of foreign red cells from the blood of aging mice. *Mech. Age. Dev.*, **2**, 23–32

34. Normann, S. J. (1973). Reticuloendothelial system function. VI. Experimental alterations influencing the correlation between portal blood flow and colloid clearance. *J. Reticuloendothel. Soc.*, **13**, 47–60

22
Liver cell turnover in man and animals during aging

H. M. RABES

The liver is a highly specialized organ which is centrally involved in anabolic and catabolic metabolism and represents an essential organ for the maintenance of the metabolic equilibrium and humoral homeostasis of the organism. The wide spectrum of differentiated functions can apparently only be provided by specialized hepatocellular subpopulations[1]. This has been demonstrated by qualitative and quantitative enzyme histochemistry[2,3], electron microscopical morphometry[4,5] and quantitative autoradiography[6]. These investigations disclosed that there are remarkable differences between hepatocytes in various parts of the liver lobule. In periportally localized hepatocytes aerobic energy transformation predominates; biosynthetic functions are more expressed in hepatocytes of the intermediary and perivenous zone[2,3]. Ultrastructurally, perivenous hepatocytes show a large number of mitochondria, peroxisomes and lysosomes and more smooth endoplasmic reticulum[4,5].

DNA measurements revealed that in adult rat liver, diploid hepatocytes prevail in the periportal zone and also binuclear diploid cells can be observed in this part which may give rise to mononuclear tetraploid cells. In the perivenous zone tetraploid hepatocytes and even higher ploid cells predominate[7,8]. It has been argued that there exists a steady flux of hepatocytes from the periportal zone of the lobule, with the periportally localized cells being most readily proliferating ones and the perivenous hepatocytes being functionally active, highly differentiated end-state cells[2,6]. However, no exact data are available to demonstrate that in the adult individuum liver cell renewal is limited to the periportal zone. Because of the slow cell turnover in the adult liver, which represents the classical example of a stabile, steady-stage organ[9,10], it is difficult to draw any firm conclusions about the cell turnover in different parts of the liver lobule. On the other side, the prevalence of cells of higher ploidy stage in the perivenous zone might be an indirect argument for an increased age of these cells. At adolescence, the ploidy changes from preferentially diploid to higher ploidy[11]. If increased ploidy is a sign of aging, the tetra- and octoploid cells of the perivenous lobular areas might indeed represent old-aged cells as compared to the diploids of the periportal regions.

One has to bear in mind that a diploid hepatocyte, as preferentially present in the liver at birth, may during the cell cycle either end up in two diploid cells, in one tetraploid, or in a single binucleated diploid hepatocyte which again in a new cycle could develop into two tetraploid hepatocytes. Analogous processes can be assumed for tetraploid cells, ending up either in two mono-nuclear tetraploid, a single binucleated tetraploid or an octoploid cell. Each new type of a hepatocyte can only be produced via DNA synthesis. This implies that changes of the ploidy or nuclearity reflect proliferative activity, whether or not cytokinesis follows DNA synthesis and G_2 of the cell cycle (Figure 22.1).

In rats the changes of nuclearity and ploidy have been thoroughly studied (see ref. 12). Although strain and sex differences may influence the cytologic pattern in the liver, an overall picture evolves which is summarized in Figure 22.2. The relative number of diploid cells high post-natally, decreases con-siderably during the early months after birth while the diploid binuclear hepatocytes show a sharp peak at about one month. Shortly thereafter, polyploid cells increase, most pronounced the tetraploid fraction which reaches a maximum at the age of around 8 months followed by a steady decline. Coincidently the number of binuclear tetraploids and octoploids rises. This indicates that there is a constant flow of cells from one compartment to the other, in order to adjust continuously to the actual functional demands of the organ. As each transit requires a round of DNA synthesis it might be concluded that the liver preserves, in principle, the capacity for cell renewal even in old age.

There are a few observations about the situation in humans. Altmann and collaborators[13] have studied ploidy and nuclearity in human livers as a function of age (Figure 22.3). In contrast to the results in rat liver, the shift of ploidy from diploid to tetraploid cells does not take place until the age of about 15 to 18 years and does not comprise a large fraction of cells. Remark-ably, the time of polyploidy development is coincident with the increase of binuclear hepatocytes the number of which decreases at old age when the tetraploid cells still increase. Though less pronounced than in rats, similar age-dependent reactions of the liver parenchyma are evident in humans. Along the line of arguments as given earlier one tends to conclude that human liver preserves until senescence a capacity for changing the cellular ploidy pattern indirectly suggesting a sustained ability for proliferation at old age, at least for a fraction of hepatocytes.

The question arises how large the fraction of cells is that does not take part in cell proliferation in senescence. An indirect indication for a decreased growth fraction with age comes from the observation of a decreasing liver weight with age[14,15], concomitantly with a decline in cell number[14].

It is evident from autoradiographic studies using tritiated thymidine as a precursor of DNA synthesis to estimate the cycling cells, that at least in rat liver, cell proliferation decreases post-natally and drops to a value of less than 0.1% of hepatocytes simultaneously in the cycle during adolescence

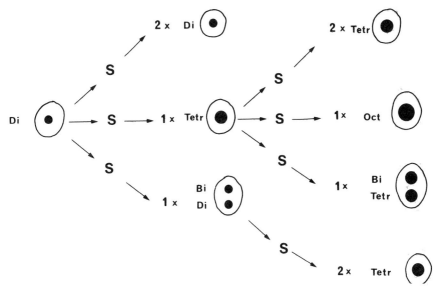

Figure 22.1 Scheme of development of hepatocellular polyploidy

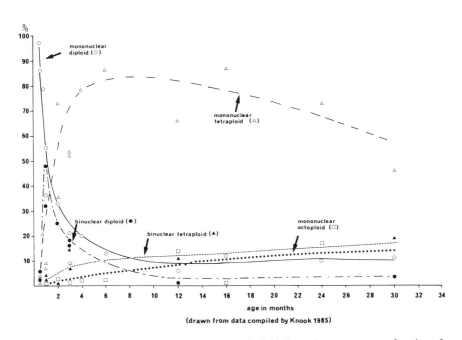

Figure 22.2 Development of binuclearity and polyploidy in rat hepatocytes as a function of age (data from ref. 12)

227

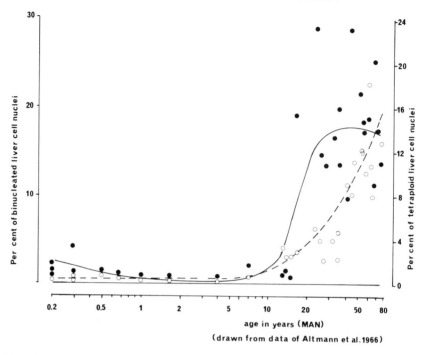

Figure 22.3 Binuclear, diploid and tetraploid hepatocytes in human liver as a function of age (date from ref. 13)

(Figure 22.4). It is difficult to quantify any possible further decrease during senescence.

A better way to comprehend the putatively changing mode of proliferation of liver cells with age is to use regenerating liver as a tool. After intoxication or resection of part of the organ, hepatocytes are triggered by a yet unknown mechanism[16] from the resting G_0 state into the cell cycle[17]. Biochemical studies using ^{14}C-thymidine as a DNA precursor revealed that there is a wave of DNA synthesis after a lag period of about 15 h after two-thirds partial hepatectomy in weanling rats, measured by the specific activity of DNA. When young adult rats were studied the increase of specific activity was delayed for about 3 h. At the age of one year or more, the start of DNA synthesis was not observed until about 23 h after the operation indicating a tendency for a delay of response to cell loss with age[18].

Autoradiographic investigation at different time intervals after two-thirds hepatectomy in young adult[19] and old rats with an age of 32 to 33 months substantiated these assumptions (Figure 22.5). The fraction of ^{3}H-thymidine-labelled hepatocytes in young adult rats reaches a maximum between 20 and 27 h after partial hepatectomy, followed by a decline and a second, smaller wave of DNA-synthesizing cells at about 56 h. In contrast, senile rats show a much reduced response: At the time of maximum DNA synthesis in the young adults, senile rat liver contains only a few S-phase cells. The peak of response is at about 34 h after partial hepatectomy, but lower by a factor of

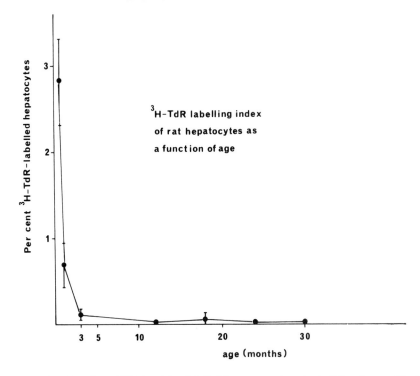

Figure 22.4 Fraction of ³H-thymidine labelled hepatocytes in rats at different ages, 60 min after a single dose of ³H-thymidine

about 2.5 as compared to the younger group. It appears that the degree of synchronization of cellular response is much lower in senile than in young adult rats.

This impression is further substantiated by comparing the auto-radiographic localization of proliferating hepatocytes after partial hepa-tectomy in young adult and senile rats. An earlier evaluation of labelling indices in different parts of the liver lobule between portal tract and branches of the vena hepatica disclosed a very peculiar pattern[6,17]. The wave of DNA synthesis starts in young adults at about 18 h after operation preferentially in those hepatocytes which are localized closely, but not immediately adjacent to the portal tract. At 20 h the wave of DNA-synthesizing cells reaches a maximum in this peculiar part of the lobule, with a steep decline towards the hepatic vein. At 27 h a high labelling index is found in all parts of the lobule except for a perivenous quarter of the lobule. In this area it takes until 40 h that a maximum of nearly 20% S-phase cells is seen, at a time interval when the majority of the other hepatocytes has already left DNA synthesis. A second wave starts at about 56 h, again with cells localized near, but not adjacent to the portal tract[6,17]. These results are in favour of the hypothesis that cell proliferation in the liver remnant after partial hepatectomy proceeds in a highly regulated pattern enabling the functionally-active organ to main-

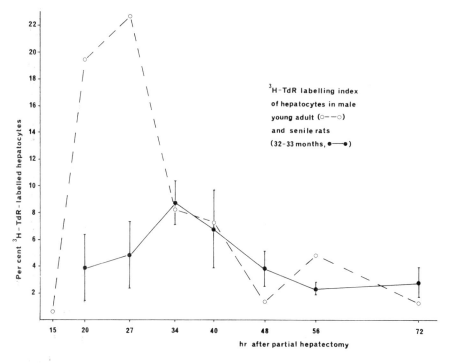

Figure 22.5 ³H-thymidine labelling index of hepatocytes at different intervals after partial hepatectomy, 60 min after a single injection of ³H-thymidine in young adult rats (data from ref. 19) and senile rats

tain its metabolic load even during the regenerative period because only a fraction of hepatocytes within the different metabolic sub-populations is simultaneously engaged in the cell cycle. The antagonism between proliferation and differentiation is taken into account during liver regeneration in a most elegant way in young adult rats.

In senile rats, this delicate antagonism does not appear to function properly. It has been demonstrated that DNA synthesizing hepatocytes are at all times after two-thirds hepatectomy located preferentially in the periportal zone, not immediately adjacent to the portal tract. The number of hepatocytes simultaneously in DNA synthesis does not exceed about 10% in any part of the lobule. This suggests that hepatocytes in old rats respond more slowly and are less synchronized to the stimulus for proliferation. The upper limit of cells permitted to proceed into DNA synthesis in a given functional unit of the liver lobule is much smaller than in young adult rats. One could speculate about the possibility that old hepatocytes might become refractory to growth stimulation because of a loss of growth factor receptors or because of a lack of the cellular metabolism to re-orient biosynthetic pathways to DNA synthesis. The exact molecular mechanisms are yet unknown.

It was the late Elmar Stöcker and his group who made evident for the first time that the growth fraction[20] of rat liver after partial hepatectomy decreases with age[21-23]. After a 10-day continuous infusion of tritiated thymidine a plateau of labelled cells was reached at 99.8% with juvenile, at 93% with young adult and 77% with old rats, aged 24 to 30 months[21,22].

Using osmotic minipumps for a continuous administration of tritiated thymidine we performed similar experiments using young adult and senile rats at an age of 33 months, the average life time of the Wistar AF/Han rat strain used being 33 ± 1 months. In these rats, determination of the cumulative G_1–S transit showed remarkable differences between the two groups (Figure 22.6). While the labelling index of young adult rats was more than 30% at 24 h continuous ³H-thymidine exposure and had reached a value of more than 80% after 48 h and increased slightly further to more than 90% at 72 h, the respective values in senile rats were only marginally increased at 24 h and showed a much less steep increase at 48 and 72 h (Figure 22.6).

Comparing the autoradiograms at equal time points after partial hepatectomy shows that in senile rats the growth fraction is limited to periportally localized hepatocytes, while in young adult rats all compartments of the lobule are involved in the regeneration except for a small rim around the branches of the hepatic vein. However, even after extended thymidine

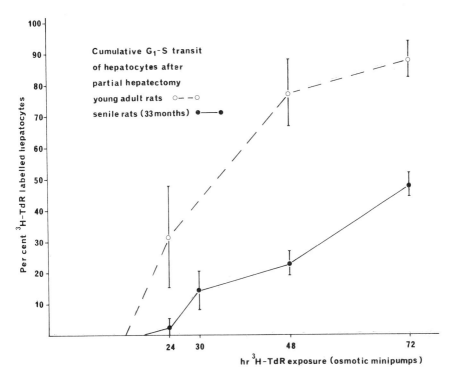

Figure 22.6 Cumulative G_1–S transit determined by the tritiated thymidine labelling index of hepatocytes after continuous ³H-thymidine exposure by intraperitoneally-implanted osmotic minipumps after partial hepatectomy

exposure, in senile rats not all hepatocytes in the periportal zone are labelled, in contrast to young adult rats, indicating that even in the sub-population most prone to respond to a growth stimulus a large portion of cells becomes refractory with age (Figures 22.7–22.10). Those cells, however, which start

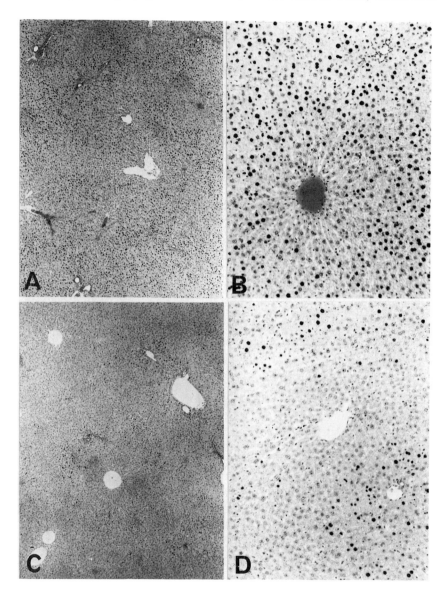

Figure 22.7 Cumulative topographical distribution of DNA-synthesizing cells in regenerating rat liver 24 h after partial hepatectomy. Autoradiograms of the liver of young adult (A, B) and senile rats (C, D) after continuous ³H-thymidine exposure with intraperitoneally-implanted osmotic minipumps for 24 h after partial hepatectomy. (A) and (C), × 21; B and D, × 70

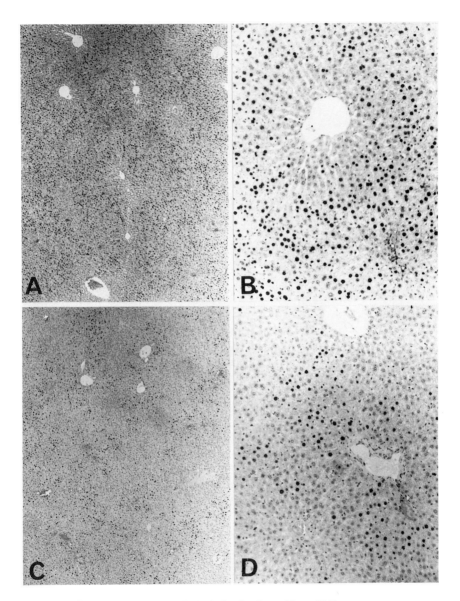

Figure 22.8 ³H-thymidine exposure for 30 h (for details see Figure 22.7)

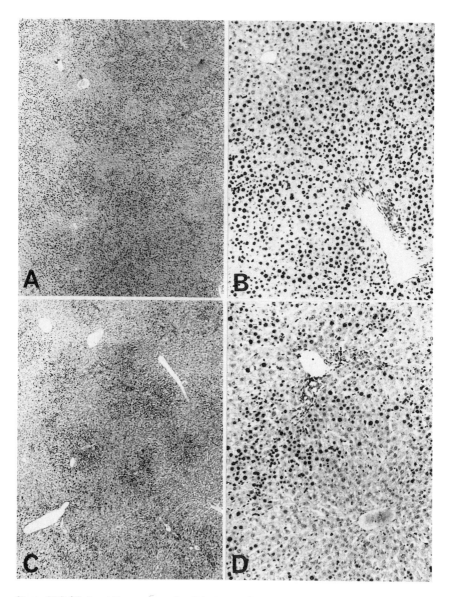

Figure 22.9 ^{3}H-thymidine exposure for 48 h (for details see Figure 22.7)

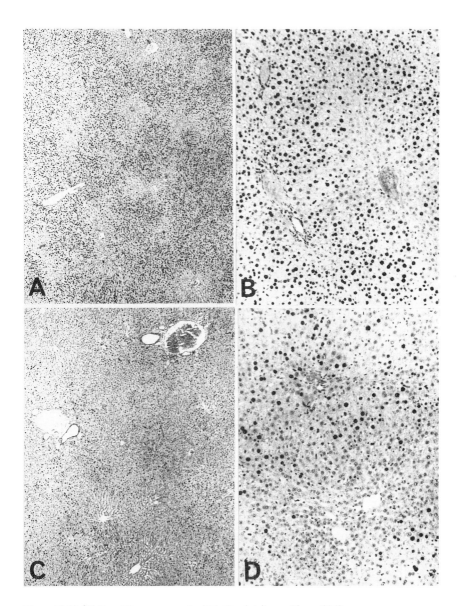

Figure 22.10 ³H-thymidine exposure for 72 h (for details see Figure 22.7)

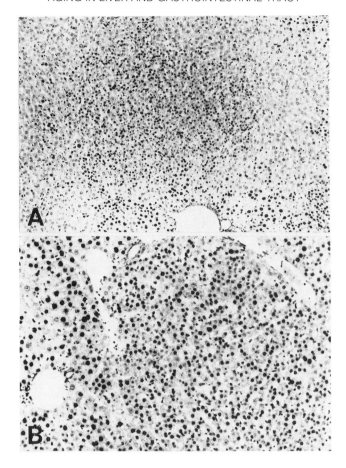

Figure 22.11 Highly-proliferating, preferentially-diploid focal sub-populations in the liver of a senile rat. Autoradiogram after ³H-thymidine exposure for 72 h after partial hepatectomy. A, × 35; B, × 70

DNA synthesis have an almost normal transit time through the cell cycle as seen in young adult rats[23].

Stöcker pointed out that non-proliferating hepatocytes of $2\frac{1}{2}$-year-old rats after partial hepatectomy might be triggered into DNA synthesis when the liver resection is repeated. In his calculation the non-growth fraction will become smaller with each round of replication induced by additional cell loss[21,22]. It is not yet certain that this hypothesis holds true also in senile rats during the last months of life. Limitation of the growth fraction in senile rats concerns all parts of the liver lobule, but most strictly the perivenous hepatocytes. However, the overall decrease of response to proliferative stimuli is counteracted by specific sub-populations seen in the regenerating liver of senile rats. They show a high ³H-thymidine labelling index after continuous infusion. Typically, these sub-populations consist almost exclusively of diploid cells (Figure 22.11), form circular foci or are more diffuse localized near the portal tracts. These foci with a high proliferative activity after partial hepatectomy might represent a population which is, in an otherwise proliferation-depressed organ, proliferation-oriented and might compensate, under normal non-stimulatory conditions, for accidental cell loss in the organ. However, it might be too speculative to label these peculiar cells as being a kind of stem-cell population for cell renewal in senile rat liver.

Another interpretation would be that these diploid populations prone to proliferation represent foci of pre-neoplastic cells in the old liver. It has been shown that carcinogen-induced enzyme-aberrant putative pre-neoplastic foci[24,25], indeed consist preferentially of pure populations of diploid hepatocytes[26,27]. Dysregulation of proliferation in old-aged liver thus might end up not only in growth inhibition, but also occasionally in enhanced growth potential of sub-populations.

This review, speculative in part, on proliferation in aging liver was aimed at demonstrating that cell turnover in the liver persists until senescence. The number of differentiated end-cells increases, but even with a reduced fraction of hepatocytes which take part in proliferation, the liver in rodents as well as in man is capable even in old-aged individuums to meet the demands of physiological cell renewal and also to compensate, in a long-lasting regenerative process, for a major cell loss of the liver cells.

Acknowledgements

The expert technical assistance of Ms Barbara Berning and Ms Monika Metzger is gratefully acknowledged. The author is indebted to Mrs Petra Tränkel for preparation of the manuscript. The work was supported by Deutsche Forschungsgemeinschaft, Bonn.

References

1. Rappaport, A. M. (1963). Acinar units and the pathophysiology of the liver. In Rouiller, C. H. (ed.) *The Liver. Morphology, Biochemistry, Physiology*. pp. 265–328. (New York: Academic Press)
2. Jungermann, K. and Sasse, D. (1978). Heterogeneity of liver parenchymal cells. *Trends Biochem. Sci.*, **3**, 198
3. Pette, D. and Brandau, H. (1966). Enzym-Histiogramme und Enzymaktivitätsmuster der Rattenleber. *Enzymol. Biol. Clin.*, **6**, 79–122
4. Loud, A. V. (1968). A quantitative stereological description of the ultrastructure of normal rat liver parenchymal cells. *J. Cell Biol.*, **37**, 27–46
5. Reith, A., Schüler, B. and Vogell, W. (1968). Quantitative und qualitative elektronenmikroskopische Untersuchungen zur Struktur des Leberläppchens normaler Ratten. *Z. Zellforsch.*, **89**, 225–40
6. Rabes, H. M. (1976). Kinetics of hepatocellular proliferation after partial resection of the liver. In Popper, H. and Schaffner, F. (eds.) *Progress in Liver Diseases, Vol. V*. pp. 83–99 (New York: Grune & Stratton)
7. Nadal, C. and Zajdela, F. (1966). Polyploidie somatique dans le foie de rat. I. Le rôle des cellules binucléées dans la genèse des cellules polyploides. *Exp. Cell Res.*, **42**, 99–116

8. Sulkin, N. M. (1943). A study of the nucleus in the normal and hyperplastic liver of the rat. *Am. J. Anat.*, **73**, 107–25

9. Altmann, H.-W. (1966). Der Zellersatz, insbesondere an den parenchymatösen Organen. *Verh. Dtsch. Ges. Path.*, **50**, 15–53

10. Bizzozero, G. (1894). An address on the growth and regeneration of the organism. *Br. Med. J.*, **1**, 728–32

11. Alfert, M. and Geschwind, I. I. (1958). The development of polysomaty in rat liver. *Exp. Cell Res.*, **15**, 230–2

12. Knook, D. L. (1985). Aging liver cells. In Cristofalo, V. J. (ed.) *CRC Handbook of Cell Biology of Aging.* pp. 229–43. (Boca Raton, Florida: CRC Press)

13. Altmann, H.-W., Loeschke, K. and Schenck, K. (1966). Über das Karyogramm der menschlichen Leber unter normalen und pathologischen Bedingungen. *Virchows Arch. Path. Anat.*, **341**, 85–101

14. Tauchi, H. and Sato, T. (1978). Hepatic cells of the aged. In Kitani, K. (ed.) *Liver and Aging.* p. 3. (Amsterdam: Elsevier/North Holland Biochemical Press)

15. Lindner, J., Grasedyck, K., Bittmann, S., Mangold, I., Schütte, B. and Ueberberg, H. (1977). Some morphological and biochemical results on liver ageing, especially regarding connective tissue. In Platt, D. (ed.) *Liver and Aging.* p. 23. (Stuttgart, New York: Schattauer-Verlag)

16. Porter, R. and Whelan, J. (1978) Hepatotrophic factors. *Ciba Foundation Symposium*, No. 55 (new series). (Amsterdam, Oxford, New York: Elsevier, Excerpta Medica, North-Holland)

17. Rabes, H. M., Wirsching, R., Tuczek, H.-V. and Iseler, G. (1976). Analysis of cell cycle compartments of hepatocytes after partial hepatectomy. *Cell Tissue Kinet.*, **9**, 517–32

18. Bucher, N. L. R., Swaffield, M. N. and DiTroia, J. F. (1964). The influence of age upon the incorporation of thymidine-2-^{14}C into the DNA of regenerating rat liver. *Cancer Res.*, **24**, 509–12

19. Rabes, H. M. and Brändle, H. (1969). Synthesis of RNA, protein, and DNA in the liver of normal and hypophysectomized rats after partial hepatectomy. *Cancer Res.*, **29**, 817–22

20. Mendelsohn, M. L. (1960). The growth fraction: a new concept applied to tumors. *Science*, **132**, 1496

21. Stöcker, E., Schultze, B., Heine, W.-D. and Liebscher, H. (1972). Wachstum und Regeneration in parenchymatösen Organen der Ratte. Autoradiographische Untersuchungen mit ^{3}H-Thymidin. *Z. Zellforsch.*, **125**, 306–31

22. Stöcker, E. (1975). Altersabhängige Proliferationskinetik in parenchymatösen Organen von Ratten. *Verh. Dtsch. Ges. Pathol.*, **59**, 78–94

23. Heine, W.-D. and Stöcker, E. (1970). Der Proliferationsmodus der Leber seniler Ratten nach Teilhepatektomie. *Verh. Dtsch. Ges. Pathol.*, **54**, 550–4

24. Rabes, H. M., Scholze, P. and Jantsch, B. (1972). Growth kinetics of diethylnitrosamine-induced, enzyme-deficient 'preneoplastic' liver cell populations *in vivo* and *in vitro*. *Cancer Res.*, **32**, 2577–86

25. Rabes, H. M. (1983). Development and growth of early preneoplastic lesions induced in the liver by chemical carcinogens. *J. Cancer Res. Clin. Oncol.*, **196**, 85–92

26. Sarafoff, M., Rabes, H. M. and Dörmer, P. (1986). Correlations between ploidy and initiation probability determined by DNA cytophotometry in individual altered hepatic foci. *Carcinogenesis*, **7**, 1191–6

27. Schwarze, P. E., Pettersen, E. O., Shoaib, M. C. and Seglen, P. O. (1984). Emergence of a population of small, diploid hepatocytes during hepatocarcinogenesis. *Carcinogenesis*, **5**, 1267–75

Section 4
Liver Drug Metabolism

23
Does aging compromise hepatic microsomal mono-oxygenase activity?

D. L. SCHMUCKER, D. A. VESSEY, R. K. WANG and A. G. MALONEY

INTRODUCTION

The elderly represent approximately 13% of the population of the United States and this figure is increasing steadily. Furthermore, the elderly present unique, yet serious, health-care problems. For example, this segment of society is the most medicated and accounts for $>25\%$ of all prescription drugs dispensed, amounting to more than \$15 billion (U.S.) annually. The average Medicare patient in an acute care hospital is a recipient of a poly-pharmacy regimen averaging 10 different medications daily. This marked increase in drug exposure has resulted in a significantly greater incidence of adverse drug reactions in geriatric subjects in comparison to young individuals (see refs. 1 and 2 for reviews). Thus, a major question confronting clinicians treating geriatric patients remains – is the prescribed drug dosage too high and will it result in adverse effects or is it too low to yield the desired therapeutic response?

There is considerable clinical evidence for an age-related decline in drug disposition and it is based largely on data depicting increased plasma $t_{1/2}$ values or reduced elimination rates for various xenobiotics (see refs. 2 and 3 for reviews). These changes may reflect (a) reduced renal clearance, (b) shifts in the volume of distribution (V_d) due to altered body composition or (c) diminished hepatic clearance and/or metabolism of drugs or their metabolites. Although there is evidence to support each of the above, most attention has been focused on the impact of aging on the hepatic mono-oxygenase system and how this may compromise drug disposition in the elderly (Figure 23.1). In spite of this emphasis, the current understanding of the impact of aging on liver drug clearance and metabolism remains confused.

Reductions in hepatic blood flow and liver volume have been implicated in the age-related decline in drug clearance. However, much of these data are subject to alternative interpretations and this issue remains unresolved (see

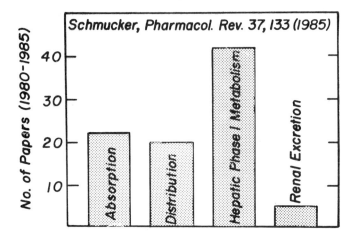

Figure 23.1 Distribution of clinical and experimental studies between 1980 and 1985 concerned with the pharmacokinetics of drug disposition in the elderly. Hepatic microsomal mono-oxygenase function(s) was the focus of more than twice the studies than any of the other contributing factors, e.g. absorption, distribution or excretion. (Data were derived from Schmucker[2])

ref. 2 for a review). Woodhouse *et al.* examined several mono-oxygenase activities in liver microsomes obtained via percutaneous needle biopsy in humans and reported no significant age-related declines, but a marked inter-individual variation in these indices (up to 6-fold)[4]. There have been *no conclusive* studies on *in vitro* hepatic mono-oxygenase activities in humans as a function of age or sex[5,6]. The general consensus is that the evidence for an age-dependent decline in hepatic cytochromes P-450 dependent drug metabolism in humans is largely circumstantial.

INBRED RODENT MODELS

On the other hand, there exists a plethora of *in vitro* studies on the hepatic mono-oxygenases in inbred male rodents as a function of age (see refs. 3 and 7 for reviews). Practically all of the data concerning *in vitro* liver mono-oxygenase activities during aging have been generated in highly inbred male rodents. Kato *et al.* are generally credited as being the first to demonstrate a negative correlation between chronological age and *in vitro* liver mono-oxygenase activities[8-10]. Subsequent studies from a number of different laboratories reported age-dependent declines in (a) non-induced activities of hepatic mono-oxygenases and (b) the inducibility of certain liver mono-oxygenases in inbred rats[11-14]. However, even in inbred rats there are considerable discrepancies regarding *in vitro* hepatic mono-oxygenase activities[15-17] (Table 23.1). Some of these conflicting data may reflect differences in animal strain, sex or maintenance (see ref. 7 for a review). Although these studies suggest an age-dependent decline in the capacity of the hepatic mono-oxy-genase system, the evidence is based on *in vitro* data from inbred rodents

Table 23.1 Effect of age on *in vitro* hepatic mono-oxygenases in male rats

Rat strain	*Age* (months)	*Control**	*PB/Control***	*Reference*
Cytochromes P-450 (nmol/mg protein)				
CFN (Wistar)	3	1.26	2.5	Birnbaum and Baird
	28–30	1.01	2.5	(1978)[12]
Fischer 344	1	0.80	2.9	Schmucker and Wang
	16	0.70	3.0	(1980)[18]
	27	0.30	4.0	
Fischer 344	2.5	1.22	2.2	Kao and Hudson (1980)[16]
	25	0.89	2.3	
Fischer 344	3–5	0.79		Rikans and Notley (1981)
	14–15	0.54		
	24	0.55		
NADPH cytochrome c reductase (nmol/mg protein/min)				
Fischer	3	137	1.3	Gold and Widnell
	24	106	1.4	(1974)[13]
CFN (Wistar)	3	59	2.3	Birnbaum and Baird
	28–30	58	1.9	(1978)[12]
Fischer 344	1	77	2.0	Schmucker and Wang
	16	112	2.5	(1980)[18]
	27	36	2.1	
Fischer 344	3–5	240		Rikans and Notley (1981)
	14–15	140		
	24	120		

* Values represent non-induced mono-oxygenases
** Values represent the ratio of phenobarbital (PB)-induced to non-induced mono-oxygenases

and does not exclude extra-hepatic influences, e.g. shifts in steroid hormones or nutrition.

Most of our rodent studies have been conducted using inbred male F344 rats. Initial studies confirmed and extended the original observations of Kato *et al.* and demonstrated significant changes (2–4 fold) in the liver mono-oxygenases, including (a) reduced NADPH cytochrome *c* (P-450) reductase activity, (b) a loss of cytochromes P-450 and (c) a decline in the rate of ethylmorphine *N*-demethylation in microsomes *in vitro* as a function of increasing age[18,19]; (Figure 23.2). Furthermore, the inducibility of these mono-oxygenase functions in response to phenobarbital was markedly inhibited by aging. Even after 6 days of phenobarbital administration, the values measured in immature and mature rats were significantly greater than those exhibited by microsomes isolated from senescent animals. However, the magnitude of the phenobarbital-induced increases was similar, e.g. 4–5-fold for the cytochromes P-450, regardless of animal age. Thus, while the actual rate of mono-oxygenase induction may not be compromised during aging, the maximum level of induction is lower in old animals. It should be noted that non-induced mono-oxygenase indices in immature rats (1 month) were quite similar to those of senescent animals (27 months). In order to avoid confusion between changes attributable to development or senescence, subsequent studies employed 3–6-month-old rats as young adult animals.

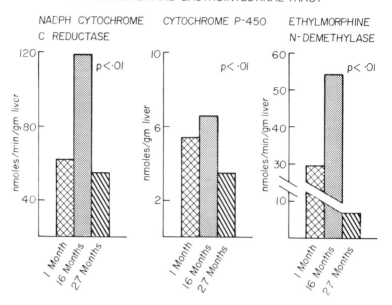

Figure 23.2 Age-related changes in the non-induced activities of several rat liver microsomal mono-oxygenases. The activity of NADPH cytochrome *c* (P-450) reductase and the rate of ethylmorphine *N*-demethylation exhibit marked increases during development/maturation and subsequent declines during senescence. There is also a significant loss of cytochromes P-450 during aging as measured by the total CO-binding difference spectrum

Other studies focused on an unrelated liver microsomal enzyme, glucose-6-phosphatase (E.C. 3.1.3.9). The specific activity of this enzyme declines gradually throughout development, maturation and senescence in male F344 rats when expressed per membrane protein or per gram of liver[20]. However, the activity per liver does not decline between maturity and senescence, suggesting that the *in vivo* enzymatic capacity of the intact organ may not be compromised during aging.

Our data on hepatic mono-oxygenases confirmed the studies reporting (a) age-related differences in either non-induced or phenobarbital-induced activities of NADPH-cytochrome *c* (P-450) reductase and (b) the absence of an age-dependent 'lag' in the initiation of hepatic reductase synthesis. Adelman *et al.* employed retired breeder rather than virgin rats for their studies demonstrating an age-dependent lag in the induction and synthesis of P-450 reductase (see ref. 15 for a review). Interestingly, previous studies in our laboratory demonstrated that this particular animal model exhibits differences in a variety of indices, including hepatic fine structure and lipid metabolism, in comparison to age-matched virgin animals of the same strain[21,22]. No significant differences in several *in vitro* indices of hepatic microsomal mono-oxygenase function were observed. On the basis of these data, we suggested that retired breeder rats may not be an appropriate model in which to study the normal aging process.

Concomitant quantitative fine structural studies revealed a 40–50% decline in the concentration of hepatic smooth-surfaced endoplasmic reticulum

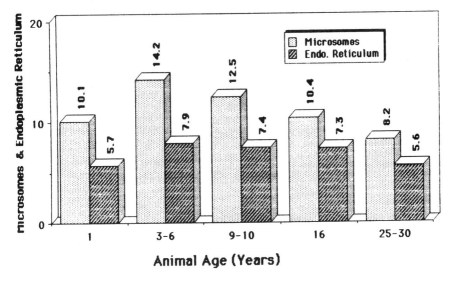

Figure 23.3 A comparison of the age-related shifts in (a) the yield of microsomal protein measured biochemically and (b) the hepatocellular content of endoplasmic reticulum determined *in situ* via stereological analysis in male Fischer rat. The yield of microsomes (mg/g tissue) declines gradually beginning in young adulthood and this loss is accompanied by a reduction in the concentration (m^2/g liver tissue) of total endoplasmic reticulum membrane

(SER), the primary locus of the microsomal mono-oxygenases, as a function of aging in the inbred male rat[23,24]. These data were confirmed by parallel changes in the hepatic concentration of microsomal protein (Figure 23.3). Both Pieri *et al.*[25] and Meihuizen and Blansjaar[26] reported age-related increases (30%) in the hepatic SER content of female rats. These conflicting data may be reconciled by considering the differences in animal strain, sex and stereological methodologies. However, a loss of SER from the livers of old rats may contribute quantitatively to *suspected* reductions in the hepatic contents of microsomal mono-oxygenases.

While a loss of SER, and its constituent enzymes, may contribute to reduced *in vivo* mono-oxygenase activities, this does not preclude qualitative changes intrinsic to the enzymes or to their microsomal milieu. Aging appears to have little impact on the protein/polypeptide composition of hepatic microsomes, but several investigators have reported alterations in the membrane's lipid domain[27,28]. Since certain phospholipids influence the efficacy of membrane-bound enzymes, e.g. phosphatidylcholine is required for optimal NADPH cytochrome P-450 reductase activity, shifts in the relative amounts of membrane phospholipids may be reflected in the metabolic capacity of the mono-oxygenases. For example, an increase in the phosphatidylethanolamine/phosphatidylcholine ratio exerts an inhibitory effect on hepatic P-450 reductase. We demonstrated a slight decline in the total phospholipid content of rat liver microsomes owing to a loss of phosphatidylcholine. A concomitant increase in the membrane cholesterol content resulted in an age-related increase in the cholesterol/phospholipid ratio and a decrease in the fluidity of the lipid domain[29]. The only other study to measure liver microsomal fluidity in the rat as a function of age reported an increase in this property and suggested that a corresponding decline in the fatty acid saturation index was responsible[30]. A number of investigators, including ourselves, have observed age-related increases in the relative concentrations of the most unsaturated fatty acid species, i.e. $C_{22:6}$, in rodent liver microsomes[29]. However, no definitive conclusions can be drawn concerning the impact of such shifts on either membrane fluidity or the efficacy of constituent enzymes (see ref. 7 for a review).

Thus, our studies demonstrated that (a) the non-induced and phenobarbital-induced activities of microsomal mono-oxygenases decline, (b) the hepatic concentration of SER is reduced, (c) the cholesterol/phospholipid ratio of the microsomes increases and (d) the fluidity of the membrane lipid domain is diminished in the livers of inbred male rats as a function of aging. While these changes are intrinsic to the hepatocytes and *may* compromise hepatic drug clearance and metabolism *in vivo,* there is no definitive evidence to support this hypothesis.

In lieu of appropriate pharmacokinetic data, we subsequently focused our studies on a specific mono-oxygenase, NADPH cytochrome P-450 reductase (E.C. 1.6.2.4), in an effort to identify changes which may be expressed *in vivo.* Since there is considerable evidence for age-dependent accumulations of 'altered' enzymes which exhibit diminished catalytic activities, we initiated studies to determine whether or not P-450 reductase undergoes a similar phenomenon (see refs. 31 and 32 for reviews). A comprehensive bisubstrate analysis of microsomal cytochrome *c* reductase did not reveal any significant age-dependent shifts in the kinetic profile[33] (Table 23.2). Subsequently, P-450 reductase was solubilized and isolated to homogeneity from the livers of young adult, mature and senescent rats. The specific activity of young adult soluble P-450 reductase was two-fold higher than that of enzyme isolated from senescent animals (Figure 23.4)[34]. Furthermore, there was (a) no change in the molecular weight, (b) a shift to a more heat-stable form and (c) a decline in immunotitratable activity (Table 23.2). Approximately 40–50% of the P-450 reductase isolated from 'senescent' microsomes, while immu-

Table 23.2 Characterization of rat cytochrome P-450 reductase

	Mean animal age (months)		
	3	9	27
Yield of soluble enzyme (%)	21	7	1
Molecular weight (kD)	74	74	74
Isoelectric point (pH)	4.8–5.2	4.8–5.2	4.8–5.2
Heat inactivation (%) (10 min; 50°C)	50	50	20
Kinetic profile (μM)			
$K_{m\ NADPH}$	6.9	6.0	6.5
$K_{m\ cytochrome\ c}$	4.0	2.9	2.2
$K_{i\ NADP}$	59		15

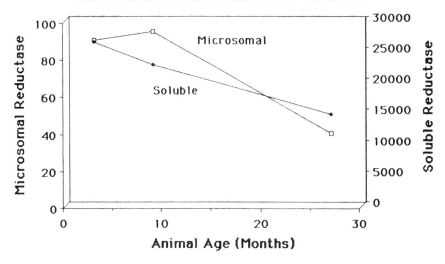

Figure 23.4 Effect of aging on the specific activity of microsome-bound and soluble NADPH cytochrome c (P-450) reductase from male Fischer rats. The activity of both enzyme preparations declines markedly from young adulthood/maturity to senescence. The enzyme activities are expressed as nmoles/mg protein/min.

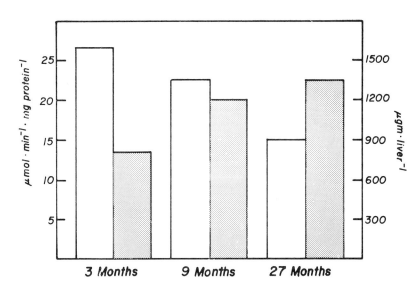

Figure 23.5 Soluble and electrophoretically homogeneous male rat liver NADPH cytochrome P-450 reductase. The specific activity of enzyme isolated from senescent rats is only half that measured in enzyme from young adults. However, the livers of old rats contain approximately twice the enzyme activity as those of the young animals. Therefore, total hepatic reductase activity is similar in all age groups, suggesting that *in vivo* enzyme function may not be impaired during aging.

noprecipitable, was catalytically inactive. The primary Lineweaver–Burke kinetic plots for both enzyme substrates, NADPH and cytochrome c, exhibited straight parallel slopes, indicative of one or, at most, two pools of reductase in the membranes of old animals, i.e. catalytically-active and inactive forms.

The yield of soluble reductase from young adult rats represented approximately 20% of the total liver pool. The recovery of enzyme from young adult and mature animals was markedly greater than that from the senescent rats. This may reflect an age-related difference in the enzyme's affinity for NADP which is not apparent from the $k_{m\ NADPH}$ or $K_{i\ NADP}$ data. Subsequent calculations based on measurements of total enzyme activity and recovered enzyme protein suggested that the livers of old rats contain more reductase as those of young adult animals (Figure 23.5). In essence, the livers of old rats contain twice the NADPH-cytochrome P-450 reductase as do those of young animals, but half of this enzyme pool consists of altered and catalytically-inactive reductase. These data support the contention that the age-related decline in *in vitro* mono-oxygenase activities results from changes intrinsic to the hepatocytes, whereas the total liver reductase activity remains unchanged during aging. Therefore, an age-related decline in *in vivo* hepatic clearance and metabolism of drugs in this animal model may not result from a change intrinsic to the hepatocyte microsomal mono-oxygenases.

OUTBRED PRIMATE MODELS

The data reviewed above demonstrate specific age-related changes in several *in vitro* properties of an important hepatic mono-oxygenase, but also suggest that such alterations may not be significant factors contributing to the decline in *in vivo* clearance and metabolism of xenobiotics. The absence of *in vivo* pharmacokinetic data in the inbred male rat to correlate with results obtained *in vitro* suggested the need for a more appropriate animal model. Since (a) there exists a plethora of clinical pharmacokinetic data and (b) access to suitable human liver tissue is limited, we initiated a series of studies using a non-human primate model, the rhesus monkey.

Initial studies demonstrated (a) the absence of change in the cytochromes P-450 content and (b) a substantial increase in the specific activity of NADPH cytochrome c (P-450) reductase in monkey liver microsomes as a function of aging and regardless of sex (Figure 23.6)[35]. The degree of inter-individual variation in these indices, as well as in the rate of ethylmorphine N-demethylation, was considerable and increased with age – an observation also reported by James *et al.* using human microsomes[4]. In the only other study to examine hepatic mono-oxygenases as a function of aging in monkeys, Sutter *et al.* reported no significant changes in the content of the cytochromes P-450 or in the activities of NADPH cytochrome c (P-450) reductase and aryl hydrocarbon hydroxylase (Figure 23.6)[36].

Subsequently, we solubilized the microsomes and purified P-450 reductase to homogeneity as demonstrated by densimetric scans of electrophoretic

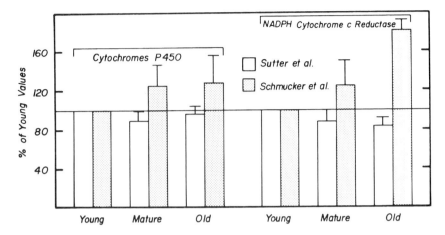

Figure 23.6 Specific activities of hepatic NADPH cytochrome *c* (P-450) reductase and the cytochromes P-450 contents in liver microsomes from female pig-tailed macaques (□) and male and female rhesus monkeys (▨) as a function of aging. All of the data are expressed as the percentage of the values obtained in the youngest animals measured. The reductase activity measured in microsomes from old rhesus monkeys is significantly higher than that in membranes from the younger age groups. (These data were obtained from refs. 35 and 36.)

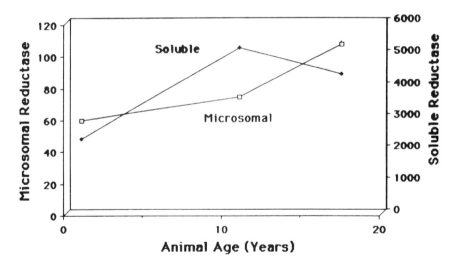

Figure 23.7 Specific activities of microsomal (membrane-bound) and of animal age. Unlike the rat liver enzyme, monkey P-450 reductase does not exhibit an age-related decline in activity regardless of the mode of data expression. The reductase activity is expressed as nmoles/mg protein/min

gels[37]. The specific activity of soluble monkey P-450 reductase increased similar to that of the membrane-bound enzyme during aging (Figure 23.7). The properties of the soluble enzyme did not exhibit any marked shifts during aging, although both the heat inactivation profile and the bisubstrate kinetic

Table 23.3 Characterization of monkey cytochrome P-450 reductase

	Mean animal age (years)		
	1.5	13.7	18.3
Yield of soluble enzyme (%)	26	29	16
Molecular weight			
major band (kD)	77	77	77
minor bands (kD)	21.58	21.58	21.58
Heat inactivation (%)	10	35	20
(40 min; 50°C)			
Kinetic profile (μM)			
$k_{m\ \text{NADPH}}$	10.5	8.5	11.4
$K_{m\ \text{cytochrome } c}$	14.7	5.8	12.4
$K_{i\ \text{NADP}}$	218	192	227

analysis suggested that reductase isolated from mature monkeys was more 'active' than that purified from either young or old animals (Table 23.3). The primary Lineweaver–Burke plots were straight and parallel, indicating that the enzyme in all three age groups examined consisted of one or, at most, two forms with respect to catalytic activity. The immunotitration profile was markedly different from that obtained with soluble rat liver reductase and suggested that more enzyme protein is required to achieve an activity level exhibited by considerably less reductase from 'old' monkeys (Figure 23.8).

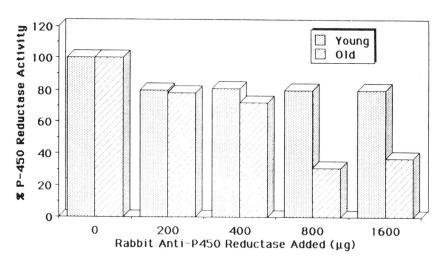

Figure 23.8 Inhibition of soluble monkey liver NADPH cytochrome c (P-450) reductase with increasing concentrations of rabbit α–rat P-450 reductase as a function of age. Initial reductase specific activities are identical, but following the addition of antibody the activity of enzyme from old monkeys is inhibited to a greater extent than reductase from young adult animals. These data support the contention that reductase from older monkeys appears to be more catalytically active than enzyme from young rhesus, i.e. the activity/immunoprecipitable enzyme ratio is greater in the former age group.

The total phospholipid, the major phospholipid species and the cholesterol concentrations in the microsomes did not exhibit significant age- or sex-related differences, although Sutter *et al.* reported moderate increases in these parameters[36]. The cholesterol/phospholipid ratio and the fluidity of the lipid domain of the membranes changed in unity with age, but there was no apparent correlation between membrane fluidity and mono-oxygenase activity.

Preliminary efforts to isolate the cytochromes P-450 fraction from solu-bilized monkey liver microsomes have been reasonably successful. We have purified this fraction to homogeneity and developed an ELISA which permits quantitation of the male (16α-hydroxylase) and female (15β-hydroxylase) specific cytochrome P-450 isozymes using intact microsomes, soluble micro-somes or the soluble cytochromes P-450 fraction. Our initial data suggest that rhesus monkey liver cytochromes P-450 are *not* characterized by age- and/or sex-related shifts in either the male or female specific isozymes.

CONCLUSIONS

Our data do not lend credence to suggestions that (a) inbred male rats correctly reflect the effects of aging on the hepatic mono-oxygenase system in humans and (b) documented age-related declines in *in vivo* pharmacokinetic indices result from 'alterations' intrinsic to the hepatocyte or the constituent mono-oxygenases. Our studies illuminate the questionable practice of extra-polating *in vitro* data generated in rodents to the *in vivo* situation in humans. Furthermore, these results suggest that inter-individual variability must be considered a significant factor in any analysis in an outbred population. These observations demand particular attention inasmuch as most of the experimental data on the subject of hepatic mono-oxygenases and aging have been derived from highly inbred male rats. The absence of any significant sex-dependent differences in mono-oxygenase activities or in the physicochemical properties of the microsomes suggests that those reported in several rodent models are not a universal phenomenon. In conclusion, the suspected con-tribution of impaired hepatic Phase I metabolism to the overall age-related decline in drug disposition requires a re-evaluation.

References

1. Schmucker, D. (1979). Age-related changes in drug disposition. *Pharmacol. Rev.,* **30,** 445–56
2. Schmucker, D. (1985). Age-related changes in drug disposition: an update. *Pharmacol. Rev.,* **37,** 133–48
3. Vestal, R. and Dawson, G. (1985). Pharmacology and aging. In Finch, C. and Schneider, E. (eds.) *Handbook of the Biology of Aging.* pp. 744–819. (New York: Van Nostrand Reinhold)
4. James, O., Rawlins, M. and Woodhouse, K. (1982). Lack of aging effect on human microsomal monooxygenase enzyme activities and on inactivation pathways for reactive metabolic intermediates. In Kitani, K. (ed.) *The Liver and Aging – 1982.* pp. 395–408. (Amsterdam: Elsevier North-Holland)

5. Pearson, M. and Roberts, C. (1984). Drug induction of hepatic enzymes in the elderly. *Age Aging*, **13**, 313–16
6. Brodie, M., Boobis, A. and Davies, D. (1981). Influence of liver disease and environmental factors on hepatic monooxygenase activity *in vitro*. *Eur. J. Clin. Pharmacol.*, **20**, 39–46
7. van Bezooijen, C. (1984). Influence of age-related changes in rodent liver morphology and physiology on drug metabolism – a review. *Mech. Ageing Develop.*, **25**, 1–22
8. Kato R. and Takanaka, A. (1968). Effect of phenobarbital on electron transport system, oxidation and reduction of drugs in liver microsomes of rats of different ages. *J. Biochem. (Tokyo)*, **63**, 406–8
9. Kato, R. and Takanaka, A. (1968). Metabolism of drugs in old rats. I. Activities of NADPH-linked electron transport and drug-metabolizing enzyme systems in liver microsomes of old rats. *Jpn. J. Pharmacol.*, **18**, 381–8
10. Kato, R. and Takanaka, A. (1968). Metabolism of drugs in old rats. II. Metabolism *in vivo* and effect of drugs on old rats. *Jpn. J. Pharmacol.*, **18**, 389–406
11. Baird, M., Samis, H. and Massie, H. (1971). Recovery from zoxazolamine paralysis and metabolism *in vitro* of zoxazolamine in aging mice. *Nature*, **233**, 565–7
12. Birnbaum, L. and Baird, M. (1978). Induction of hepatic mixed function oxidases in senescent rodents. *Exp. Gerontol.*, **13**, 299–303
13. Gold, G. and Widnell, C. (1975). Response of NADPH cytochrome *c* reductase and cytochrome P-450 in hepatic microsomes to treatment with phenobarbital-differences in rat strains. *Biochem. Pharmacol.*, **24**, 2105–6
14. McMartin, D., O'Connor, J., Fasco, M. and Kaminsky, L. (1980). Influence of aging and induction on rat liver and kidney microsomal mixed function oxidase systems. *Toxicol. Appl. Pharmacol.*, **54**, 411–19
15. Adelman, R. (1975). Impaired hormonal regulation of enzyme activity during aging. *Fed. Proc.*, **34**, 179–82
16. Kao, J. and Hudson, P. (1980). Induction of the hepatic cytochrome P-450 dependent monooxygenase system in young and geriatric rats. *Biochem. Pharmacol.*, **29**, 1191–4
17. Player, T., Mills, D. and Horton, A. (1977). Age-dependent changes in rat liver microsomal and mitochondrial NADPH-dependent lipid peroxidation. *Biochem. Biophys. Res. Commun.*, **78**, 1397–1402
18. Schmucker, D. and Wang, R. (1980). Age-related changes in liver drug-metabolizing enzymes. *Exptl. Gerontol.*, **15**, 321–9
19. Schmucker, D. and Wang, R. (1981). Effects of aging and phenobarbital on the rat liver microsomal drug-metabolizing system. *Mech. Ageing Develop.*, **15**, 189–202
20. Schmucker, D. and Wang, R. (1980). Effects of animal age and phenobarbital on rat liver glucose-6-phosphatase activity. *Exptl. Gerontol.*, **15**, 7–13
21. Schmucker, D. (1976). Age-related changes in hepatic fine structure: a quantitative analysis. *J. Gerontol.*, **31**, 135–43
22. Anthony, L., Schmucker, D., Mooney, J. and Jones, A. (1978). A quantitative analysis of fine structure and drug metabolism in livers of clofibrate-treated young adult and retired breeder rats. *J. Lipid Res.*, **19**, 154–65
23. Schmucker, D., Mooney, J. and Jones, S. (1977). Age-related changes in hepatic endoplasmic reticulum: a quantitative analysis. *Science*, **197**, 1005–8
24. Schmucker, D., Mooney, J. and Jones, A. (1978). Stereological analysis of hepatic fine structure in the Fischer 344 rat. Influence of sublobular location and animal age. *J. Cell Biol.*, **78**, 319–37
25. Pieri, C., Nagy, Z., Mazzufferi, G. and Guili, C. (1975). The aging rat liver as revealed by electron microscopic morphometry. I. Basic parameters. *Exptl. Gerontol.*, **10**, 291–304
26. Meihuizen, H. and Blansjaar, N. (1980). Stereological analysis of liver parenchymal cells in young and old rats. *Mech. Ageing Develop.*, **13**, 111–18
27. Vlasuk, G. and Walz, F. (1982). Liver microsomal polypeptides from Fischer 344 rats affected by age, sex and xenobiotic induction. *Arch. Biochem. Biophys.*, **214**, 248–59
28. Hawcroft, D., Jones, T. and Martin, P. (1982). Studies on age-related changes in cytochrome P-450, cytochrome b_5, and mixed function oxidase activity in mouse liver microsomes in relation to their phospholipid composition. *Arch. Gerontol. Geriatr.*, **1**, 55–74
29. Schmucker, D., Wang, R., Vessey, D., James, J. and Maloney, A. (1984). Age-dependent alterations in the physicochemical properties of rat liver microsomes. *Mech. Ageing Develop.*, **27**, 207–17

30. Armbrecht, J., Birnbaum, L., Zenser, T. and Davis, B. (1982). Changes in hepatic microsomal membrane fluidity with age. *Exptl. Gerontol.,* **17**, 41–8
31. Rothstein, M. (1979). The formation of altered enzymes in aging animals. *Mech. Ageing Develop.,* **9**, 197–202
32. Gershon, D. (1979). Current status of age-altered enzymes: alternative mechanisms. *Mech. Ageing Develop.,* **9**, 189–96
33. Schmucker, D. and Wang, R. (1983). The effect of aging on the kinetic profile of rat liver microsomal NADPH cytochrome *c* reductase. *Exptl. Gerontol.,* **18**, 313–21
34. Schmucker, D. and Wang, R. (1983). Age-dependent alterations in rat liver microsomal NADPH cytochrome *c* (P-450) reductase: a qualitative and quantitative analysis. *Mech. Ageing Develop.,* **21**, 137–56
35. Maloney, A., Schmucker, D., Vessey, D. and Wang, R. (1986). The effects of aging on the hepatic microsomal mixed function oxidase system of male and female monkeys. *Hepatology,* **6**, 282–7
36. Sutter, M., Wood, G., Williamson, L., Strong, R., Pickham, K. and Richardson, A. (1985). Comparison of the hepatic mixed function oxidase systems of young, adult and old non-human primates. *Biochem. Pharmacol.,* **34**, 2983–7
37. Schmucker, D. and Wang, R. (1987). Effects of aging on the properties of rhesus monkey liver microsomal NADPH cytochrome *c* (P-450) reductase. *Drug Metab. Disp.,* **15**, 225–32

24
Phase 1 drug metabolism in aging

K. W. WOODHOUSE, F. WILLIAMS, E. MUTCH, H. WYNNE, M. RAWLINS and O. F. W. JAMES

INTRODUCTION

Most surveys indicate that the incidence of adverse drug reactions increases steadily with age[1]. While this may be due to increased prescribing, altered pharmacokinetics may contribute. Many studies have shown that the systemic clearance of a variety of drugs, particularly those metabolised by the hepatic microsomal mono-oxygenase (MMO) enzyme system decreases with advancing years in man[2].

Many of the early studies of phase 1 drug-metabolising enzymes *in vitro* focused on aging animals, and demonstrated a significant reduction in the specific activity of hepatic MMO enzymes with age in male rats[3]. These findings were widely extrapolated, and statements appeared in the literature to the effect that hepatic drug-metabolising enzymes showed a similar decline with age in humans. However it is now clear that the changes observed in geriatric male rats may well be species- and sex-specific, and extrapolation of these findings to humans or indeed any other primate is dangerous[4-6].

Until recently[4] virtually no information was available concerning the effect of ageing on the specific activities of phase 1 drug-metabolising enzymes (particularly MMO enzymes) in humans. We therefore undertook a series of studies to:

(a) investigate the effect of age on the *in vitro* activity of MMO enzymes in histologically normal human liver;
(b) to investigate the effect of age on the affinity of the enzymes for their substrate;
(c) to investigate the effect of disease, age, and frailty, on phase 1 drug-metabolising enzymes in man; and
(d) to investigate the effect of age on liver size and blood flow in humans.

THE EFFECT OF AGE ON HEPATIC MICROSOMAL MONOOXYGENASE ACTIVITY IN HUMAN LIVER

Patients and methods

Liver tissue was obtained by Menghini needle biopsy during diagnostic work-up in subjects subsequently shown to have normal liver histology, or from histologically normal wedge biopsies obtained at laparotomy (usually for cholecystectomy) after informed consent. These measures had been approved by the Local Ethical Committee. No subject was taking drugs known to influence MMO enzyme activity, alcohol consumption was trivial, and history of cigarette smoking was obtained. Biopsies were stored at $-18°C$ until analysis and microsomal preparations were prepared as previously described[7]. Because of the sensitivity required, probe substrates were used, namely aldrin epoxidation and 7-ethoxycoumarin O-deethylation (low-affinity form). The methodology has previously been described in detail[8,9].

Results

Smoking had no effect on the specific activity of either enzyme and there was no correlation between age and either aldrin epoxidase or 7-ethoxycoumarin O-deethylase activity, but inter-individual variation was considerable (Figures 24.1 and 24.2). Furthermore, the recovery of microsomal protein (which contains the drug-metabolising enzyme) also bore no correlation whatsoever to age.

AFFINITY OF MICROSOMAL MONO-OXYGENASE ENZYMES FOR SUBSTRATE

For drugs metabolised with first-order kinetics, the affinity of the enzyme for substrate is a very important determinant of reaction rate. A fall in enzyme affinity, manifested by a rise in the Michaelis constant (K_m), would lead to a significant reduction in the rate of metabolism of a foreign compound.

We have therefore undertaken a careful enzyme kinetic analysis of the metabolism of 7-ethoxyresorufin and aldrin in rat liver microsomes with respect to age, and of 7-ethoxycoumarin in histologically normal human liver with respect to age.

Animal studies

Using young (168 days) and old (903 days) rats, the kinetics of aldrin and 7-ethoxyresorufin (another probe substrate) metabolism was measured in liver microsomes as previously described[9,10]. K_m values were calculated using the direct linear plot[11].

The results are shown in Figures 24.3 and 24.4, and show that the affinity of these enzymes for their substrate does not alter with ageing in animals[12].

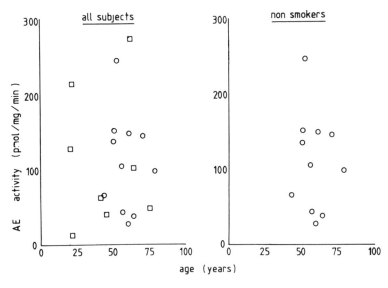

Figure 24.1 Age and specific activity of microsomal aldrin epoxidase (AE) in human liver microsomes. □ = Smokers; ○ = non-smokers

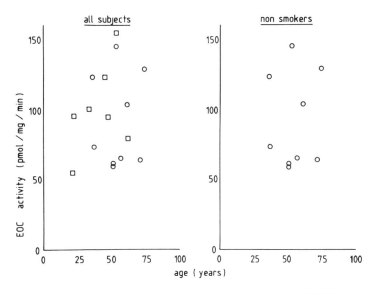

Figure 24.2 Age and specific activity of 7-ethoxycoumarin O-deethylase (EOC) in human liver microsomes. □ = Smokers; ○ = non-smokers

Human studies

Histologically normal liver was obtained as described above. The enzyme kinetics of 7-ethoxycoumarin O-deethylation was measured using a wide

257

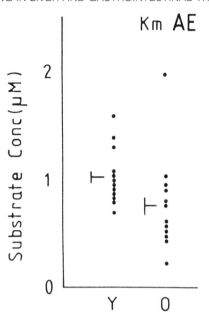

Figure 24.3 Affinity of rat liver microsomal aldrin epoxidase (AE) for substrate (measured as K_m). Y = Young rats, 168 days; O = old rats, 903 days. All animals were male

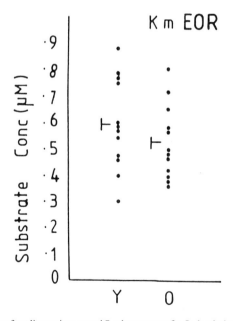

Figure 24.4 Affinity of rat liver microsomal 7-ethoxyresorufin O-deethylase (EOR) for substrate (measured as K_m). Y = Young rats, 168 days; O = old rats, 903 days. All animals were male

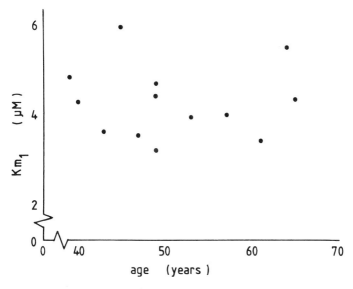

Figure 24.5 The effect of age on the affinity of the high affinity form (K_{m1}) of 7-ethoxycoumarin O-deethylation for substrate in liver microsomes prepared from histologically normal human liver

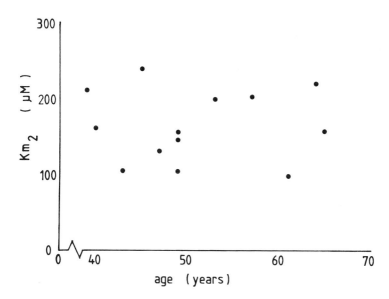

Figure 24.6 The effect of age on the affinity of the low affinity form (K_{m2}) of 7-ethoxycoumarin O-deethylation for substrate in liver microsomes prepared from histologically normal human liver

substrate range. The metabolism of this substrate is mediated by at least two kinetic components (high and low affinity) in human liver microsomes; the K_m values of both components can be determined using Eadie–Hofstee analysis as previously described[9].

The results are shown in Figures 24.5 and 24.6. There was no change in the affinity of either component of 7-ethoxycoumarin O-deethylation for the substrate with advancing years.

THE INFLUENCE OF DISEASE, AGE AND FRAILTY ON PHASE 1 DRUG METABOLISM

It has been postulated that disease and frailty rather than age are responsible for impaired drug metabolism. Because of the difficulty in obtaining liver tissue from frail subjects, we have used plasma esterase activities (an important phase 1 drug-metabolising enzyme) as a marker.

Patients and methods

Blood samples (5 ml) were taken from 3 groups of patients, namely fit young patients, fit ambulant elderly patients, and frail geriatric in-patients. Plasma aspirin esterase activities were measured *in vitro* as previously described[13].

Results

The results are shown in Figures 24.7 and 24.8. Serum albumin concentrations were significantly lower in both groups of elderly patients compared to the

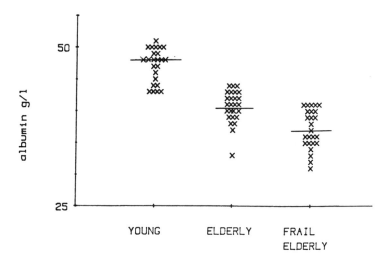

Figure 24.7   Serum albumin concentrations in young, fit elderly, and frail elderly patients

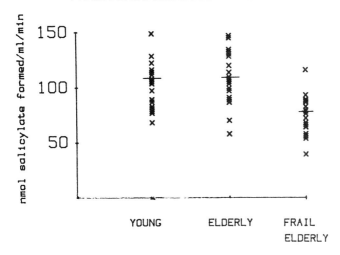

Figure 24.8   Plasma aspirin esterase activity in young, fit elderly, and frail elderly patients

young controls. Although the mean albumin level was lower in debilitated than fit elderly patients, this difference was not statistically significant.

Plasma aspirin esterase activity, however, was similar in the young control, and in fit elderly patients. In contrast, enzyme activity was significantly reduced in debilitated elderly patients.

LIVER SIZE AND BLOOD FLOW

Although it is widely stated that both liver size and blood flow[14,15] fall with advancing years in man, this statement is based on relatively scanty data. Furthermore, no study has previously investigated the effect of age upon both liver volume and blood flow in the same subjects. We therefore performed a systematic study to examine the extent of changes of both liver volume and blood flow in healthy subjects over a wide age range. Such changes, if they did occur, could account for impaired *in vivo* elimination of both low and high extraction drugs, without having to resort to suggestions that enzyme activity *per se* is altered.

Patients and Methods

65 healthy volunteers (33 females) between the ages of 24 and 91 years were recruited from colleagues and from local social clubs. None was taking medication that could influence drug metabolism, and all had normal blood count, renal function and liver function tests.

Liver size was determined using a modification of a previously published ultrasound method[17], and was shown to correlate well ($r = 0.97$) with volumes measured at CT in 6 patients. Liver blood flow was measured by estimating the clearance of indocyanine green[18].

261

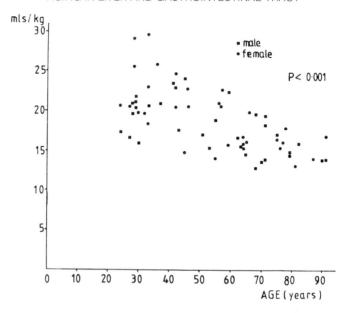

Figure 24.9 The effect of age on liver volume in healthy human subjects standardised for body weight

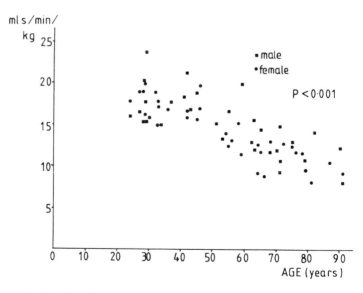

Figure 24.10 The effect of age on liver blood flow in fit human subjects standardised for body weight

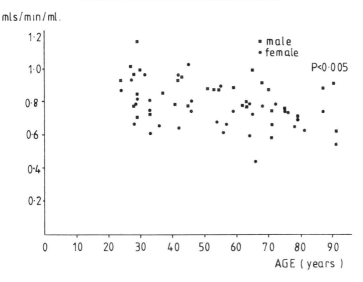

Figure 24.11 The effect of age on liver perfusion (expressed as ml of blood flow per minute per ml of liver) in fit human subjects

Results

The results are shown in Figures 24.9–24.11. There was a significant correlation between age and both liver volume and liver blood flow. Furthermore, liver volume still declined with age even when correction was made for changes in body weight. Interestingly the blood flow per unit of liver volume also decreased significantly with age.

DISCUSSION

When Kato and colleagues demonstrated that the activity of the important drug-metabolising enzymes, the hepatic microsomal mono-oxygenases, fell with advancing years in male rats, it appeared that this provided a simple and easy explanation of the reduced *in vivo* clearance of many oxidized drugs which has been described in humans. These results in rats were widely quoted, and careless extrapolations were made by some authors to the human. It would now appear, however, that the changes described by Kato may well be sex- and species-specific[6]. The studies described here clearly show that in human liver, there is no obvious age-related decline in the specific activity of MMO enzymes, at least as far as the two probe substrates studied are concerned. It is interesting to note that other authors have also failed to notice an age-related decline in MMO enzymes using a primate model[5]. It is therefore necessary to examine other mechanisms by which drug clearance *in vivo* may be impaired in elderly subjects.

The hypothesis that the affinity of the MMO enzymes for their substrate may fall with advancing years (reflected in a rise in K_m values) was attractive.

263

Such a change if it did occur would undoubtedly lead to reduction in drug elimination in the elderly patient. However our studies have clearly failed to demonstrate such age-related changes in both rat liver (where one may have expected it to be most apparent), or indeed in histologically normal human liver.

The effect of disability and disease has been widely discussed as a cause of impaired drug elimination in geriatric patients, and is well known to be a confounding factor in geriatric pharmacological studies[6]. Our studies using plasma aspirin esterase, have clearly shown that frailty and disease are much more important determinants of the activity of this enzyme at least than age. Whilst it is not possible to directly extrapolate from these plasma enzymes to the microsomal mono-oxygenase enzymes, indirect evidence suggests that similar factors also apply here[6].

Finally, a reduction in liver size, and in liver blood flow, could by themselves account for decreased drug elimination in the elderly patient. Our studies clearly demonstrate that even in otherwise healthy subjects, there is a progressive and marked decline in liver size (expressed per kilogram body weight) and liver blood flow (both in absolute terms, and expressed per unit of liver tissue), with age.

In summary therefore it would appear, in contrast to previous widely held views, that the major determinants of impaired drug elimination in the elderly are reduced liver size and blood flow and concurrent disease and frailty. Alterations in drug-metabolising enzymes, would not appear to be a function of ageing *per se*.

References

1. Hurwitz, N. (1969). Predisposing factors in adverse reactions to drugs. *Br. Med. J.*, **1**, 536–9
2. Greenblatt, D. J., Sellers, E. M. and Shader, R. I. (1982). Drug disposition in old age. *N. Engl. J. Med.*, **306**, 1081–8
3. Kato, R., Vassanelli, P. and Frontino, G. (1964). Variation in the activity of liver microsomal drug metabolizing enzymes in rats in relation to the age. *Biochem. Pharmacol.*, **13**, 1037–51
4. Woodhouse, K. W., Mutch, E., Williams, F. M. and James, O. F. W. (1984). The effect of age on pathways of drug metabolism in human liver. *Age Ageing*, **13**, 328–34
5. Maloney, A. G., Schmucker, D. L., Vessey, D. S. and Wang, R. K. (1986). The effects of aging on the hepatic microsomal mixed-function oxidase system of male and female monkeys. *Hepatology*, **6**, 282–7
6. Kitani, K. (1986). Hepatic drug metabolism in the elderly. *Hepatology*, **2**, 316–19
7. Woodhouse, K. W., Williams, F. M., Mutch, E., Wright, P., James, O. F. W. and Rawlins, M. D. (1983). The effects of alcoholic cirrhosis on the activities of microsomal aldrin epoxidase, 7-ethoxycoumarin O-deethylase and epoxide hydrolase, and on the concentrations of reduced glutathione in human liver. *Br. J. Clin Pharmacol.*, **15**, 667–72
8. Williams, F. M., Woodhouse, K. W., Middleton, D., Wright, P., James, O. F. W. and Rawlins, M. D. (1982). Aldrin epoxidation in small samples of human liver. *Biochem. Pharmacol.*, **31**, 3701–3
9. Woodhouse, K. W., Williams, F. M., Mutch, E., Wright, P., James, O. F. W. and Rawlins, M. D. (1984). The effect of alcoholic cirrhosis on the two kinetic components (high and low affinity) of the microsomal O-deethylation of 7-ethoxycoumarin in human liver. *Eur. J. Clin. Pharmacol.*, **26**, 61–4
10. Williams, F. M., Mutch, E., Woodhouse, K. W., Lambert, D. and Rawlins, M. D. (1986).

Ethoxyresorufin O-deethylation by human liver microsomes. *Br. J. Clin. Pharmacol.*, **22,** 263–86

11. Eisenthal, R. and Cornish-Bowden, P. (1974). The direct linear plot. *Biochem J.*, **139,** 715–20

12. Wynne, H., Mutch, E., James, O. F. W., Rawlins, M. and Woodhouse, K. W. (1987). Effect of age on monooxygenase enzyme kinetics in rat liver microsomes. *Age Ageing,* **16,** 153–8

13. Williams, F. M., Asad, S. I., Lessof, M. H. and Rawlins, M. D. (1987). Plasma esterase activity in patients with aspirin sensitive asthma or urticaria. *Eur. J. Clin. Pharmacol.* (In press)

14. Thompson, E. N. and Williams, R. (1965). Effect of age on liver function with particular reference to bromosulphalein excretion. *Gut,* **6,** 266–9

15. Tauchi, H. and Sato, T. (1978). Hepatic cells of the aged. In Kitani, K. (ed.) *Liver and Ageing.* pp. 3–19. (Amsterdam: Elsevier/North-Holland)

16. Tauchi, H. (1984). Cytomorphological studies of aging. *Asian Med. J.,* **27,** 741–60

17. Firtschy, P., Robotti, G., Schneekloth, G. and Vock, P. (1983). Measurement of liver volume by ultrasound and computed tomography. *J. Clin. Ultrasound,* **11,** 299–303

18. Caesar, J., Shaldon, S., Chiandussi, L., Guevena, L. and Sherlock, S. (1961). The use of indocyanine green in the measurement of hepatic blood flow and as a test of hepatic function. *Clin. Sci.,* **21,** 43–57

25
Class II reactions in aging

J. FEVERY

INTRODUCTION

Class II reactions comprise a heterogeneous group of conjugations whereby chemical moieties, derived from so-called donor substrates, are coupled to the acceptor substrates (Table 25.1). The enzymes catalysing these reactions can reside in the various compartments of liver parenchymal cells. Several enzymes are also present in other tissues such as kidney, intestine, lung or skin. They frequently are characterized by a great heterogeneity ('isoforms') with a quite high substrate-specificity. The class II reactions lead to production of more hydrophilic compounds. Some substrates undergo at first a class I reaction whereby, for example, a hydroxyl group was incorporated to yield a substance suitable for conjugation.

Table 25.1   Class II reactions

Conjugation	Location	Substrates
1. Sugar moiety		
glucuronic acid		bilirubin, steroids, thyroxine,
glucose	endoplasmic reticulum	*p*-nitrophenol, morphine, harmol,
xylose		paracetamol (acetaminophen)
2. Aminoacids		
glycine		
taurine	endoplasmic reticulum	bile acids, benzoic acids
glutathione		
	cytosol	bromsulfophthalein (BSP), DNCB, ethacrynic acid
3. Sulphate	cytosol	steroids, adrenaline, morphine, harmol, paracetamol (acetaminophen)
4. Acetyl	cytosol	INH, sulphonamides
Methyl		adrenaline

Are these reactions under influence of aging? In clinical medicine, the general impression holds that drug toxicity is more frequently encountered in the old age group. However, recent reports suggest that this might result

267

primarily from the more frequent intake of drugs by the elderly[1,2]. In addition, the aged person might be more susceptible to drug actions and toxicity because of altered pharmacokinetics or pharmacodynamics[3-5]. This does not imply that the rate of class I and/or class II reactions is decreased. Several other factors are involved in the *in vivo* handling of drugs. Indeed, in contrast to the situation in paediatric medicine, dosages administered in adult and geriatric clinics are usually not adapted to body weight or surface. Furthermore, the fat content of the human body increases with age, and serum albumin tends to drop; this might greatly influence uptake, storage and distribution volume of drugs. Hepatic blood flow can be decreased in the elderly, owing to atherosclerosis or to reduced cardiac output secondary to arteriosclerotic heart disease, myocardiopathy, to systemic diseases or infection or to β-blockade. This can hamper hepatic uptake of several drugs. Age-related alterations of hepatic parenchymal cell sinusoidal or canalicular membranes have not been studied in great detail. They might alter uptake and secretion processes. Glomerular filtration rate decreases slightly, again resulting in prolonged half-life times of some drugs.

In animal experiments, class II reactions undergo alterations when protein deficiency is induced. Furthermore, conjugation reactions can be enhanced in man and animals by enzyme-inducing agents such as barbiturates, glutethimide, clofibrate, spironolactone, rifampicin etc. or be depressed by enzyme inhibition due to drug therapy with for example, novobiocin, triphenylacetic acid or allopurinol. The concentrations of donor substrate and/or cofactors might decrease owing to diet or disease or to age as observed in some animals[6,7]. This can markedly affect the *in vivo* conjugation rate. Several enzyme activities are highly influenced by sex or sex steroid hormones[8]. The question thus remains whether class II reactions *per se* are influenced by aging, if one takes care of species differences and environmental factors.

In most species investigated, the foetal or neonatal period is characterized by low enzyme activities. They rise progressively in young animals even to reach levels above adult values. Less information is available concerning possible changes in older age, as will be evidenced from the literature reviewed.

GLUTATHIONE-S-TRANSFERASES

Glutathione-S-transferases are dimers of two homologous or heterologous subunits. Their heterogeneity has now firmly been established by separation studies[9-14] (Table 25.2) and recently also by molecular biology and establishment of mRNAs and cDNAs[15]. This heterogeneity necessitates the use of a great variety of substrates when assaying enzyme activity. Enzyme activities are low in the neonatal rat[16] and monkey[17] and increase till puberty. GSH-S-transferase activity towards 1-chloro-2,4-dinitrobenzene (CDNB), a substrate for several subunits, did not show age-related changes[18-20]. In the male rat, activity towards 1,2-dichloro-4-nitrobenzene (DCNB) is exerted mainly by subunit 3 and increases after puberty till a maximum at age 6–12 months followed by a gradual decline in old rats (28 months), whereas the activity

Table 25.2 Heterogeneity of rat hepatic glutathione-S-transferases

Denomination*				'Marker' substrates for the given subunit structure**
Current	Previous			
1–1	B or ligandins	L2	YaYa	Δ^5-androstenedione
1–2		BL	YaYa	
2–2	AA	B2	YcYc	cumene hydroperoxide, thiocyanates
3–3	A	A2	Yb1Yb1	halogenated aryl derivatives, e.g. DNCB, bromsulfophthalein (BSP) and p-nitrobenzyl chloride
3–4	C	AC	Yb1Yb2	
4–4	D	C2	Yb2Yb2	4-hydroxynonenal, ethacrynic acid
5–5	E	E2		1,2-epoxy-3-(p-nitrophenoxy)propane iodomethane
6–6	M	M2	YmYm	
7–7	P			

* The current denomination (refs. 9 and 10) refers to the subunit composition; previous names (refs. 11 and 13) related to separation characteristics of the dimeric enzymes in various systems used by different investigators
** Summarized from refs. 10, 11 and 20

towards BSP (also subunit 3) rather remained constant over the period $1\frac{1}{2}$ to 12 months with a decrease till low values in rats of age 28 months[21]. Alterations in female rats were in general very small or absent.

The pronounced heterogeneity of glutathione-S-transferases is also obvious from the marked species differences observed as well as from the inducibility by pretreatment with phenobarbital, *trans*-stilbene oxide and butylated hydroxyamisole[22]. This also precludes prediction of the human situation from animal experiments.

UDP-GLUCURONOSYLTRANSFERASES AND SULPHATASE

The UDP-glucuronosyltransferases are also characterized by a great functional and structural heterogeneity and by species differences[23–26]. Marked late-foetal (p-nitrophenol group) or post-natal (e.g. bilirubin) developmental changes are present in most animal species[23]. Several isoforms, respectively active versus 3-OH-steroids, p-nitrophenol or 3-OH-bile salts and testosterone, have been isolated[27–31] and for some the mRNA coding has been outlined[32].

The induction by pretreatment with phenobarbitone, clofibrate, spironolactone, 3-methylcholanthrene etc. varies greatly according to the acceptor substrate and the animal species investigated[24,27,33,34]. Furthermore, activation by *in vitro* addition of detergents or UDP-N-acetylglucosamine also can vary with the substrate and the species investigated[26,33]. A pronounced effect of sex and sex hormones has been observed with enhancement of enzyme activity towards bilirubin by progesterone and inhibition by testosterone; opposite effects were noted towards p-nitrophenol[8]. Again all these variables should be taken into account when studying the effect of old age. Several authors did not find significant alterations in UDP-glucuronosyltransferase activities toward p-nitrophenol or phenolphthalein in male Fischer 344 rats whereas a mild (10–20%) decrease was described in male Wistar rats[35–38].

Sulfation of acetaminophen (paracetamol) by isolated hepatocytes was reported to be slightly decreased in old rats but not in old mice when compared to young adults[39].

MECHANISMS POSSIBLY INVOLVED

These usually mild alterations of enzyme-specific activities should be interpreted in relation to changes in liver and body weight. In male and female Fischer 344 rats body weight increases progressively with age[18] but the liver-to-body weight ratio also increased in the male rat possibly compensating for the mild decrease in specific activity. Total liver activity, which is more relevant for the *in vivo* situation, may thus remain unchanged. In females the liver-to-body weight ratio remains unaltered as well as does specific enzyme activity.

The mild decreases in some enzyme activities observed in male rats might be related to age-induced alterations in membrane composition. Nokubo[40] observed a progressive increase of the apparent microviscosity of liver plasma membrane preparations in male but not in female rats whereas others[41] documented an increase with age of the protein:phospholipid and the cholesterol:phospholipid ratio, whereas the protein:cholesterol ratio remained constant. More specifically, the phosphatidylcholine content of the membranes decreased.

DATA IN MAN

In man the liver volume as well as the liver volume per body surface decreased in the elderly[42,43]. Acetylation, measured by the plasma half-life of isoniazid showed no significant[44] or a small increase[45] with age. However, when the groups were sub-divided according to sex, Paulsen and Nilsson[46] reported a

Table 25.3 Acetylation of INH in older age (data summarized from ref. 46)

| Age | Mean plasma half-life (min) | | | |
	Males	Females	Total group	n
<45	153	139	146	111
46–65	162	141	151	109
>65	179	137	157	90

progressive increase of the INH plasma half life with age in males; no change was observed in the already lower values of females (Table 25.3). The data on glucuronidation in man are discussed by Schenker and Hoyumpa in Chapter 26[47].

CONCLUSION

Class II reactions are characterized by marked species differences and by a pronounced heterogeneity of the enzymes (existence of multiple isoforms). Some are membrane-bound and thus subject to membrane alterations and perturbations. The effect of sex and sex hormones is more important than previously thought. In general, specific enzyme activities remain rather constant with increasing age in female animals but show a slight decrease in the males. When relating the *in vitro* results to the *in vivo* situation, it should be noted that the liver in male rats increases with age, probably compensating for the mild decrease in enzyme activity.

In man, *in vitro* assays are very scarce. Acetylation *in vivo* seems to decrease in males with increasing age but not in females. Other factors seem more important for the *in vivo* situation, such as liver size and blood flow, distribution volume and albumin concentration, decreasing glomerular filtration and the effect of sex, sex hormones, alcohol, smoking and enzyme-inducing or -inhibiting medication. More data are clearly needed in man.

References

1. Weber, J. C. P. and Griffin, J. P. (1986). Prescriptions, adverse reactions, and the elderly. *Lancet*, **1**, 1220
2. Woodhouse, K. W., Mortimer, O. and Wiholm, B-E. (1986). Hepatic adverse drug reactions: the effect of age. In Kitani, K. (ed.) *Liver and Aging – 1986*. pp. 75–9. (Amsterdam: Elsevier Science Publishers)
3. James, O. F. W. (1985). Drugs and the ageing liver. *J. Hepatol.*, **1**, 431–5
4. Vestal, R. E., Wood, A. J. J., Branch, R. A., Wilkinson, G. W. and Shand, D. G. (1978). Studies of drug disposition in the elderly using model compounds. In Kitani, K. (ed.) *Liver and Aging – 1978*. pp. 343–57. (Amsterdam: Elsevier/North Holland Biomedical Press)
5. Kitani, K. (1986). Hepatic drug metabolism in the elderly. *Hepatology*, **6**, 316–19
6. Stohs, S. J. and Lawson, T. (1986). The role of glutathione and its metabolism in aging. In Kitani, K. (ed.) *Liver and Aging – 1986*. pp. 59–70. (Amsterdam: Elsevier Science Publishers)
7. Hazelton, G. A. and Lang, C. A. (1980). Glutathione contents of tissue in the aging mouse. *Biochem. J.*, **188**, 25–30
8. Muraca, M. and Fevery, J. (1984). Influence of sex and sex steroids on bilirubin uridine diphosphate-glucuronosyltransferase activity of rat liver. *Gastroenterology*, **87**, 308–13
9. Habig, W. H., Pabst, M. J. and Jakoby, W. B. (1976). Glutathione S-transferase AA from rat liver. *Arch. Biochem. Biophys.*, **175**, 710–16
10. Habig, W. H. and Jakoby, W. B. (1981). Assays for differentiation of glutathione S-transferases. *Methods Enzymol.*, **77**, 398–405
11. Mannervik, B. and Jensson, H. (1982). Binary combinations of four protein subunits with different catalytic specificities explain the relationship between six basic glutathione S-transferases in rat liver cytosol. *J. Biol. Chem.*, **257**, 9909–12
12. Meuwissen, J. A. T. P. and Heirwegh, K. P. M. (1982). Aspects of bilirubin transport. In Heirwegh, K. P. M. and Brown, S. B. (eds.) *Bilirubin*. pp. 39–83. (Boca Raton, Florida: CRC Press)

13. Sugiyama, Y., Yamada, T. and Kaplowitz, N. (1983). Newly identified bile acid binders in rat liver cytosol. Purification and comparison with glutathione S-transferases. *J. Biol. Chem.*, **258**, 3602–7

14. Jakoby, W. B., Ketterer, B. and Mannervik, B. (1984). Glutathione transferases: nomenclature. *Biochem. Pharmacol.*, **33**, 2539–40

15. Tu C.-P.D., Lai, H.-C.J., Li,N.-q., Weiss, M. J. and Reddy, C. C. (1984). The Y_c and Y_a subunits of rat liver glutathione S-transferases are the products of separate genes. *J. Biol. Chem.*, **259**, 9434–9

16. Eidne, K. A., Sherman, B. A., Millar, R. P. and Kirsch, R. E. (1984). Ligandin concentrations in the steroidogenic tissues of the rat during development. *Biochim. Biophys. Acta*, **801**, 424–8

17. Levi, A. J., Gatmaitan, Z. and Arias, I. M. (1970). Deficiency of hepatic organic anion-binding protein, impaired organic anion uptake by liver and 'physiologic' jaundice in newborn monkeys. *N. Engl. J. Med.*, **283**, 1136

18. Fujita, S., Kitagawa, H., Ishizawa, H., Suzuki, T. and Kitani, K. (1985). Age-associated alterations in hepatic glutathione-S-transferase activities. *Biochem. Pharmacol.*, **34**, 3891–4

19. Spearman, M. E. and Leibman, K. C. (1984). Effects of aging on hepatic and pulmonary glutathione S-transferase activities in male and female Fischer 344 rats. *Biochem. Pharmacol.*, **33**, 1309–13

20. Spearman, M. E. (1986). Interaction of endogenous and exogenous chemicals with rat glutathione S-transferases: implications of age-related changes. In Kitani, K. (ed.) *Liver and Aging – 1986*. pp. 45. (Amsterdam: Elsevier Science Publishers)

21. Kanai, S., Kitani, K., Fujita, S. and Kitagawa, H. (1985). The hepatic handling of sulfobromphthalein in aging Fischer-344 rats: *in vivo* and *in vitro* studies. *Arch. Gerontol. Geriatr.*, **4**, 73–85

22. Gregus, Z., Varga, F. and Schmelas, A. (1985). Age-development and inducibility of hepatic glutathione S-transferase activities in mice, rats, rabbits and guinea-pigs. *Comp. Biochem. Physiol.*, **80C**, 85–90

23. Wishart, G. J. (1978). Functional heterogeneity of UDP-glucurocuronosyltransferase as indicated by its differential development and inducibility by glucocorticoids. *Biochem. J.*, **174**, 485

24. Lillienblum, W., Walli, A. K. and Bock, K. W. (1982). Differential induction of rat liver microsomal UDP-glucuronosyl transferase activities by various inducing agents. *Biochem. Pharmacol.*, **31**, 907

25. Leakey, J. A., Althaus, Z. R., Bailey, J. R. *et al.* (1983). UDP-glucuronosyltransferase activity exhibits two developmental groups in liver from foetal rhesus monkeys. *Biochem. J.*, **214**, 1007

26. Fevery, J., van de Vijver, M., Michiels, R. and Heirwegh, K. P. M. (1977). Comparison in different species of biliary bilirubin-IX conjugates with the activities of hepatic and renal bilirubin-IX–uridine diphosphate glycosyltransferases. *Biochem. J.*, **164**, 737–46

27. Bock, K. W., Josting, D., Lilienblum, W. *et al.* (1979). Purification of rat liver microsomal UDP-glucuronosyl transferase. Separation of two enzyme forms inducible by 3-methylcholanthrene or phenobarbital. *Eur. J. Biochem.*, **98**, 19

28. Tukey, R. H. and Tephley, T. R. (1981). Purification and properties of rabbit liver estrone and *p*-nitrophenol UDP-glucuronosyltransferase. *Arch. Biochem. Biophys.*, **209**, 565

29. Falany, C. N. and Tephly, T. R. (1983). Separation, purification and characterization of three isozymes of UDP-glucuronosyltransferase from rat liver microsomes. *Arch. Biochem. Biophys.*, **227**, 248

30. Matern, H., Matern, S. and Gerok, W. (1982). Isolation and characterization of rat liver microsomal UDP-glucuronosyltransferase activity toward chenodeoxycholic acid and testosterone as a single form of enzyme. *J. Biol. Chem.*, **257**, 7422

31. Kirkpatrick, R. B., Falany, C. N. and Tephly, T. R. (1984). Glucuronidation of bile acids by rat liver 3-OH androgen UDP-glucuronosyltransferase. *J. Biol. Chem.*, **259**, 6176

32. MacKenzie, P. I., Gonzalez, F. J. and Owens, I. S. (1984). Cell-free translation of mouse liver mRNA coding for two forms of UDP-glucuronosyltransferase. *Arch. Biochem. Biophys.*, **230**, 676

33. Winsner, A. (1971). Age and sex dependent variability of the activation characteristics of UDP-glucuronyltransferase *in vitro*. *Biochem. Pharmacol.*, **20**, 1249–58

34. Siest, G., Antoine, B., Fournel, S., Magdalou, J. and Thomassin, J. (1987). The glucuronosyltransferases: what progress can pharmacologists expect from molecular biology and cellular enzymology? *Biochem. Pharmacol., 36*, 983–9

35. Ali, M., Nicholls, P. J. and Yoosuf, A. (1979). The influence of old age and of renal failure on hepatic glucuronidation in the rat. *Proceedings of the B.P.S.,* April 4–6, pp. 498–9

36. Jayaraj, A., Hardwick, J. P., Diller, T. W. and Richardson, A. G. (1985). Metabolism, covalent binding, and mutagenicity of aflatoxin B_1 by liver extracts from rats of various ages. *J. Natl. Cancer Inst., 74*, 95–103

37. Borghoff, S. J. and Birnbaum, L. S. (1985). Age-related changes in glucuronidation and deglucuronidation in liver, small intestine, lung, and kidney of male Fischer rats. *Drug Metab. Disp., 13*, 62–7

38. van Bezooijen, C. F. A. (1984). Influence of age-related changes in rodent liver morphology and physiology on drug metabolism – A review. *Mech. Ageing Develop., 25*, 1–22

39. Sweeny, D. J. and Weiner, M. (1985). Metabolism of acetaminophen in hepatocytes isolated from mice and rats of various ages. *Drug Metab. Disp., 13*, 377–9

40. Nokubo, M. (1985). Physical-chemical and biochemical differences in liver plasma membranes in aging F-344 rats. *J. Gerontol., 40*, 409–14

41. Spinedi, A., Rufini, S. and Luly, P. (1985). Age-dependent changes of rat liver plasma membrane composition. *Experientia, 41*, 1141–3

42. Bach, B., Hansen, J. M., Kampmann, J. P., Rasmussen, S. N. and Skovsted, L. (1981). Disposition of antipyrine and phenytoin correlated with age and liver volume in man. *Clin. Pharmacokinet., 6*, 389–96

43. Swift, C. G., Homeida, M., Halliwell, M. and Roberts, C. J. C. (1978). Antipyrine disposition and liver size in the elderly. *Eur. J. Clin. Pharmacol., 14*, 149–52

44. Farah, F., Taylor, W., Rawlins, M. D. and James, O. (1977). Hepatic drug acetylation and oxidation: effects of aging in man. *Br. Med. J., 2*, 155–56

45. Gachaly, B., Vas, A., Hajos, P. and Kaldor, A. (1984). Acetylator phenotypes: effect of age. *Eur. J. Clin. Pharmacol., 26*, 43–5

46. Paulsen, O. and Nilsson, L. G. (1985). Distribution of acetylator phenotype in relation to age and sex in Swedish patients. *Eur. J. Clin. Pharmacol., 28*, 311–15

47. Schenker, S. and Hoyumpa, A. (1988). Benzodiazepines in the elderly as a model drug. In Bianchi *et al.* (eds.) Falk Symposium, No. 47, *Aging in the Liver and Gastrointestinal Tract.* pp. 275–82. (Lancaster: MTP Press)

26
Benzodiazepines in the elderly as a model drug

S. SCHENKER and A. HOYUMPA

INTRODUCTION

Consideration of drug metabolism and elimination in the aged is important, not only to optimize clinical prescribing of therapeutic agents, but also to improve overall understanding of drug metabolism with advancing age. In the clinical area, it is well-appreciated that the elderly consume a disproportionate number of drugs, often in combination, and account for a substantial percentage of drug-induced adverse reactions[1,2]. This does not necessarily imply a special predilection of the aged to such side effects[5] and may simply reflect greater drug usage, increased incidence of combined organ disease which renders prescribing more difficult, and possibly poorer compliance. Nevertheless, as the population is aging increasingly, it behooves us to consider the problem as a clinically relevant issue.

In the basic science area, some aspects of drug pharmacokinetics in the aged are well-defined, while others dealing especially with hepatic drug elimination are still uncertain. Thus, it is well-agreed that drug absorption is little, if any, altered in the aged, that drug binding in plasma tends to be decreased and that the volume of drug distribution tends to reflect the greater fat content as percentage of body weight in aging[2]. Thus, for lipid-soluble drugs, the volume of drug distribution increases and, for water-soluble agents, it tends to decrease[2-4]. Perhaps, most important, it is clear that with aging renal function falls. Thus, drugs excreted principally by the kidneys are eliminated more slowly in the aged.

As stated earlier, the pharmacokinetic role of the liver in the aged is much less clear. It is believed that liver blood flow, both in absolute terms and as a percentage of cardiac output, falls with aging[2]. This should result in reduced clearance of flow-dependent (high extraction) drugs eliminated by the liver. Indeed, propranolol clearance falls with aging, but this effect is not universally documented. Likewise, there is evidence that the overall mass of the liver decreases in the aged[6]. This should ensue in impaired clearance of all drugs metabolized by the liver in the aged, an effect clearly not seen. It is in the hepatic enzymatic machinery for biotransforming drugs, however, that the data for aging are least clear. In rodents, especially males, drug oxidation generally falls with aging. Studies in aged primates, however, show no alteration of the cytochrome P-450 system and no change in a limited assessment of hepatic *in vitro* drug oxidation[7]. In man, there are few studies of the hepatic drug oxidizing system *in vitro* in aged liver, while pharmacokinetic *in vivo* data are not uniform. Thus, the subject of drug disposition by the aged human liver clearly is of interest to basic scientists committed to the area of drug metabolism.

BENZODIAZEPINES AS MODEL DRUGS

In considering drug disposition in aged man, benzodiazepines are excellent model drugs[8,9]. The reasons are as follows. First, the metabolic biotransformation pathways of these agents are well worked out and the parent drugs and their metabolites are easy to assay. Second, the kinetics of these agents are clearly defined both in young and elderly people. They are low extraction agents and their elimination is primarily dependent only on hepatic metabolism. Furthermore, they are highly bound to plasma proteins, permitting an assessment of this in the aged on drug distribution and elimination. Third, some benzodiazepines are metabolized by oxidation and other by conjugation to ether glucuronides. The biotransformation products of oxidation have significant pharmacologic properties resulting in prolonged drug action. By contrast, the glucuronides are pharmacologically inactive and, thus, the duration of sedation is brief. Comparison of the handling of both groups of drugs permits assessment of oxidation versus glucuronidation in aging. Finally, the end-point of the pharmacologic action of this group of drugs is fairly easily measurable, i.e. assessment of sedation. In addition, the sedative effect of the drugs on the brain is known to be mediated by specific cerebral receptors[10,11]. These are susceptible to study. For these reasons, benzodiazepines are good model drugs to examine the effects of aging on hepatic drug elimination.

EFFECTS OF AGING IN MAN ON BENZODIAZEPINE DISPOSITION

Benzodiazepines metabolized by oxidation

Few data are available on the effect of aging on the absorption of these drugs. Although gastric hypoacidity and hypomotility may be expected with older age, diazepam absorption appears to be similar in the young and old[12]. The time of peak serum bromazepam in the two groups was also comparable[13]. This is consistent with their lipophilic characteristics. By contrast, most studies report decreased serum albumin and a lower binding of benzodiazepines with old age[2,3,14]. Theoretically, this lower binding of these drugs could contribute to a larger volume of distribution, more rapid penetration of the drug into the brain and more rapid access of the free drug to the metabolizing systems in the liver, hence more rapid elimination. Indeed, the volume of drug distribution of the lipid-soluble benzodiazepines (i.e. diazepam, chlordiazepoxide) is substantially higher in the aged, especially in females[15,16]. Where this has been corrected for the amount of drug bound to protein, the change persisted. This suggests that the increased volume of distribution for lipid soluble benzodiazepines with aging is due primarily to the higher percentage of body fat in the elderly, especially in females. This interpretation is consistent with the reports of greater volume of distribution of lipophilic benzodiazepines in the obese[17,18] and of a good correlation between the fat uptake of these drugs and their *in vitro* lipid/water partition coefficient[4]. By contrast, the volume of distribution of the relatively non-lipophilic drugs, antipyrine and acetaminophen, actually declines with aging[19,20]. The larger volume of distribution in the elderly (and the obese) may have clinical implications. Thus, for single dosing, blood levels and the intensity and duration of action of the drug will be influenced by the drug's volume of distribution (V_d)[21]. With chronic drug use, a higher V_d will influence the drug half-life and thus a proper dosing interval[2].

With protracted use, clearance determines steady state drug levels[2,14]. In general, a lower clearance has been reported with aging for benzodiazepines biotransformed by oxidation, i.e. hydroxylation or dealkylation[2,15,22]. This is especially true for males[2]. The list of benzodiazepines thus affected includes diazepam, chlordiazepoxide, desmethyldiazepam, desalkylflurazepam, clobazam, alprazolam, triazolam, midazolam and brotizolam. Interestingly, two benzodiazepines which are metabolized by nitro-reduction, nitrazepam and flunitrazepam, undergo only negligible age-related changes in clearance[23]. The mechanism(s) of the decreased clearance of some of these drugs with aging is uncertain. It clearly is not related to liver blood flow (which may fall with aging) as most of these benzodiazepines exhibit relatively low extraction and thus their elimination depends primarily on hepatic metabolism. Likewise, decreased liver mass seen with aging cannot readily account for these findings since some drugs are affected while others metabolized by nitro-reduction and glucuronidation (see below) are not. It may be, however, that the reserve in the liver for the latter two enzymatic processes (especially glucuronidation) versus oxidation is sufficient even with a lower functional liver mass or that there is extra-hepatic compensatory metabolism for these drugs. The most logical explanation would be demonstration of decreased hepatic oxidizing machinery (i.e. cytochrome P-450) with aging. Fluidity of organelles with aging in rodents tends to decrease and thus may contribute to altered microsomal oxidation[24]. Unfortunately, there are virtually no data for man in this area, although in sub-human primates no consistent change in microsomal fluidity with aging was seen[7]. One small study, studying ethoxycoumarin O-deethylase and aldrin epoxidase dealt with mixed sexes and only 11 normal individuals. There was no significant relationship of age with the enzymatic activity which varied greatly among subjects[25]. Thus, this area remains essentially unstudied in man. It is also uncertain why a lower clearance is seen, especially in males. It is of interest, however, that in rodents, males exhibit a great depression of drug metabolism for some agents with aging[6]. This has been attributed to feminization of the drug oxidizing system[26-28]. It is possibly of interest in this regard that female sex hormones (i.e. oral contraceptives) may depress the oxidation of some drugs (i.e. caffeine, antipyrine), including some benzodiazepines such as chlordiazepoxide[29,30]. Further research in this specific area is warranted.

Half-life ($t_\frac{1}{2}$) of a drug is a hybrid kinetic parameter which is directly proportional to drug volume of distribution and inversely dependent on clearance. With aging, drug V_d increases for lipophilic drugs (most benzodiazepines), especially in women. Clearance of these drugs falls, especially in males. Thus, $t_\frac{1}{2}$ with aging tends to increase for both reasons. Clearly this kinetic parameter, therefore, is not an optimal expression of altered drug disposition with aging, unless the other variables are known[2,8]. Moreover, it does not usually take into account drug binding in plasma.

Benzodiazepines metabolized by glucuronidation

By contrast with the oxidized benzodiazepines, those inactivated by glucuronidation (oxazepam, lorazepam, temazepam, lormetazepam) are little or not at all affected by aging[31-34]. More specifically their volume of distribution, $t_\frac{1}{2}$ and clearance are usually not significantly altered. Similar findings are noted with acetaminophen (largely de-toxified by glucuronidation), although one study reported a decrease in clearance of borderline significance[20]. The reason(s) for this relative preservation of glucuronidation with aging is uncertain. Interestingly, a similar phenomenon is seen with liver disease wherein oxidation of drugs tends to be more selectively depressed[33,35-37]. Moreover, glucuronidation is not depressed by the H_2-receptor antagonist cimetidine[38], by disulfiram[39] or oral contraceptives[40,41]. The latter drugs, in fact, may enhance the glucuronidation of some agents. (The relative induction with aging of drugs oxidized versus those glucuronidated will not be discussed here.) The differences in inhibition of oxidized versus glucuronidated benzodiazepines is probably owing to the more specific effects of these inhibitors on the cytochrome P-450 system (i.e. cimetidine). Why should glucuronidation be relatively 'immune', both to aging and liver disease? Explanations may be forthcoming from the different microsomal location and constraint of glucuronidating enzymes. Ample evidence based on older studies with trypsin[42] and modern cloning techniques[43] suggest that glucuronyltransferases are located deep in the microsome behind a lipophilic barrier. Furthermore, these enzymes tend to be present in excess capacity in latent form, and apparently may be functionally released by appropriate stimuli[44]. Extrahepatic reserves have already been alluded to[45]. These theoretic explanations as to aging and glucuronidation need to be corroborated with specific studies.

Predictive studies of benzodiazepines pharmacokinetics

To the extent that aging may depress the clearance of certain drugs and with those of narrow therapeutic index may result in adverse side effects over a period of time, it would be helpful to develop specific predictive tests for prescribing correctly such drugs. There is, unfortunately, no creatinine clearance for hepatic drug elimination in aging. It does appear, however, that reasonable correlations exist over a large age group among clearances of drugs metabolized by oxidation and by glucuronidation, but not between the two groups[19,46]. Thus, for oxidized drugs, good correlations of elimination half-life between antipyrine and diazepam ($r = 0.73$), desmethyldiazepam ($r = 0.83$) and between diazepam and desmethyldiazepam ($r = 0.77$) have been obtained. For drugs glucuronidated (without a decrease in clearance with aging) good correlations have been obtained between acetaminophen and oxazepam clearance ($r = 0.87$), lorazepam clearance ($r = 0.70$), temazepam clearance ($r = 0.63$) and between lorazepam and oxazepam clearances ($r = 0.72$). By contrast no correlation was seen between antipyrine and conjugated drug clearances on the one hand and acetaminophen and oxidized drug clearances. Interestingly, nitrazepam, whose elimination by nitro-reduction is not reduced with aging did not correlate with antipyrine elimination across a large age range ($r = 0.23$)[23]. Likewise, the elimination half-life of triazolam, which is quite rapid, did not correlate with that of antipyrine[47]. Thus, despite some exceptions, this overall correlation attests to some generality in the metabolic pathways affected by aging. However, the predictive value of these correlations is at best of the order of 65%, too low to be of value in the individual patient.

Pharmacodynamics of benzodiazepines in aging

There is reasonably good evidence that the brain in the elderly is more sensitive to the sedative effects of benzodiazepines, independent of their blood levels[2,48-51]. The mechanism(s) of this effect is uncertain. Part of the effect could be owing to decreased drug binding with more unbound drug reaching cerebral receptors. Intrinsic alterations in cerebral benzodiazepine receptors in the aged also have been suggested. In experimental animals, the data are conflicting, but it is generally felt that no major differences occur with aging[52]. In man few data are available, but preliminary studies with positron emission tomography (PET) suggest a decrease in receptor density with aging, although altered blood–brain permeability also could account for the findings reported[53]. No solid information on receptor affinity is available. One parallel situation may be patients with liver disease, wherein sensitivity to benzodiazepines has also been suggested[54]. In this instance, however, preliminary data with PET imply an increase in benzodiazepine receptors[55], more consistent with greater sensitivity. Whatever the mechanism(s) of such sensitivity of the aged to benzodiazepines, caution in administering such drugs to the elderly (independent of pharmacokinetics) is warranted.

PRESCRIBING PRACTICES

Benzodiazepines, in general, have a high therapeutic index, hence, serious toxicity is unlikely. However, summation with other drugs and concerns about impaired performance in the elderly when the attention span may be important (as in driving) are significant issues. It would appear that many oxidized benzodiazepines and their active metabolites will tend to accumulate over time, whereas glucuronidated drugs will not. Also, the latter agents have a short half-life and their metabolites are not pharmacologically active. Thus, for compliant patients, the glucuronidated benzodiazepines would appear less likely to cause side effects on pharmacokinetic grounds. However, lack of compliance with these agents is likely to result in uneven drug action. Even given these pharmacokinetic differences, the aged are apparently more sensitive to benzodiazepines and thus careful titration to desired clinical response, with periodic follow up, seems safest. In the final analysis, it is not *which* drug is used but *how* it is used that is the key to optimal drug therapy of the elderly.

Acknowledgement

Supported by Veterans Administration (Research Service, Audie Murphy Memorial Veterans' Hospital).

References

1. Clinical depression of the central nervous system due to diazepam and chlordiazepoxide in relation to cigarette smoking and age: a report from the Boston Collaborative Drug Surveillance Program, Boston University Medical Center. (1973). *N. Engl. J. Med.*, **288**, 277–80
2. Greenblatt, D. J., Sellers, E. M. and Shader, R. I. (1982). Drug disposition of old age. *N. Engl. J. Med.*, **306**, 1081–8
3. Greenblatt, D. J., Abernethy, D. R. and Shader, R. I. (1986). Pharmacokinetic aspects of drug therapy in the elderly. *Ther. Drug Monitor.*, **8**, 249–55
4. Scavone, J. M., Friedman, H., Greenblatt, D. J. and Shader, R. I. (1987). Effect of age, body composition, and lipid solubility on benzodiazepine tissue distribution in rats. *Arzneim.-Forsch./Drug Res.*, **37**, 2–6
5. Woodhaus, K. W., Mortimer, O. and Wiholm, B. E. (1986). Hepatic adverse drug reactions: the effect of age. In Kitani, K. (ed.) *Liver and Aging: Liver and Brain*, pp. 75–80. (Amsterdam: Elsevier)
6. Kitani, K. (1986). Hepatic drug metabolism in the elderly. *Hepatology*, **6**, 316–19
7. Maloney, A. G., Schmucker, D. L., Vessey, D. S. and Wang, R. K. (1986). The effect of aging on the hepatic microsomal mixed-function oxidase system of male and female monkey. *Hepatology*, **6**, 282–7
8. Greenblatt, D. J., Divoll, M., Abernethy, D. R., Ochs, H. R. and Shader, R. I. (1983). Benzodiazepine kinetics: implications for therapeutics and pharmacogeriatrics. *Drug Metab. Rev.*, **14**, 251–92
9. Salzman, C., Shader, R. I., Greenblatt, D. J. and Harmatz, J. S. (1983). Long vs. short half-life benzodiazepines in the elderly. *Arch. Gen. Psychiatry*, **40**, 293–7
10. Braestrup, C. and Squires, F. (1977). Specific benzodiazepine receptors in rat brain characterized by high-affinity [³H]diazepam binding. *Proc. Natl. Acad. Sci. USA*, **74**, 3805–9
11. Mohler, H. and Okada, T. (1977). Benzodiazepine receptor: demonstration in the central nervous system. *Science*, **198**, 849–51

12. Ochs, H. R., Otten, H., Greenblatt, D. J. and Dengler, H. J. (1982). Diazepam absorption: effects of age, sex and Billroth gastrectomy. *Dig. Dis. Sci.*, **27**, 225–30
13. Ochs, H. R., Greenblatt, D. J., Friedman, H., Burstein, E. S., Locniskar, A., Harmatz, J. S., and Shader, R. I. (1987). Bromozepam pharmacokinetics: influence of age, gender, oral contraceptives, cimetidine and propranolol. *Clin. Pharmacol. Ther.*, **41**, 567–70
14. Divoll, M. and Greenblatt, D. J. (1982). Effect of age and sex on lorazepam protein binding. *J. Pharm. Pharmacol.*, **34**, 122–3
15. Klotz, U., Avant, G. R., Hoyumpa, A., Schenker, S. and Wilkinson, G. R. (1975). The effects of age and liver disease on the disposition and elimination of diazepam in adult man. *J. Clin. Invest.*, **55**, 347
16. Ochs, H. R., Greenblatt, D. J., Divoll, M., Abernethy, D. R., Feyerabend, H. and Dengler, H. J. (1981). Diazepam kinetics in relation to age and sex. *Pharmacology*, **23**, 24–30
17. Greenblatt, D. J., Abernethy, D. R., Locniskar, A., Harmatz, J. S., Limjuco, R. A. and Shader, R. I. (1984). Effect of age, gender, and obesity on midazolam kinetics. *Anesthesiology*, **61**, 27–35
18. Abernethy, D. R., Greenblatt, D. J., Divoll, M. and Shader, R. I. (1983). Enhanced glucuronide conjugation of drugs in obesity: studies of lorazepam, oxazepam, and acetaminophen. *J. Lab. Clin. Med.*, **101**, 873–80
19. Greenblatt, D. J., Divoll, M., Abernethy, D. R., Harmatz, J. S. and Shader, R. I. (1982). Antipyrine kinetics in the elderly: prediction of age-related changes in benzodiazepine oxidizing capacity. *J. Pharmacol. Exp. Ther.*, **220**, 120–6
20. Divoll, M. Abernethy, D. R., Ameer, B. and Greenblatt, D. J. (1982). Acetaminophen kinetics in the elderly. *Clin. Pharmacol. Ther.*, **31**, 151–6
21. Greenblatt, D. J. (1980). Pharmacokinetic comparisons. *Psychosomatics*, **21**, 9–14
22. Roberts, R. K., Wilkinson, G. R., Branch, R. A. and Schenker, S. (1978). Effect of age and parenchymal liver disease on the disposition and elimination of chlordiazepoxide (Librium®). *Gastroenterology*, **75**, 479–85
23. Greenblatt, D. J., Abernethy, D. R., Locniskar, A. *et al.* (1985). Age, sex and nitrazepam kinetics: relation to antipyrine disposition. *Clin. Pharmacol. Ther.*, **38**, 697–703
24. Schmucker, D. L., Vessey, D. A., Wang, R. K. *et al.* (1984). Age-dependent alterations in the physicochemical properties of rat liver microsomes. *Mech. Ageing. Devel.*, **27**, 207–17
25. James, O. F. W., Rawlins, M. D. and Woodhouse, K. (1982). Lack of aging effect on human microsomal monooxygenase enzyme activities and on inactivation pathways for reactive metabolic intermediates. In *Liver and Aging, Liver and Drugs.* pp. 395–406. (Amsterdam: Elsevier)
26. Kamataki, T., Maeda, K., Shimada, M. *et al.* (1985). Age-related alteration in the activities of drug-metabolizing enzymes and contents of sex-specific forms of cytochrome P-450 in liver microsomes from male and female rats. *J. Pharmacol. Exp. Ther.*, **233**, 222–8
27. Fujita, T., Kitagawa, H., Chiba, M. *et al.* (1985). Age- and sex-associated differences in the relative abundance of multiple species of cytochrome P-450 system. *Biochem. Pharmacol.*, **34**, 1861–4
28. Suzuki, T., Fujta, S. and Kitani, K. (1985). The mechanism of senescence associated loss of sex difference in drug metabolizing enzyme activities in rats. In Vereczkey, L. and Magyar, K. (eds.) *Cytochrome P-450: Biochemistry, Biophysics and Induction.* pp. 231–34. (Budapest: Akademia Kiado)
29. Patwardhan, P. V., Desmond, P. V., Johnson, R. F. and Schenker, S. (1980). Impaired elimination of caffeine by oral contraceptive steroids. *J. Lab. Clin. Med.*, **95**, 603–8
30. Roberts, R. K., Desmond, P. V., Wilkinson, G. R. and Schenker, S. (1979). Disposition of chlordiazepoxide: sex differences and effects of oral contraceptives. *Clin. Pharmacol. Ther.*, **25**, 826–31
31. Ochs, H. R., Greenblatt, D. J. and Otten, H. (1981). Disposition of oxazepam in relation to age, sex and cigarette smoking. *Klin. Wochenschr.*, **59**, 899–903
32. Greenblatt, D. J., Divoll, M., Harmatz, J. S. and Shader, R. I. (1980). Oxazepam kinetics: effects of age and sex. *J. Pharmacol. Exp. Ther.*, **215**, 86–91
33. Kraus, J. W., Desmond, P. V., Marshall, J. P., Johnson, R. F., Schenker, S. and Wilkinson, G. R. (1978). Effects of aging and liver disease on disposition of lorazepam. *Clin. Pharmacol. Ther.*, **24**, 411–19
34. Divoll, M., Greenblatt, D. J., Harmatz, J. S. and Shader, R. I. (1981). Effect of age and gender on disposition of temazepam. *J. Pharmaceut. Sci.*, **70**, 1104–7

35. Shull, H. J. Jr, Wilkinson, G. R., Johnson, R. F. and Schenker, S. (1976). Normal disposition of oxazepam in acute viral hepatitis and cirrhosis. *Ann. Intern. Med.*, **84**, 420–5
36. Patwardhan, R. V., Johnson, R. F., Hoyumpa, A. M. Jr, Sheehan, J. J., Desmond, P. V., Wilkinson, G. R., Branch, R. A. and Schenker, S. (1981). Normal metabolism of morphine in cirrhosis. *Gastroenterology*, **81**, 1006–11
37. Ochs, H. R., Greenblatt, D. J., Verburg-Ochs, B. and Matlis, R. (1986). Temazepam clearance unaltered in cirrhosis. *Am. J. Gastroenterol.*, **81**, 80–3
38. Patwardhan, R. V., Yarborough, G. W., Desmond, P. V., Johnson, R. F., Schenker, S. and Speeg, K.V. Jr. (1980). Cimetidine spares the glucuronidation of lorazepam and oxazepam. *Gastroenterology*, **79**, 912–16
39. Sellers, E. M., Giles, H. G., Greenblatt, D. J. and Naranjo, C. A. (1980). Differential effects on benzodiazepine disposition by disulfiram and ethanol. *Arzneim.-Forsch./Drug Res.* **30**, 882–6
40. Patwardhan, R. V., Mitchell, M., Johnson, R. F. and Schenker, S. (1983). Differential effects of oral contraceptive steroids on the metabolism of benzodiazepines. *Hepatology*, **3**, 248–53
41. Mitchell, M. C., Hanew, T., Meredith, C. G. and Schenker, S. (1983). Effects of oral contraceptive steroids on acetaminophen metabolism and elimination. *Clin. Pharmacol. Ther.*, **34**, 48–53
42. Wilkinson, J. and Hallinan, T. (1977). Trypsin-susceptibility of UDP-glucuronosyltransferase. *FEBS Lett.*, **75**, 138–40
43. Jackson, M. R., McCarthy, L. R., Harding, D., Wilson, S., Coughtrie, M. W. H. and Burchell, B. (1987). Cloning of a human liver microsomal UDP-glucuronosyltransferase cDNA. *Biochem. J.*, **242**, 581–8
44. Desmond, P. V., James, R., Schenker, S., Gerkens, J. F. and Branch, R. A. (1981). Preservation of glucuronidation in carbon tetrachloride-induced acute liver injury in the rat. *Biochem. Pharmacol.*, **30**, 993–9
45. Gerkins, J., Desmond, P. V., Schenker, S. and Branch, R. A. (1981). Hepatic and extrahepatic glucuronidation of lorazepam in the dog. *Hepatology*, **1**, 329–35
46. Greenblatt, D. J., Abernethy, D. R., Divoll, M. and Shader, R. I. (1983). Close correlation of acetaminophen clearance with that of conjugated benzodiazepines but not oxidized benzodiazepines. *Eur. J. Clin. Pharmacol.*, **25**, 113–15
47. Greenblatt, D. J., Divoll, M., Abernethy, D. R., Moschitto, L. J., Smith, R. B. and Shader, R. I. (1983). Reduced clearance of triazolam in old age: relation to antipyrine oxidizing capacity. *Br. J. Clin. Pharmacol.*, **15**, 303–9
48. Pomara, N., Stanley, B., Block, R., Guido, J., Stanley, M., Greenblatt, D. J., Newton, R. E. and Gershon, S. (1984). Diazepam impairs performance in normal elderly subjects. *Psychopharmacol. Bull.*, **20**, 137–9
49. Stevenson, I. H., Hochings, N. F. and Surft, C. G. (1982). Pharmacokinetics and pharmacodynamics of single doses of hypnotic drugs in healthy elderly subjects. In Kitani, K. (ed.), *Liver and Aging: Liver and Drugs.* pp. 317–28. (Amsterdam: Elsevier)
50. Castleden, C. M., George, C. F., Marcer, D. and Hallet, C. (1977). Increased sensitivity to nitrazepam in old age. *Br. Med. J.*, **1**, 10–12
51. Reidenberg, M. M., Levy, M., Warner, H., Coutinho, C. B., Schwartz, M. A., Yu, G. and Chripko, J. (1978). Relationship between diazepam dose, plasma level, age and central nervous system depression. *Clin. Pharmacol. Ther.*, **23**, 371–4
52. Meyers, M. B. and Komiskey, H. L. (1985). Aging: effect on the interaction of ethanol and pentobarbital with the benzodiazepine-GABA receptor-ionophore complex. *Brain Res.*, **343**, 262–7
53. Yamasaki, T., Inoue, O., Shinotoh, H., Itoh, T., Iyo, M., Teteno, Y., Suzuki, K., Kashida, Y., Hashimoto, K., and Tadokoro, H. (1986). Benzodiazepine receptor study in the elderly using PET and clinical application of a new tracer, [11]Cα-methyl-N-methylbenzylamine. In Kitani, K., (ed.) *Liver and Aging: Liver and Drugs.* pp. 265–77. (Amsterdam: Elsevier)
54. Branch, R. A., Morgan, M. C., James, J. and Read, A. E. (1976). Intravenous administration of diazepam in patients with chronic liver disease. *Gut*, **17**, 975–83
55. Samson, Y., Bernuau, J., Pappata, S., Chavoix, G., Baron, J. C. and Maziere, M. A. (1987). Cerebral uptake of benzodiazepine measured by positron emission tomography in hepatic encephalopathy. *N. Engl. J. Med.*, **316**, 414–15

27
Oxygen radicals and liver injury

D. V. PARKE, N. E. PREECE AND L. J. KING

INTRODUCTION

Autoxidative injury and oxygen radicals

Autoxidative injury, produced by the toxic effects of reactive oxygen radicals, is now known to be a fundamental mechanism implicated in many degenerative disease states, including tumour promotion and malignancy[1,2], atherosclerosis and myocardial infarction[3,4], diabetes[5], rheumatoid arthritis[6], gastric ulceration[7], cataract[8] and hepatic disease[9,10]. It is also believed to be the major cause of aging, and lifespan appears to be inversely related to the extent of free-radical damage[11,12]. The production of these reactive oxygen species, including peroxide (O_2^{--}), superoxy anion (O_2^{-}), the hydroxyl radical (OH') and singlet oxygen ($^1O_2$), occurs by reduction of tissue oxygen[13] via a variety of enzymic and non-enzymic reactions including the action of xanthine oxidase[14], NADPH-cytochrome P-450 reductase[15] and the cytochromes P-450[16,17], redox cycling involving quinone intermediates[18], trans-oxygenation in the synthesis of the prostanoids[19], and the chemical reduction of oxygen in aqueous solution by ferrous iron[20]. Indeed, iron is critical to these mechanisms of oxygen radical production, especially the formation of hydroxyl radicals and singlet oxygen[21]. The normal physiological roles of these reactive oxygen radicals are considered to be the prevention of infection[22], the acute inflammatory response to injury, and the turnover of intracellular components, such as the membranes of the endoplasmic reticulum and enzymic proteins[23]. Prevention of undesirable tissue destruction and cellular injury by these highly cytotoxic reactive oxygen species is achieved by an effective defence system which includes the redox buffer glutathione, the enzymes glutathione peroxidase, glutathione reductase, the glutathione transferases, superoxide dismutase, and catalase, and anti-oxidants and radical scavengers, including ascorbic acid, tocopherols, ubiquinones, and retinoids[5,21,24-26].

Oxygen radicals in liver injury from alcohol, drugs, ischaemia and re-perfusion

Alcohol, drugs, and many toxic chemicals are known to manifest adverse effects, especially on the liver and gastrointestinal tract, by augmenting the production of oxygen radicals. For example, alcohol is known to exert its toxicity on the gastric mucosa[27] and the liver[28] by the production of oxygen radicals formed by an isozyme of cytochrome P-450 induced by ethanol. The anthracycline antibiotics, doxorubicin, daunorubicin and actinomycin D[29], and to some extent, the analgesic paracetamol, are thought to exert their hepatotoxic effects by the production of oxygen radicals by redox cycling of quinone metabolites[30]. The halocarbon, carbon tetrachloride, manifests its marked hepatotoxicity by the generation of oxygen-containing radicals and lipid peroxides consequent upon its reductive de-halogenation by cytochrome P-450 to the CCl_3^- radical[31]. Other chemicals evoking hepatotoxicity through an increased production of oxygen radicals include chloroform[32], benzene[33], and the carcinogen, benzidine[34], and oxygen radicals are also considered to be the mediators of aromatic amine carcinogenesis[35]. However, possibly the most toxic of all chemicals in this respect is inorganic iron, and administration of a number of chelated complexes of iron, e.g. ferric-EDTA or ferric diethylenetriamine pentaacetic acid, have been shown to be potent promoters of hydroxyl radical production[36]. The complex of ferric iron with nitrilotriacetate (iron-NTA) administered intraperitoneally has also been shown to be an unusually potent inducer of lipid peroxidation *in vivo*, as monitored by determination of exhaled alkanes[37].

In recent years, a number of anti-hyperlipidaemic drugs, such as clofibrate and ciprofibrate, and certain highly lipophilic, slowly-metabolized esters, such as di(2-ethylhexyl)phthalate and other phthalate ester plasticisers, have been shown to give rise to the production of hydrogen peroxide in the liver, with consequent proliferation of the peroxisomes, induction of a novel cytochrome P-450, hepatotoxicity and carcinogenicity[38]. Whether the production of peroxide involves electron leakage from the cytochromes of the endoplasmic reticulum[39], or from the mitochondrial cytochromes, or is generated by the peroxisomal enzymes themselves, is not yet fully understood, but this chemically-induced production of peroxide and the consequent hepatotoxicity and hepatocarcinogenicity, is an important mechanism of liver injury, at least in small rodents. This phenomenon may be of considerable significance to public health as there is an increasing number of non-metabolisable, highly lipophilic chemicals being manufactured for use as detergents, plasticisers, lubricants, etc., which will accumulate in the environment and in the animal body, resulting in the generation of peroxide and other reactive oxygen species in the liver by uncoupling microsomal oxidation[39], leading to an increase in degenerative disease and of the aging processes, as exemplified by the Spanish toxic oil disaster[40].

Liver injury may also be induced by ischaemia, re-perfusion[41], trauma (haemorrhage) and inflammation (killed *Corynebacterium parvum* with or without endotoxin i.v.)[42]. Oxygen radical-induced damage has again been implicated, resulting from the generation of superoxide anion by xanthine oxidase, which is formed from xanthine dehydrogenase during anoxia; xanthine oxidase also liberates iron from ferritin, thereby enhancing the production of hydroxyl radicals and exacerbating the consequent tissue necrosis[41].

Quantitative determination of autoxidative injury

One of the past difficulties in studying autoxidative damage has been the lack of specificity and reproducibility of the quantitative techniques available, such as the earlier colorimetric determination of malondialdehyde, a breakdown product of lipid hydroperoxides and other autoxidized tissue products. However, during the past decade, a number of more specific and reliable methods have been developed, including the determination of lipid peroxidation from the exhalation of alkanes in the expired air – a valuable method for studying lipid peroxidation in intact animals by a non-invasive technique[43–45]. Other methods include, new colorimetric[46] and HPLC[47] methods for the determination of malondialdehyde and other breakdown products of lipid hydroperoxides in tissues and urine[47], spectrophotometric determination and gas chromatography–mass spectrometry analysis of 4-hydroxynonenal and other 4-hydroxyalkenals[48,49], and the determination of singlet oxygen and hydroxyl radical by chemiluminescence[50].

Before embarking on a comprehensive programme of study of autoxidative injury of the liver, to examine the effects of diet, drugs and toxic chemicals, possible protective agents, and the mechanism of liver injury associated with ischaemia, re-perfusion, trauma, and inflammation, it became necessary to optimize the experimental procedures available. This required the determination of the most appropriate animal species, the most susceptible tissues, and the most sensitive and reproducible analytical methodology for *in vivo* studies, since *in vitro* experiments are of little value owing to rapid depletion of components of the endogenous anti-oxidant defence system, thereby exaggerating the possible cytotoxic effects. Lastly, the various chemicals which produce autoxidative injury of the liver were studied to select an appropriate chemical model.

EXPERIMENTAL

Chemicals

Cumene hydroperoxide and *tert.*-butyl hydroperoxide (Sigma Chemicals Ltd., Poole, Dorset, UK), buthionine sulphoximine (Chemical Dynamics Corp., S. Plainfield, NJ, USA), bromotrichloromethane, carbon tetrachloride, disodium nitrilotriacetate and iron acetylacetonate (Aldrich Chemicals Ltd., Gillingham, Dorset, UK), and 2-thiobarbituric acid and 1,1,3,3-tetraethoxypropane (BDH Chemicals Ltd., Poole, Dorset, UK) were purchased. Cylinder gases were obtained from the British Oxygen Company Ltd., Brentford, Middlesex, UK and hydrocarbon standards and chromatography equipment from Chromatography Services Ltd., Hoylake, Merseyside, UK. Iron nitrilotriacetate was freshly prepared according to the method of Goddard et al.[37].

Animals

Male, Wistar albino rats, 4–12 weeks old and 100–300 g body weight (University of Surrey Breeding Unit), and male CD-1 mice, 8 weeks old and 30 g body weight (Charles River Ltd., Margate, UK) were allowed rodent diets and water *ad libitum*. Chemicals were administered intraperitoneally in appropriate solvents, at various doses.

Methods

Alkanes were determined by gas chromatography coupled to a specially designed metabolic chamber[51]. Optimization of the method indicated that ethane was the most suitable alkane for determination as an index of lipid peroxidation[51].

Animals were dosed and placed in the metabolic chamber, for determination of ethane, for various periods of time. The animals were then killed by cervical dislocation, the livers and kidneys rapidly removed, samples of tissue homogenized in cold 0.1 M potassium phthalate buffer, pH 3.5, and thiobarbituric acid-reactive materials (malondialdehyde or MDA) determined by the method of Gutteridge[46], using 1,1,3,3-tetraethoxypropane to prepare standards.

Glutathione[52], glutathione peroxidase[53], hepatic cytochrome P-450[54], benzphetamine N-demethylase[55] and 7-ethoxyresorufin O-deethylase[56] activities were determined in tissue preparations by the published methods.

RESULTS

Model toxic chemicals

Of the many different chemicals studied for their ability to cause lipid peroxidation *in vivo* in rodents, as measured by ethane exhalation, relatively few were particularly effective. The most active compounds in the mouse are shown in Table 27.1, where it can be seen that the halocarbons CCl_4 and $CBrCl_3$ were less effective than the hydroperoxides, *tert.*-butyl and cumene hydroperoxides, and these were less effective than the iron complexes, iron acetylacetonate and iron nitrilotriacetate (FeNTA).

Using FeNTA as the model autoxidizing compound, linear dose–responses were obtained when the compound was administered intraperitoneally to rats or mice. Furthermore, good correlations were obtained between the different methods of quantification, alkane production correlating with tissue lipid peroxidation as measured by the thiobarbituric acid method (MDA), and

Table 27.1 Ethane exhalation as a measure of autoxidation after administration of various toxic chemicals to mice. Ethane exhalation was determined over 30 min, with groups of 4 male mice, before and after intraperitoneal administration of various toxic chemicals. Values are test–control $\pm$ SEM

Chemical	Dose (mmol)	Ethane exhaled	
		(nmol/kg body wt.)	(nmol/nmol chemical)
Carbon tetrachloride	2.9	12 ± 5	4 ± 2
Bromotrichloromethane	2.2	18 ± 7	8 ± 3
tert-Butyl hydroperoxide	1.1	22 ± 10	20 ± 9
Cumene hydroperoxide	1.1	55 ± 22	50 ± 20
Iron acetylacetonate	0.22	13 ± 6	59 ± 27
Iron nitrilotriacetate	0.07	150 ± 40	2140 ± 570

both of these agreeing with semi-quantitative histopathological assessments of tissue damage, manifested as hepatic and renal necrosis (results not shown).

Species differences

The rat and mouse responded differently to increasing i.p. doses of FeNTA. As may be seen from Figure 27.1, the mouse showed a greater response than the rat in the production of ethane and, at the higher doses of FeNTA, this was the most sensitive index of lipid peroxidation in mouse, whereas liver MDA was the most sensitive index in rat.

Tissue susceptibility to lipid peroxidation induced by FeNTA also differs in the two rodent species, with the kidney being more vulnerable than the liver to autoxidative damage in the mouse, and the liver being the more vulnerable in the rat (see Figure 27.1).

Effects of acute and chronic treatment with FeNTA on rat liver enzymes

After acute treatment of rats with the model autoxidizing chemical, FeNTA, at doses of 12 mg Fe/kg body weight, which causes 50% mortality, the total cytochrome P-450 was 50% decreased, benzphetamine N-demethylase a cytochrome P-450 marker enzyme activity was 40% decreased, but ethoxyresorufin O-deethylase (EROD) a specific marker for cytochrome P-448 activity was unchanged (see Table 27.2). Glutathione peroxidase activity was also unchanged.

After chronic treatment with FeNTA (10 doses of 5×6 mg Fe/kg and 5×12 mg Fe/mg over 14 days) mortality was 30%, total cytochromes P-450 and benzphetamine N-demethylase were only 25% decreased, while ethoxyresorufin O-deethylase, the P-448 marker, was actually increased by 150%. Glutathione peroxidase was also significantly decreased, by 25%. This

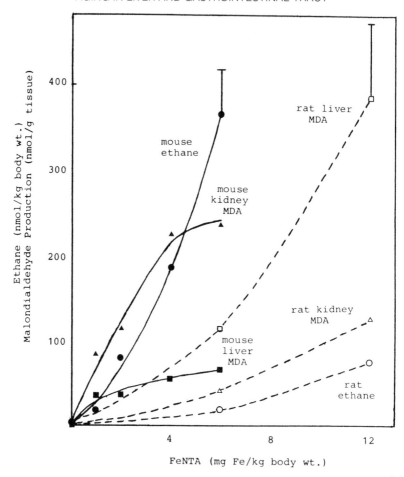

Figure 27.1 Dose–response of ethane exhalation and tissue malondialdehyde production after iron nitrilotriacetate administration. Ethane exhalation was measured over 30 min, and tissue malondialdehyde formation was determined within 50 min, after intraperitoneal administration of varying doses of iron nitrilotriacetate (FeNTA) to groups of 6 male mice or 4 male rats. For clarity, SEM values are shown only at the maximum values

indicates that prolonged treatment with an autoxidizing chemical is liable to change the isoenzyme composition of the cytochromes P-450, favouring an increase in the cytochromes P-448. The significant loss in glutathione peroxidase activity indicates that this protective enzyme is not induced by chronic treatment, but nevertheless remains at an effective level.

Table 27.2 Effect of acute and chronic treatment with iron nitrilotriacetate (NTA) on rat liver glutathione peroxidase activity, cytochrome P-450 content, and mixed-function oxidase activities*

Enzymic parameter	Control	Chronic	Acute
Glutathione peroxidase (nmol NADPH oxidized/mg protein per min)	170 ± 10	123 ± 13	180 ± 13
Cytochrome P-450 (nmol/mg protein)	0.36 ± 0.03	0.27 ± 0.04	0.19 ± 0.01
Benzphetamine N-demethylase (nmol HCHO formed/mg protein per min)	3.3 ± 0.3	2.6 ± 0.3	2.1 ± 0.3
Ethoxyresorufin O-deethylase (nmol resorufin formed/mg protein per min)	0.05 ± 0.01	0.13 ± 0.01	0.08 ± 0.01

* Acute treatment was a single dose of iron NTA (12 mg Fe/kg body weight) 48 h before death. Chronic treatment was 10 doses of iron NTA over 14 days the last dose being 24 h before death (5×6 mg Fe and 5×12 mg Fe/kg body weight). Mortality was 50% in the acute dosed rats and 30% in the chronically dosed rats. 4-week-old rats were used. Values are mean $\pm$ SEM using H_2O_2 as substrate for glutathione peroxidase activity, and benzphetamine and ethoxyresorufin as substrates for cytochromes P-450 and P-448 respectively

Effect of glutathione depletion on autoxidative injury in rats and mice

Male rats pretreated with buthionine sulphoximine (2 mmol/kg body weight), an inhibitor of glutathione biosynthesis, then given an i.p. dose of FeNTA (6 mg Fe), showed marked increases, over animals given FeNTA alone, in ethane exhalation (280% control), liver malondialdehyde production (190%) and kidney malondialdehyde production (210%), with marked decreases in liver glutathione (by 75%) and kidney glutathione (by 80%) (see Table 27.3). Similarly, male mice pretreated with buthionine sulphoximine (2 mmol/mg body weight), then with FeNTA (2 mg Fe) i.p. showed marked increases in ethane exhalation (10-fold) and kidney malondialdehyde production (3-fold), but with no significant increase in liver malondialdehyde formation; kidney glutathione was decreased some 75% but liver glutathione was decreased only by 50% (see Table 27.3). These studies show the marked protective effect of tissue glutathione against oxygen radical production, lipid peroxidation and tissue autoxidative damage.

DISCUSSION

The finding that the halocarbons were effective, but not the most potent, chemicals to give rise to oxygen radical production and lipid peroxidation, was somewhat surprising considering the prolonged and extensive studies given these compounds, but also reassuring in that carbon tetrachloride has been widely used in the treatment of human subjects for liver fluke and other

Table 27.3 Effect of iron nitrilotriacetate (NTA) in glutathione-depleted rodents*

Dose of FeNTA (mg Fe/kg body wt.)	Buthionine sulphoximine treatment	Ethane exhalation (nmol/kg body wt.)	Liver MDA (nmol/g)	Liver GSH (μmol/g)	Kidney MDA (nmol/g)	Kidney GSH (μmol/g)
Mice						
0	none	14 ± 3	29 ± 2	6.6 ± 1.1	35 ± 4	2.7 ± 0.2
0	+	9 ± 2	39 ± 11	4.7 ± 1.4	43 ± 11	$0.5 \pm 0.2**$
2	none	28 ± 2	28 ± 3	7.3 ± 0.5	71 ± 14	2.3 ± 0.5
2	+	$277 \pm 53**$	33 ± 4	$3.6 \pm 0.5**$	$217 \pm 49**$	$0.6 \pm 0.1**$
6	none	431 ± 120	52 ± 2	5.5 ± 0.3	234 ± 29	0.9 ± 0.3
Rats						
0	none	11 ± 2	23 ± 4	7.1 ± 0.5	14 ± 2	4.0 ± 1.0
0	+	12 ± 2	19 ± 2	$3.0 \pm 0.3**$	13 ± 2	$0.9 \pm 0.1*$
6	none	74 ± 32	89 ± 34	9.0 ± 0.3	27 ± 5	4.4 ± 0.3
6	+	$205 \pm 59**$	167 ± 52	$2.2 \pm 0.4**$	$62 \pm 12**$	$0.9 \pm 0.1**$
12	none	188 ± 63	172 ± 75	7.4 ± 0.5	56 ± 14	5.2 ± 0.5

* Male animals were given iron NTA intraperitoneally, and ethane exhalation was determined over 30 min and tissue MDA measured 35 min after dosing for mice, and over 45 min and after 50 min, respectively, for rats. Some animals were depleted of GSH by treating with buthionine sulphoximine (2 mmol/kg body weight) intraperitoneally 2 h before treating with FeNTA for mice, and 4 h before with rats. Results are mean values ± SEM of 4 to 8 animals.
** Significantly different from animals not treated with buthionine sulphoximine ($P < 0.01$)

parasitic infestations of the liver and gastrointestinal tract. That the iron complexes were the most potent, particularly iron nitrilotriacetate, is in accord with the continued emphasis that has been placed on the role of iron in oxygen radical production by Gutteridge and others[21,36,37].

The satisfactory correlation of ethane exhalation with tissue malondialdehyde production and morphological changes quantified by histopathology validates the quantitative methodology, and the dose–response obtained with FeNTA confirms the role of iron in oxygen radical production and the ability of these radicals to cause lipid peroxidation, autoxidative damage and, finally, tissue necrosis. There now remains a similar need to correlate these parameters with quantification of the formation of hydroxy-alkenals and of the chemiluminescence associated with the production of hydroxy radicals and singlet oxygen.

The stimulation of lipid peroxidation, alkane exhalation, and malondialdehyde formation in rodent tissues by administration of FeNTA shows a dose–response, although this is diminished at low doses, especially in the rat (see Figure 27.1), and is probably owing to the natural protection of the animal by the anti-oxidant defence system of glutathione, anti-oxidants and radical scavengers, and the associated enzymes[11,24–26]. More recently, the role of bilirubin as an anti-oxidant and radical scavenger has been highlighted, and this once-considered toxic waste product of haem degradation is now acknowledged to be a powerful biological chain-breaking anti-oxidant, especially in the blood and liver, major sites of oxygen radical production, where bilirubin is present in effective concentrations[57].

Figure 27.1 also shows the different dose–responses of rat and mouse to FeNTA, the latter being 2–6 times more susceptible to oxygen radical formation and autoxidation than the former, undoubtedly owing to the higher basal metabolism of the mouse and hence its greater tissue oxygen uptake. The greater damage to mouse kidney than liver, and the reverse situation in the rat, may be owing to the lower glutathione concentration in mouse kidney than liver, and to its more extensive depletion by FeNTA, or to a greater excretion of FeNTA via the kidney in the mouse (Table 27.3). Moreover, the greater lipid peroxidation in the mouse than in rat will result in a greater excretion of the cytotoxic and mutagenic malondialdehyde and other tissue breakdown products via the kidney[47].

The effects of acute and chronic treatments of rats with FeNTA show only minor difference (Table 27.2), with reduction in liver glutathione peroxidase activity and a selective decrease of cytochrome P-450 together with a slight increase in cytochrome P-448, after chronic dosage. This is in agreement with previous work using immunohistochemical techniques, that the pheno-barbital-inducible forms of cytochrome P-450 are more susceptible to carbon tetrachloride-induced hepatotoxicity than were the 3-methylcholanthrene- or β-naphthoflavone-inducible forms of cytochrome P-448[58]. Furthermore, in paracetamol-induced lipid peroxidation in mice, methylcholanthrene pre-treatment led to a 28-fold increase over control in ethane exhalation, while phenobarbital pretreatment resulted in only a 10-fold increase, indicating that the cytochromes P-448 may be more effective oxygen-radical generators than the cytochromes P-450 or the cytochrome P-450 reductase[59]. Furthermore, the cytochromes P-448 are known to selectively activate toxic chemicals and carcinogens, whereas the phenobarbital-induced cytochromes P-450 lead preferentially to detoxication[60].

The depletion of liver and kidney glutathione (GSH) contents correlate well with the tissue malondialdehyde production after treatment of both rats or mice with FeNTA, with or without prior treatment with the inhibitor of GSH biosynthesis, buthionine sulphoximine (Table 27.3) although, as expected, the summated effect is greater than the effect of FeNTA alone. This confirms the protective role of tissue GSH, in both kidney and liver, of both rats and mice, and the protective effects of the anti-oxidant BHT have been similarly demonstrated. The natural anti-oxidant defence system is subject to impairment from nutritional deficiencies[5,59] (e.g. vitamin E, selenium, sulphur amino acids) and genetic abnormalities of one or more of the enzymes involved[5] (e.g. glucose-6-phosphate dehydrogenase, glutathione peroxidase), and to loss of efficacy owing to aging, which is believed to lead to increased de-coupling of cytochrome P-450 from its reductase, with consequent increase in oxygen radical production[16,59].

In conclusion, liver injury resulting from oxygen radicals and lipid peroxidation may arise from (i) the ingestion of drugs and chemicals which accelerate production of oxygen radicals overwhelming the natural anti-oxidant protective mechanisms[40], (ii) ischaemia and re-perfusion, trauma or inflammation, accelerating oxygen radical formation[5], and (iii) impairment of the tissue protective mechanisms, owing to malnutrition, aging or genetic aberrations[5]. Sensitive and specific analytical methods are now available to objectively quantify these different aspects of autoxidative liver injury and thereby to elucidate the molecular mechanisms involved, with the ultimate objectives of prevention or treatment.

Acknowledgement

This work was financially supported by the Ministry of Agriculture, Food, and Fisheries, UK.

References

1. Totter, J. R. (1980). Spontaneous cancer and its possible relationship to oxygen metabolism. *Proc. Natl. Acad. Sci. USA*, **77**, 1763–7
2. Kensler, T. W. and Trush, M. A. (1984). Role of oxygen radicals in tumour promotion. *Environ. Mutagenesis*, **6**, 593–616
3. Harman, D. (1984). Free radical theory of aging: the 'free radical' diseases. *Age*, **7**, 111–31
4. Werns, S. W. and Lucchesi, B. R. (1987). Inflammation and myocardial infarction. *Br. Med. Bull.*, **43**, 460–71
5. Clark, I. A., Cowden, W. B. and Hunt, N. H. (1985). Free radical-induced pathology. *Med. Res. Rev.*, **5**, 297–332
6. Blake, D. R., Allen, R. E. and Lunec, J. (1987). Free radicals in biological systems – a review orientated to inflammatory processes. *Br. Med. Bull.*, **43**, 371–8
7. Perry, M. A., Wadhwa, S., Parks, D. A., Pickard, W. and Granger, D. N. (1986). Role of oxygen radicals in ischaemia-induced lesions in the cat stomach. *Gastroenterology*, **90**, 362–7
8. Bhuyan, K. C., Bhuyan, D. K. and Podos, S. M. (1986). Lipid peroxidation in cataract of the human. *Life Sci.*, **38**, 1463–71
9. Moscarella, S., Laffi, G., Buzzelli, G., Mazzanti, R., Caramelli, L. and Gentilini, P. (1984). Expired hydrocarbons in patients with chronic liver disease. *Hepatogastroenterology*, **31**, 60–3
10. Comporti, M. (1985). Biology of disease. Lipid peroxidation and cellular damage in toxic liver injury. *Lab. Invest.*, **53**, 599–623
11. Harman, D. and Eddy, D. E. (1979). Free radical theory of aging: beneficial effect of adding antioxidants to the maternal mouse diet on life span of offspring; possible explanation of the sex difference in longevity. *Age*, **2**, 109–22
12. Brizzee, K. R., Eddy, D. E., Harman, D. and Ordy, J. M. (1984). Free radical theory of aging: effect of dietary lipids on lipofuscin accumulation in the hippocampus of rats. *Age*, **7**, 9–15
13. Halliwell, B. and Gutteridge, J. M. C. (1984). Oxygen toxicity, oxygen radicals, transition metals and disease. *Biochem. J.*, **219**, 1–14
14. Winterbourn, C. C. and Sutton, H. C. (1986). Iron and xanthine oxidase catalyze formation of an oxidant species distinguishable from ˙OH: comparison with the Haber–Weiss reaction. *Arch. Biochem. Biophys.*, **244**, 27–34
15. Winston, G. W. and Cederbaum, A. J. (1983). NADPH-dependent production of oxy radicals by purified components of the rat liver mixed-function oxidase system. *J. Biol. Chem.*, **258**, 1508–13
16. Ekström, G. and Ingelman-Sundberg, M. (1984). Cytochrome P-450-dependent lipid peroxidation in reconstituted membrane vesicles. *Biochem. Pharmacol.*, **33**, 2521–3
17. Ingelman-Sundberg, M. and Johansson, I. (1984). Mechanisms of hydroxyl radical formation and ethanol oxidation of ethanol-inducible and other forms of rabbit liver microsomal cytochromes P-450. *J. Biol. Chem.*, **259**, 6447–58
18. Younes, M., Cornelius, S. and Siegers, C.-P. (1985). Fe^{2+}-supported *in vivo* lipid per-

oxidation induced by compounds undergoing redox cycling. *Chem. Biol. Interactions*, **54**, 97–103

19. Kadlubar, F. F., Frederick, C. B., Weiss, C. C. and Zenser, T. V. (1982). Prostaglandin endoperoxide synthetase-mediated metabolism of carcinogenic aromatic amines and their binding to DNA and protein. *Biochem. Biophys. Res. Commun.*, **108**, 253–8

20. Braughler, J. M. Duncan, L. A. and Chase, R. L. (1986). The involvement of iron in lipid peroxidation. *J. Biol. Chem.*, **261**, 10 282–9

21. Halliwell, B. and Gutteridge, J. M. C. (1986). Iron and free radical reactions: two aspects of antioxidant protection. *TIBS*, **11**, 372–5

22. Babior, B. M. (1978). Oxygen-dependent microbial killing by phagocytes. Part 1. *N. Engl. J. Med.*, **298**, 659–68

23. Del Maestro, R. F. (1984). Free radical injury during inflammation. In Armstrong, D. *et al.* (eds.) *Free Radicals in Molecular Biology, Aging and Disease.* pp. 87–102. (New York: Raven Press)

24. Siegers, C.-P., Hübscher, W. and Younes, M. (1982). Glutathione S-transferase and GSH-peroxidase activities during the state of GSH-depletion leading to lipid peroxidation in rat liver. *Res. Commun. Chem. Path. Pharmacol.*, **37**, 163–9

25. Sies, H. (1986). Biochemistry of oxidative stress. *Angew. Chem.*, **25**, 1058–71

26. McCay, P. B. (1985). Vitamin E: Interactions with free radicals and ascorbate. *Annu. Rev. Nutr.*, **5**, 323–40

27. Mizui, T. and Doteuchi, M. (1986). Lipid peroxidation: A possible role in gastric damage induced by ethanol in rats. *Life Sci.*, **38**, 2163–7

28. Ekström, G., Cronholm, T. and Ingelman-Sundberg, M. (1986). Hydroxyl-radical production and ethanol oxidation by liver microsomes isolated from ethanol-treated rats. *Biochem. J.*, **233**, 755–61

29. Doroshow, J. H. (1983). Anthracycline antibiotic-stimulated superoxide, hydrogen peroxide, and hydroxyl radical production by NADH dehydrogenase. *Cancer Res.*, **43**, 4543–51

30. Kappus, H. (186). Overview of enzyme systems involved in bioreduction of drugs and in redox cycling. *Biochem. Pharmacol.*, **35**, 1–6

31. Younes, M. and Siegers, C.-P. (1985). The role of iron in the paracetamol- and CCl$_4$-induced lipid peroxidation and hepatotoxicity. *Chem. Biol. Interactions*, **55**, 327–34

32. Ekström, T., Ståhl, A., Sigvardsson, K. and Högberg, J. (1986). Lipid peroxidation *in vivo* monitored as ethane exhalation and malondialdehyde excretion in urine after oral administration of chloroform. *Acta Pharmacol. Toxicol.*, **58**, 289–96

33. Greenlee, W. F., Sun, J. D. and Bus, J. S. (1981). A proposed mechanism of benzene toxicity: formation of reactive intermediates from polyphenol metabolites. *Toxicol. Appl. Pharmacol.*, **59**, 187–95

34. Manno, M., Ioannides, C. and Gibson, G. G. (1985). The modulation by arylamines of the *in vitro* formation of superoxide anion radicals and hydrogen peroxide by rat liver microsomes. *Toxicol. Lett.*, **25**, 121–30

35. Nakayama, T., Kimura, T., Kodama, M. and Nagata, C. (1983). Generation of hydrogen peroxide and superoxide anion from active metabolites of naphthylamines and amino azo dyes: its possible role in carcinogenesis. *Carcinogenesis*, **4**, 765–9

36. Winston, G. W., Feierman, D. E. and Cederbaum, A. I. (1984). The role of iron chelates in hydroxyl radical production of rat liver microsomes, NADPH-cytochrome P-450 reductase and xanthine oxidase. *Arch. Biochem. Biophys.*, **232**, 378–90

37. Goddard, J. G., Basford, D. and Sweeney, G. D. (1986). Lipid peroxidation by iron nitrilotriacetate in rat liver. *Biochem. Pharmacol.*, **35**, 2381–7

38. Elliott, B. M., Dodd, N. J. F. and Elcombe, C. R. (1986). Increased hydroxyl radical production in liver peroxisomal fractions from rats treated with peroxisome proliferators. *Carcinogenesis*, **7**, 795–9

39. Bast, A. (1986). Is formation of reactive oxygen by cytochrome P-450 perilous and predictable? *TIPS*, **7**, 266–70

40. Aldridge, W. N. (1985). Toxic oil syndrome. *Human Toxicol.*, **4**, 231–5

41. Biemond, P., Swaak, A. J. G., Beindorff, C. M. and Koster, J. F. (1986). Superoxide-dependent and -independent mechanisms of iron mobilization from ferritin by xanthine oxidase. *Biochem. J.*, **239**, 169–73

42. Arthur, M. J. P., Bentley, I. S., Tanner, A. R., Kowalski Saunders, P., Millward-Sadler,

G. H. and Wright, R. (1985). Oxygen-derived free radicals promote hepatic injury in the rat. *Gastroenterology*, **89**, 1114–22

43. Lawrence, G. D. and Cohen, G. (1982). Ethane exhalation as an index of *in vivo* lipid peroxidation: concentrating ethane from a breath collection chamber. *Anal. Biochem.*, **122**, 283–90

44. Filser, J. G., Bolt, H. M., Muliawan, H. and Kappus, H. (1983). Quantitative evaluation of ethane and *n*-pentane as indicators of lipid peroxidation *in vivo*. *Arch. Toxicol.*, **52**, 153–47

45. Wade, C. R. and van Rij, A. M. (1985). *In vivo* peroxidation in man as measured by the respiratory excretion of ethane, pentane and other low-molecular-weight hydrocarbons. *Anal. Biochem.*, **150**, 1–7

46. Gutteridge, J. M. C. (1982). Free-radical damage to lipids, amino acids, carbohydrates and nucleic acids determined by thiobarbituric acid reactivity. *Int. J. Biochem.*, **14**, 649–53

47. Draper, H. H., Polensek, L., Hadley, M. and McGirr, L. G. (1984). Urinary malondialdehyde as an indicator of lipid peroxidation in the diet and in the tissues. *Lipids*, **19**, 836–43

48. Esterbauer, H., Zollner, H. and Lang, J. (1985). Metabolism of the lipid peroxidation product 4-hydroxynonenal by isolated hepatocytes and by liver cytosolic fractions. *Biochem. J.*, **228**, 363–73

49. van Kuijk, F. J. G. M., Thomas, D. W., Stephens, R. J. and Dratz, E. A. (1986). Occurrence of 4-hydroxyalkenals in rat tissues determined as pentafluorobenzyloxime derivatives by gas chromatography–mass spectrometry. *Biochem. Biophys. Res. Commun.*, **139**, 144–9

50. Miura, T. and Ogiso, T. (1985). Luminol chemiluminescence and peroxidation of unsaturated fatty acid induced by the xanthine oxidase system: effect of oxygen radical scavengers. *Chem. Pharm. Bull.*, **33**, 3402–7

51. Preece, N. E. (1986). Studies on Chemical Induced Autoxidation *in vivo*. Ph.D. thesis, University of Surrey, UK

52. Eyer, P. and Podhradsky, D. (1986). Evaluation of the micro method for the determination of glutathione using enzymatic cycling and Ellman's reagent. *Anal. Biochem.*, **153**, 57–66

53. Paglia, D. E. and Valentine, W. N. (1967). Studies on the quantitative and qualitative characterisation of erythrocyte glutathione peroxidase. *J. Clin. Med.*, **70**, 158–69

54. Omura, T. and Sato, R. (1964). The carbon monoxide pigment of liver microsomes. I. Evidence for its haemoprotein nature. *J. Biol. Chem.*, **239**, 2370–8

55. Lu, A. Y. H., Strobel, H. W. and Coon, M. J. (1970). Properties of a solubilized form of the cytochrome P-450 containing mixed-function oxidase of liver microsomes. *Mol. Pharmacol.*, **6**, 213–20

56. Burke, M. D. and Mayer, R. T. (1974). Ethoxyresorufin: direct fluorimetric assay of microsomal O-dealkylation which is preferentially inducible by 3-methylcholanthrene. *Drug Metab. Disp.*, **2**, 583–8

57. Stocker, R., Yamamoto, Y., McDonagh, A. F., Glazer, A. N. and Ames, B. N. (1987). Bilirubin is an antioxidant of possible physiological importance. *Science*, **235**, 1043–6

58. Moody, D. E., Taylor, L. A. and Smuckler, E. A. (1986). Immunohistochemical evidence for alterations in specific forms of rat hepatic microsomal cytochrome P-450 during acute carbon tetrachloride intoxication. *Drug Metab. Disp.*, **14**, 709–13

59. Wendel, A. and Feuerstein, S. (1981). Drug induced lipid peroxidation in mice. I. Modulation by monooxygenase activity, glutathione and selenium status. *Biochem. Pharmacol.*, **30**, 2513–20

60. Ioannides, C., Lum, P. Y. and Parke, D. V. (1984). Cytochrome P-448 and the activation of toxic chemicals and carcinogens. *Xenobiotica*, **14**, 119–37

Section 5
Aging in the Gastrointestinal Tract: Clinical Aspects

28
Malabsorption and aging

R. M. RUSSELL

There have been relatively few studies performed on humans with regard to the effect of aging on digestive and absorptive processes. From several longitudinal and cross-sectional studies, it is known that caloric intakes decline throughout the adult age span. For example, in the Longitudinal Study on Aging done under the auspices of United States' National Institutes of Aging, the average caloric intake in a 28-year-old White male is 2700 calories[1]. However, caloric intake declines to about 2100 calories in White males by the age of 80. Socioeconomic and other factors, such as psychological depression, influence dietary intakes with age, and in some elderly individuals caloric and nutrient intakes drop to sub-optimal levels for health maintenance. Even if the declines in caloric intake are appropriate for the elderly, declines in the intakes of certain nutrients whose requirements are absolute, rather than calorie linked, may not be appropriate.

Effects of age on nutrient digestion and absorption could influence the nutritional status of the elderly. As with other organ systems, it is difficult to separate out effects of aging which are physiologic from changes which are pathologic, and studies that have been published using human subjects must be viewed with this in mind. Furthermore, elderly people are frequently taking multiple medications which could interfere with digestive and absorptive processes, and this is a further confounding factor. In this paper digestion and absorption data derived from elderly human subjects will be reviewed. Insofar as possible data from studies performed on healthy elderly will be considered – realizing that the 'health' in many research papers is defined as 'free-living' and the absence of overt disease. Topics on which the data are minimal, conflicting or inconclusive will not be discussed.

It has been quite well documented in various animal models that there is decreased stimulated and unstimulated secretion of pancreatic enzymes with advancing age[2-4]. In humans there are only scattered and inconclusive reports in the literature with regard to pancreatic function[5-9]. It has been reported that amylase, trypsin and lipase activities in fasting duodenal juice decline with advancing age[8]. In one study among institutionalized elderly, faecal fat was found to be elevated in 17 of 43 individuals[10]. In 10 of these 17 individuals in whom faecal fats were elevated, faecal free fatty acids were diminished, which is consistent with decreased pancreatic lipase activity.

It has recently been demonstrated that dietary fibre adsorbs pancreatic enzymes and makes them unavailable for participation in digestive processes[11]. High-fibre diets are frequently prescribed for the elderly to prevent constipation. It is conceivable that dietary fibre could effectively reduce free digestive enzyme concentrations within the intestinal lumen and result in malabsorption. The effect might be greatest in the elderly whose levels of enzymes are purported to be borderline–adequate to begin with. However, Southgate and Durnen were unable to find a significant change in the apparent digestibility of fat between young and elderly women on high-fibre diets, which would argue against an important effect of dietary fibre on reducing fat absorption via adsorption of pancreatic enzymes[12].

A possible reason to hypothesize fat malabsorption in the elderly is a decreased bile salt pool. In a series of studies carried out by Hellemans *et al.*, radioactive carbon dioxide in breath during bile salt breath tests was found to be increased in terms of areas under timed curves in elderly versus young adult subjects[13]. This increase in radioactive breath CO_2 is owing to an increased exposure of bile salts to bacteria. Since none of the elderly individuals was clinically malabsorbing fat, it is presumed that this increase in radioactive CO_2 was owing to decreased re-absorption of bile salts by the terminal ilieum and greater dumping of bile salts into the colon.

We have been unable to demonstrate any effect of age on faecal fat levels[14]. Thus despite a possible diminution in pancreatic enzyme output, it appears that fat digestion and absorption remains intact up to age 90. However, if greatly increased dietary fat loads are given to elderly individuals, malabsorption can be induced[15]. For example, among 6 individuals aged 34–42, the faecal fat level on a 85–90 g fat diet was 3.3–7 g/24 h. Similar results were found in 8 elderly individuals aged 67–72. However, when the elderly individuals were put on a diet of 115–120 g of fat per day, they began to malabsorb fat (50% of the elderly individuals malabsorbed greater than 12 g fat/day) whereas in the younger group faecal fat levels remained within the normal range of 3–9 g/day. Thus, it appears that when the system is greatly stressed with very high (unphysiological) dietary fat intakes, age related fat malabsorption can be demonstrated owing to a diminished pancreatic and/or intestinal reserve capacity.

Similar findings have been demonstrated for faecal nitrogen, in that faecal nitrogen levels in individuals aged 67–71 on a 1 g/kg dietary protein intake were not elevated above the normal values seen in young adults[15]. However, when protein intake was increased to 1.5 g/kg/day, faecal nitrogen increased in the elderly to 2.1–4.4 g/day whereas in the younger group (aged 34–42) faecal nitrogen ranged from 1.9–2.2 g/day. Once again there appears to be a diminished intestinal or digestive reserve capacity for dietary protein as for fat.

It is well accepted that brush-border lactase levels diminish with age which results in lactose maldigestion and may result in lactose intolerance[16–17]. There is also an apparent decrease of D-xylose absorption with age, in that D-xylose urinary excretion after an oral load of the sugar is decreased[18–20]. In a series of patients studied by us we have demonstrated a linear decrease in D-xylose excretion with age which is significant at the $p < 0.01$ level. However, by partial correlation analysis the decrease in D-xylose excretion can be shown to be totally accounted for by an age-related decline in creatinine clearance. Thus, any test of intestinal function which is based on urinary excretion data must be interpreted cautiously in the elderly until normal age-specific values are derived.

One of the more interesting studies on age effects on intestinal carbohydrate metabolism was carried out by Feibusch and Holt[21]. These investigators fed elderly and young individuals meals of varying carbohydrate content and measured breath hydrogen outputs. Young individuals did not show an increase in breath hydrogen levels of greater than 20 parts per million (p.p.m.) even after meals with carbohydrate contents as high as 200 g. However, in elderly individuals, normal breath hydrogen tests became more scarce as the

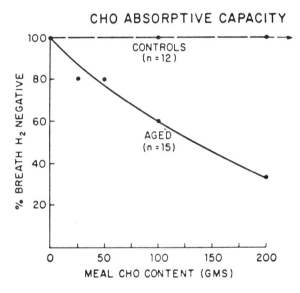

Figure 28.1 Carbohydrate absorptive characteristics of aged and young control subjects. Data are presented as percentage of total study group demonstrating a negative breath hydrogen excretion test after a meal containing the amount of carbohydrate (CHO) shown. A positive breath hydrogen excretion test is defined as production of excess hydrogen concentration of 20 p.p.m. over baseline. [Published with permission from *Digestive Disease and Science*, (1982), **27**, 1095–100][21]

amount of carbohydrate was increased in the meal (Figure 28.1). When 200 g of carbohydrate were fed, only 20% of individuals had negative breath hydrogen test results (that is breath hydrogen excretions less than 20 p.p.m.). The increase in breath hydrogen in these elderly individuals is owing to an increased exposure of the carbohydrate to bacteria in the gut lumen. This could reflect carbohydrate malabsorption with increased exposure of the unabsorbed carbohydrate to colonic bacteria. Alternatively, if elderly people have greater numbers of bacteria residing in their proximal small intestine this also could produce greater breath hydrogen excretion.

There is an interesting physiologic change in the gastrointestinal tract with age which could influence the absorption and bioavailability of several micronutrients: atrophic gastritis. Serum pepsinogens serve as good blood markers for identifying individuals with atrophic gastritis and gastric atrophy[22–24]. Serum pepsinogens I and II can be measured by radio-immunoassay. Samloff *et al.* have demonstrated a good correlation between serum pepsinogen I and II ratio and both gastric secretory function and histology[22–24]. A PGI:PGII ratio of less than 2.9 is indicative of atrophic gastritis[22–25]. A ratio of less than 2.9 accompanied by an absolute value for serum pepsinogen I of less than 2.0 μg/L defines severe gastric atrophy. The prevalence of atrophic gastritis in a Bostonian population age group 60–69 is 24%, at age 70–79 is 32% and at age > 80 is almost 40%.

The physiologic consequences of atrophic gastritis are: (1) decreased intrinsic factor secretion (although in most cases the degree of parietal cell disappearance is not severe enough to produce total lack of intrinsic factor and therefore pernicious anaemia does not develop); (2) bacterial overgrowth, owing to diminished gastric acid output and diminished killing of bacteria; (3) a higher proximal small intestinal pH which could affect nutrient absorption for particular nutrients whose absorption processes are pH dependent, or by diminishing the dissociation of micronutrients from food complexes such as dietary fibre. For example, calcium and other divalent cations are only released from dietary fibre in an acid milieu[26]. If the dietary fibre–micronutrient complex is never bathed in acid, dissociation may not take place, and the cation will be carried along with fibre into the colon.

We have studied proximal small intestinal pH in a series of individuals with atrophic gastritis and a series of age-matched individuals without atrophic gastritis. In the former we found the proximal small bowel pH at the ligament of Treitz to be 7.1 versus 6.7 in normal aged-matched subjects[27]. This seemingly small change in intestinal pH may greatly influence the absorption of certain micronutrients. One micronutrient whose absorption is pH sensitive is folic acid and another is nicotinic acid[28,29]. It should be noted that folate malabsorption owing to age alone has not been demonstrated in either animals or humans. However, we have shown that folic acid uptake by rat intestinal rings is optimal at pH 6.3 with a fall in folate uptake by the rings when the pH is either raised or lowered[28]. The proximal small intestine absorbs folic acid by a saturable energy transport system at physiologic folate concentrations[30]. It is the active transport process which has been shown to be pH sensitive[30]. Owing to the pH sensitivity of folate absorption, we studied folic acid absorption in elderly human subjects with gastric atrophy and in normal age matched controls without gastric atrophy[27].

Folate absorption tests were carried out using tritium-labelled pteroylmonoglutamic acid (PGA), one test being administered with water and a second test being administered with 0.1 N hydrochloric acid. The tests were carried out in a mixed-design, random order. Basal gastric pH measurements were carried out on all subjects using a Cecar electrode. On day 1 of each test, the subject received an intramuscular loading dose of 15 mg of unlabelled folic acid. On day 3 an oral dose of tritium-labelled PGA was administered and a 24-h urine collection was started. At 4 h after receiving the radioactive folate, a 15-mg flushing dose of unlabelled folic acid was given intra-muscularly and the subjects were then allowed to eat normally. At the end of the urine collection, 1-ml aliquots of urine were counted in triplicate and the percentage of the dose excreted over the 24 h was calculated as the measure of absorption. In normal elderly, gastric pH values were, as expected, low $(1.6 \pm 0.1 = $ mean $\pm$ SEM) with no change in the gastric pH upon hydrochloric acid administration. Mean $\pm$ SEM gastric pH in the subjects with gastric atrophy was 6.4 ± 0.4 and fell with hydrochloric acid administration to 1.4 ± 0.2. Folic acid absorption ranged between 40% and 70% in the normal individuals when given with water and did not change with hydrochloric acid (Figure 28.2). However, in the individuals with atrophic gastritis there was a marked depression in folate absorption when given with water (mean $\pm$ SEM $= 32 \pm 4\%$) which corrected to $54 \pm 4\%$ when the folic acid was administered with 0.1 N hydrochloric acid. Thus, folate malabsorption occurred in atrophic gastritis, apparently owing to the change in proximal small intestinal pH, since malabsorption of folic acid was totally corrected by giving it along with 0.1 N hydrochloric acid.

Because of diminished folic acid absorption in elderly atrophic gastritis

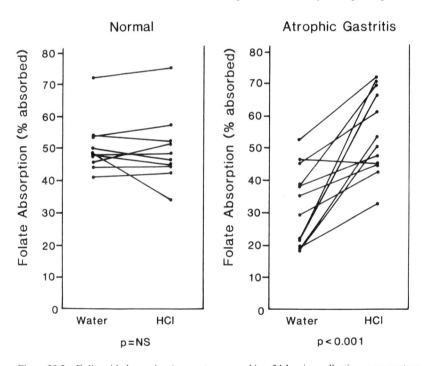

Figure 28.2 Folic acid absorption (amount recovered in a 24-h urine collection as percentage of oral dose) in normal elderly controls and in subjects with atrophic gastritis when [³H]folic acid was given with 120 ml of either water or 0.1 NHCl. [Published with permission from *Gastroenterology*, (1986), **91**, 1476–82][27]

individuals, one would expect to see more folate malnutrition among individuals with atrophic gastritis than in non-atrophic gastritis subjects. However, in the Boston elderly survey this was not seen[25]. In fact, serum folate levels were found to be significantly *higher* in atrophic gastritis individuals than in non-atrophic gastritis individuals. The explanation for this appears to be the greater number of bacteria residing in the proximal small bowel in individuals with atrophic gastritis (10^6–10^9) versus 10^2–10^3 in elderly individuals without atrophic gastritis[27]. These bacteria have been shown to synthesize folic acid *in vitro*. Thus, there appears to be a built-in mechanism (i.e. folate synthesis by bacteria) to insure normal folate nutriture in individuals with atrophic gastritis despite folate malabsorption.

By a different mechanism, atrophic gastritis may also affect the bioavailability of vitamin B_{12}. Dietary vitamin B_{12} is associated with food proteins which must be digested off the B_{12} molecule before it is able to bind with endogenous R binders or with intrinsic factor. This digestion takes place in the stomach under the influence of acid and pepsin. King *et al.* have described a group of 5 individuals with gastric atrophy who had diminished absorption of vitamin B_{12} if the vitamin were bound to chicken serum protein[31]. This malabsorption could not be corrected by giving intrinsic factor with the protein-bound vitamin B_{12} (Figure 28.3). However, giving acid along with the protein-bound vitamin B_{12} increased its absorption to within the normal range in 2 individuals, and giving acid along with pepsin (with or without intrinsic factor) further increased the absorption in the others. Thus, it

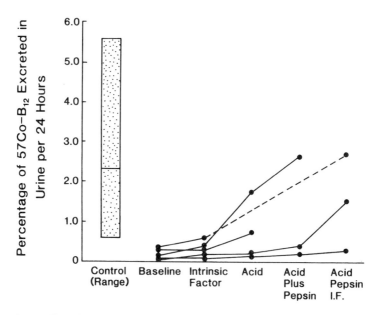

Figure 28.3 Effect of intrinsic factor, acid, pepsin or a combination thereof on protein-bound vitamin B_{12} absorption in 5 vitamin B_{12} deficient subjects. [Published with permission from *Digestive Diseases and Science*, (1979), **24**, 397–402][31]

appears that gastric atrophy may result in reduced bioavailability of protein-bound vitamin B_{12} because of lack of acid pepsin digestion of dietary protein from the vitamin B_{12} molecule, in addition to the relative lack of intrinsic factor. In terms of human nutrition this is an important issue since crystalline vitamin B_{12} is not what is normally eaten by individuals, but rather it is protein or food-associated B_{12} which is consumed. Similar findings have recently been reported for albumen-bound pyridoxine in an everted gut sac system[32]. Lowering the pH of the milieu decreased the binding of vitamin B_6 to albumen and resulted in an increased uptake of the vitamin by the gut epithelial cells[32].

A second mechanism whereby vitamin B_{12} bioavailability may be reduced in atrophic gastritis is by bacterial binding of the vitamin. We have recently demonstrated that the bioavailability of vitamin B_{12} can be increased in elderly subjects with mild to moderate atrophic gastritis by the administration of tetracycline[33].

When discussing atrophic gastritis, one should also consider iron and calcium bioavailability. Decreased iron absorption has been reported in old age; however, many studies were not well controlled for iron status or the presence of gastrointestinal disease. It has been shown that the absorption of ferric iron is diminished in achlorhydric subjects[34-36]. Acid serves to keep the ferric iron in solution until reaching the absorptive sites of the duodenal mucosa. Ferric iron is insoluble above pH 5, although ferrous iron and heme iron remain in solution at neutral or slightly alkaline pH values[36,37]. Substances which ligand ferric iron, such as ascorbate, increase the absorption of ferric iron at a neutral or slightly alkaline pH range; however, chelation must occur when the iron is in solution – that is, when the iron is in an acid milieu. Thus, acidity is needed for the chelation of ferric iron to take place, which will then be kept in solution at the higher pH of the proximal small intestine so that iron will be available for absorption. Heme iron does not appear to be affected by lack of acid and thus is normally absorbed in individuals with atrophic gastritis[36,38,39]. There may be other factors in gastric juice in addition to acid which promote the absorption of iron as well.

The elderly show reduced absorption of calcium[40]. In addition, elderly individuals show a reduced ability to adapt to low calcium diets by increasing the efficiency of calcium absorption, whereas younger individuals are able to make such an adaptation[41].

As previously mentioned, atrophic gastritis can affect calcium absorption, in that calcium must be disassociated from food complexes (e.g. fibre) at an acid pH[26]. Moreover, calcium carbonate reacts with hydrochloric acid to form soluble calcium chloride which is subsequently absorbed in the proximal small bowel. Recker recently showed in achlorhydric individuals that calcium carbonate is markedly malabsorbed as compared to normal subjects[42]. This finding contrasts with the finding of Bo-Linn et al. who studied individuals with gastric pH values which were not as high as Recker's patients (i.e. in the range of 5.0 versus 7.0)[43]. In addition, different methodology was used in Bo-Linn's study which could have influenced the solubility of calcium carbonate.

Another change which takes place in the gastrointestinal tract with age, is a change in the character of the unstirred water layer[44]. Hollander *et al.* have shown that this change may result in an increase in vitamin A absorption with advancing age. In human studies we have shown that vitamin A tolerance curves in elderly individuals using physiologic amounts of vitamin A have significantly higher peaks and greater areas under the curve than in younger adults[46]. Tolerance curves after oral vitamin A are influenced both by an absorptive component and an uptake component by peripheral tissues (e.g. liver). Thus, an elevated area under the curve could be owing to either increased absorption or decreased peripheral tissue uptake. The significance of increased vitamin A absorption and/or decreased vitamin A uptake by peripheral tissue with age should not be taken lightly. In illustrating the point, Figures 28.4 and 28.5 show two frequency distribution curves. The first is a frequency distribution curve for serum retinol levels among normal elderly subjects who are users and non-users of vitamin supplements containing vitamin A in physiologic amounts. The users of vitamins in this study were defined as taking a vitamin supplement containing vitamin A three or more times a week. Figure 28.4 shows the serum retinol frequency distributions of users versus non-users to be virtually superimposable. However, when one looks at serum retinyl ester frequency distributions (Figure 28.5) one sees that some elderly users of vitamin A supplements achieve retinyl ester levels as high as $50\,\mu g/dl$. Retinyl esters are taken as indicators of vitamin A toxicity since they may be converted to free retinol, which is unbound to retinol binding protein and thus non-specifically delivered to biologic membranes. Therefore, an increased absorption and/or decreased clearance of this vitamin

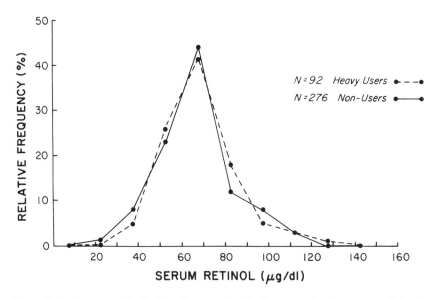

Figure 28.4 Frequency distribution of serum retinol in 'heavy users' and non-users of vitamin supplements containing vitamin A in doses of 1–2 times the United States Recommended Dietary Allowance for males. A heavy user is defined as taking the vitamin supplement 3 or more times a week

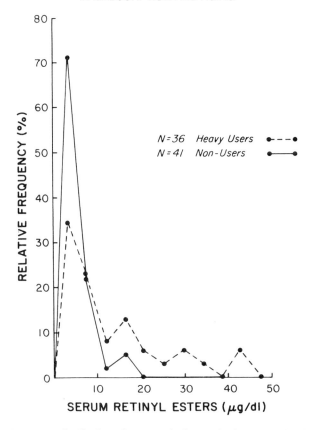

Figure 28.5 Frequency distribution of serum retinyl esters in 'heavy users' and non-users of vitamin supplements containing vitamin A in doses of 1–2 times the United States Recommended Dietary Allowance for males. A heavy user is defined as taking the vitamin supplement 3 or more times a week

due to age could be detrimental to elderly individuals who take the vitamin in excess amounts.

In summary, it appears that the aging gastrointestinal tract has a large reserve capacity *vis-à-vis* both digestive and absorptive processes. Only when that reserve capacity is overwhelmed by unphysiologic amounts of fat, protein, or carbohydrate does a clinical problem normally ensue. However, there are certain aging changes within the gastrointestinal tract which could influence the absorption of micronutrients. One such change is atrophic gastritis wherein the alteration in proximal small bowel pH and bacterial overgrowth could greatly affect the bioavailability of micronutrients such as folic acid and vitamin B_{12}. Also, the change in character of the unstirred water layer could allow more easy penetration of lipid-soluble substances across the small intestinal membrane and thus produce enhanced absorption of fat-soluble substances. It is only with further study of these intricate mechanisms that we will be able to understand the role that the aging gastrointestinal tract plays in maintaining the nutritional status of the elderly.

References

1. McGandy, R. B., Barrows, C. H., Spanias, A., Meredith A., Stone, J. L. and Norris, A. H. (1966). Nutrient intakes and energy expenditures in men of different ages. *J. Gerontol.*, **21**, 581–7
2. Khalil, T., Fujimura, M., Townsend, Jr., C. M., Greeley, Jr., G. H. and Thompson, J. C. (1985). Effect of aging on pancreatic secretion in rats. *Am. J. Surg.*, **149**, 120–5
3. Greenberg, R. E. and Holt, P. R. (1986). Influence of aging upon pancreatic digestive enzymes. *Digest. Dis. Sci.*, **9**, 970–7
4. Hollander, D. and Dadufalza, V. D. (1984). Aging-associated pancreatic exocrine insufficiency in the unanesthetized rat. *Gerontology*, **30**, 218–22
5. Bartos, V. and Groh, J. (1968). The effect of repeated stimulation of the pancreas on the pancreatic secretion in young and aged men. *Gerontol. Clin.*, **11**, 56–62
6. Rosenberg, I. R., Friedland, N., Janowitz, H. D. and Dreiling, D. A. (1966). The effect of age and sex upon human pancreatic secretion of fluid and bicarbonate. *Gastroenterology*, **50**, 191–4
7. Necheles, H., Plotke, F. and Meyer, J. (1942). Studies on old age. *Am. J. Dig. Dis.*, **9**, 157–9
8. Meyer, B., Spier, E. and Neuwelt, F. (1940). Basal secretion of digestive enzymes in old age. *Arch. Intern. Med.*, **65**, 171–7
9. Gullo, L., Ventrucci, M., Naldoni, P. and Pezzilli, R. (1986). Aging and exocrine pancreatic function. *J. Am. Geriatrics Society*, **34**, 790–2
10. Pelz, K. S., Gottfried, S. P. and Soos, E. (1968). Intestinal absorption studies in the aged. *Geriatrics*, 149–53
11. Dutta, S. K. and Hlasko, J. (1985). Dietary fiber and pancreatic disease: effect of high fiber diet on malabsorption and pancreatic insufficiency and *in vitro* enzymes. *Am. J. Clin. Nutri.*, **41**, 517–25
12. Southgate, D. A. T. and Durnin, J. V. G. A. (1970). Calorie conversion factors. An experimental reassessment of the factors used in the calculation of the energy value of human diets. *Br. J. Nutr.*, **24**, 517–35
13. Hellemans, J., Joosten, E., Ghoos, Y., Carchon, H., Vantrappen, G., Pelemans, W. and Rutgeerts, P. (1984). Positive $^{14}CO_2$ bile acid breath test in elderly people. *Age Ageing*, **13**, 138–43
14. Arora, S., Russell, R. M., Kassarjian, Z., Krasingski, S. and Kaplan, M. (1987). Evaluation of absorptive and hepatobiliary function in the aging digestive tract. Presented at the *28th Annual American College of Nutrition*, September 20–22, St Charles, Illinois
15. Werner, I. and Hambraeus, L. (1972). The digestive capacity of elderly people. In Carlson, L. A. (ed.) *Nutrition in Old Age*, pp. 55–60. (Uppsala: Almqvist and Wiksell)
16. Welsh, J. D., Russell, L. C. and Walker, Jr., A. W. (1974). Changes in intestinal lactase and alkaline phosphatase activity with age in the baboon (*Papio papio*). *Gastroenterology*, **66**, 993–7
17. Donaldson, Jr., R. M. and Gryboski, J. D. (1973). Carbohydrate intolerance. In Sleisenger, M. H. and Fordtran, J. S. (eds.) *Gastrointestinal Disease*. Ch. 76, pp. 1015–30
18. Kendall, M. J. (1970). The influence of age on the xylose absorption test. *Gut*, **11**, 548–51
19. Guth, P. H. (1968). Physiologic alterations in small bowel function with age. *Am. J. Dig. Dis.*, **13**, 565–71
20. Webster, S. G. P. and Leeming, J. T. (1975). Assessment of small bowel function in the elderly using a modified xylose tolerance test. *Gut*, **16**, 109–13
21. Feibusch, J. M. and Holt, P. R. (1982). Impaired absorptive capacity for carbohydrate in the aging human. *Digest. Dis. Sci.*, **27**, 1095–100
22. Samloff, I. M., Varis, K., Ihamaki, T., Siurala, M. and Rotter, J. H. (1982). Relationships among serum pepsinogen 1, serum pepsinogen 2, and gastric mucosal histology. *Gastroenterology*, **83**, 204–9

23. Samloff, I. M., Secrist, D. M. and Passaro, Jr., I. (1975). A study of the relationship between serum group 1 pepsinogen levels and gastric acid secretion. *Gastroenterology*, **69**, 1196–200

24. Varis, K., Samloff, I. M., Ihamaki, T. and Siurala, M. (1979). An appraisal of tests for severe atrophic gastritis in relatives of patients with pernicious anemia. *Digest. Dis. Sci.*, **24**, 187–91

25. Krasinski, S. D., Russell, R. M., Samloff, I. M., Jacob, R. A., Dallal, G. E., McGandy, R. B. and Hartz, S. C. (1986). Fundic atrophic gastritis in an elderly population. *J. Am. Geriatric Society*, **34**, 800–6

26. James, W. P. T., Branch, W. J. and Southgate, D. A. T. (1978). Calcium binding by dietary fibre. *Lancet*, **1**, 638–9

27. Russell, R. M., Krasinski, S. D., Samloff, I. M., Jacob, R. A., Hartz, S. C. and Brovender, S. R. (1987). Folic acid malabsorption in atrophic gastritis. *Gastroenterology*, **91**, 1476–82

28. Russell, R. M., Dhar, G. J., Dutta, S. K. and Rosenberg, I. H. (1979). Influence of intra-luminal pH on folate absorption: studies in control subjects and in patients with pancreatic insufficiency. *J. Lab. Clin. Med.*, **93**, 428–36

29. Elbert, J., Daniel, H. and Rehner, G. (1985). Intestinal uptake of nicotinic acid as a function of microclimate-pH. *Int. J. Vit. Nutr. Res.*, **56**, 85–93

30. Selhub, J., Powell, G. M. and Rosenberg, I. H. (1984). Intestinal transport of 5-methyl-tetrahydrofolate. *Am. J. Physiol. (Gastrointest. Liver Physiol.)*, **246**, G515–20

31. King, C. E., Leibach, J. and Toskes, P. P. (1979). Clinically significant vitamin B_{12} deficiency secondary to malabsorption of protein-bound vitamin B_{12}. *Digest. Dis. Sci.*, **24**, 397–402

32. Middleton, III, H. M. (1986). Intestinal hydrolysis of pyridoxal 5'-phosphate *in vitro* and *in vivo* in the rat. *Gastroenterology*, **91**, 343–50

33. Russell, R. M., Suter, P. M. and Golner, B. (1987). Decreased bioavailability of protein bound vitamin B_{12} in mild atrophic gastritis: reversal by antibiotics. *Gastroenterology*, **92**, 1606

34. Choudhurry, M. R. and Williams, J. (1959). Iron absorption and gastric operations. *Clin. Sci.*, **18**, 527

35. Goldberg, A., Lochhead, A. C. and Dagg, J. H. (1963). Histamine-fast achlorhydria and iron absorption. *Lancet*, **1**, 848–50

36. Jacobs, P., Bothwell, T. and Charlton, R. W. (1964). Role of hydrochloric acid in iron absorption. *J. Appl. Physiol.*, **19**, 187–8

37. Chaberek, S. and Martell, A. E. (1959). *Organic Sequesting Agents*, pp. 187–98. (New York: Wiley)

38. Biggs, J. C., Bannerman, R. M. and Callender, S. T. (1962). *Proc. 8th Congr. Eur. Soc. Haematol. (1961)*, **1**, 236

39. Bjorn-Rasmussen, E., Hallberg, L., Isaksson, B. and Arvidsson, B. (1974). Food iron absorption in man. Applications of the two-pool extrinsic tag method to measure heme and non-heme iron absorption from the whole diet. *J. Clin. Invest.*, **53**, 247–55

40. Bullamore, J. R. (1970). Effects of age on calcium absorption. *Lancet*, **2**, 535–7

41. Ireland, P. and Fordtran, J. S. (1973). Effect of dietary calcium and age on jejunal calcium absorption in humans studied by intestinal perfusion. *JCI*, **52**, 2672–81

42. Recker, R. R. (1985). Calcium absorption and achlorhydria. *N. Engl. J. Med.*, **313**, 70–3

43. Bo-Linn, G. W., Davis, G. R., Buddrus, D. J., Morawski, S. G., Santa Ana, C. and Fordtran, J. S. (1984). An evaluation of the importance of gastric acid secretion in the absorption of dietary calcium. *J. Clin. Invest.*, **73**, 640–7

44. Hollander, D. and Dadufalza, V. D. (1983). Aging: its influence on the intestinal unstirred water layer thickness, surface area, and resistance in the unanesthetized rat. *Canad. J. Physiol. Pharmacol.*, **61**, 1501–8

45. Hollander, D. and Morgan, D. (1979). Aging: its influence on vitamin A intestinal absorption *in vivo* by the rat. *Exp. Gerontol.*, **14**, 301–5

46. Krasinski, S. D., Russell, R. M. and Dallal, G. E. (1985). Aging changes vitamin A absorption characteristics. *Gastroenterology*, **88**, 1715

29
Zinc deficiency in old age: the place of supplementation

G. C. STURNIOLO, A. MARTIN, M. C. MONTINO, M. SANZARI, E. MARCHIORI, B. FINCO AND R. NACCARATO

Zinc is an essential trace element: it is a necessary constituent of more than 70 metalloenzymes and is involved in the biosynthesis and catabolism of DNA and RNA. Since zinc may also play a role in the maintenance of polynucleotide structure, zinc deficiency may be responsible for various clinical manifestations.

ZINC DEFICIENCY IN THE ELDERLY

Some clinical manifestations such as delayed wound-healing[1], immunological impairment[2] or alterations of taste and smell[3] are often present in the elderly[4] and may be caused by zinc deficiency.

Slow wound-healing appears to be frequent in the elderly and healing has been accelerated by zinc treatment[5]. Aging is also associated with progressive alterations of immune competence.

The impairment of T-lymphocyte functions can be a cause of increased incidence of autoimmune phenomena, increased susceptibility to some infections, paraproteinemia and amyloidosis. This impairment may be demonstrated by a reduced number of T-lymphocytes, delayed skin reactions to purified protein derivatives and reduced thymic hormone (*facteur timique serique*)[6]. Animal experiments have shown that zinc deficiency can result in reduction in the size and functions of the thymus as well as T-cell dependent immune response. These alterations can be reverted by zinc repletions and similar observations have been reported in humans[2].

In patients with quiescent Crohn's Disease, we have found an increased percentage of Ia-like lymphocytes, which was corrected by zinc administration ($ZnSO_4$ 220 mg thrice daily)[7].

Taste and smell alterations, in some cases, may be zinc dependent, but the taste reduction demonstrated in healthy elderly in comparison to young adults does not correlate to serum zinc levels and does not respond to zinc supplementation[8].

In the elderly, reduced food intake is also very common, and it may therefore be supposed that the zinc intake is also reduced. The existing Recommended Dietary Allowances (R.D.A.) for Zinc and Safe and Adequate Dietary Intake for the Elderly is about 12–15 mg/day and it is extrapolated from studies on young adults. However, it has recently been demonstrated[9] that zinc in the diet of pensioners living at home with a self-chosen diet was of 8–10 mg/day, and this amount of zinc appears to be sufficient for good health in the group studied. The low amount of zinc found in the diet of this elderly population may be sufficient because of the reduced energy requirements or metabolic functions of old people[10,11].

In the elderly, drug consumption, possibly reduced absorption and sub-liminal intake might cause a marginal zinc deficiency. That could become clinically or biochemically evident, only when the need for zinc is increased.

These are assumptions which may support the idea that a slight zinc deficiency might exist in old people[12].

ASSESSMENT OF ZINC DEFICIENCY

The demonstration of zinc deficiency is difficult, because so far no single biochemical test exists which is able to demonstrate a poor zinc status. The only positive proof is the correction of alterations, induced by zinc administration. Notwithstanding the absence of a zinc deficiency test, information may be collected by carrying out various tests.

Serum zinc

This has been reported to be reduced or normal in healthy elderly subjects in comparison to young adults[12]. In our experience a reduction of serum zinc was apparent in 15 healthy elderly and a further significant reduction in 30 elderly with gastrointestinal diseases (Figure 29.1).

Tissue zinc

Leukocytes, red-blood cells, hair and nails could theoretically represent the zinc status better than serum zinc, but none of the results with these tissues demonstrated a clear difference and we found no difference in comparing the red-blood cell zinc concentrations of young adults and the elderly (Figure 29.2).

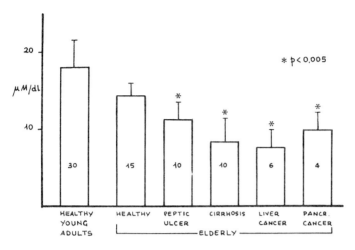

Figure 29.1 Serum zinc in elderly patients with gastrointestinal diseases

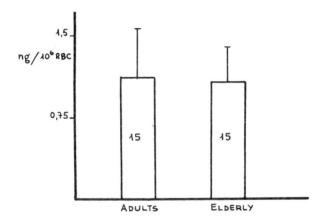

Figure 29.2 Zinc in red-blood cells

Urinary excretion

This could be the cause of zinc depletion, but it only slightly increased in our older subjects (Figure 29.3).

Intestinal absorption

The measurement of intestinal absorption is another important way of assessing zinc[13] and can be studied by various methods:

● Balance studies[15].

311

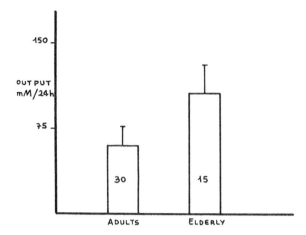

Figure 29.3 Urinary excretion of zinc

- Serum zinc concentrations after oral load[14].

- Isotopic methods with long- or short-lived isotopes[16].

Balance studies are difficult to perform because they involve, among other requirements, a metabolic room, strictly controlled diets and large availability of laboratory time.

The *isotopic methods* expose the subjects to the risk of radiation and are very expensive. The more commonly used isotope is ^{65}Zn, which is long-lived ($t_{\frac{1}{2}} = 264$ days) and a total body counter is necessary. Measurement of radioactive zinc in the faeces is an alternative. The short-lived ($t_{\frac{1}{2}} = 14$ h) isotope ^{69}Zn needs a double administration at an interval of 1 week (oral and intravenous) and the deconvolution of the two curves obtained will measure the net intestinal absorption of zinc.

A simpler though less precise method is the measurement of *plasma zinc* levels after an oral load in the Zinc Tolerance Test (ZnTT). This method can be repeated, is safe, inexpensive, well-tolerated, and can be used in the clinical routine, particularly when a physiological dosage is employed. Valberg and co-workers[14] found that the absorption measured by ZnTT correlates with that calculated by the ^{65}Zn method. In 15 elderly subjects we found a significant reduction of the area under the serum Zn curve (Figure 29.4), after the administration of 55 mg of zinc sulphate equivalent to 12.5 mg of elemental zinc, which is a physiological dose. Four subjects had a flat curve: all possible explanations for malabsorption were ruled out and the subjects were not different from the others, as regards the parameters checked (serum, urinary, red blood cell zinc, nutritional and immunological status).

According to the data reported in the literature and our own results, it does not seem possible to confirm the suspicion that a reduced zinc status exists, even when expressed by a low, but not significantly so, serum zinc level and by a markedly reduced zinc absorption.

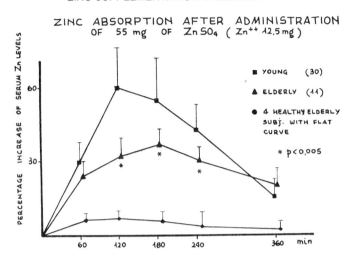

Figure 29.4 Zinc absorption after administration of 55 mg ZnSO$_4$ (Zn^{2+} = 12.5 mg)

Biochemical evidence of zinc deficiency is not necessarily paralleled by clinical signs.

In order to exclude indirectly a reduced intake of zinc, we studied several nutritional indices (ideal body weight, albumin, prealbumin, retinol binding protein, fibronectin, triceps skinfold, subscapular skinfold thickness, arm circumference) in our elderly subjects, but all the parameters were within the normal range.

Although it is relatively simple to demonstrate the effect of zinc in influencing several *immune functions in vitro*[17,18] or in experimental animals[19], it is very difficult to obtain clear-cut results as regards the effects of zinc supplementation on human immunity. The first problem is to evaluate the existence of zinc deficiency, the second problem is that no single parameter which expresses an immune impairment exists and consequently the effect of zinc can be masked by other factors. Many authors have reported that cell-mediated immunity is impaired in patients with zinc deficiency and it is frequently compromised in the elderly; immunity can be studied, in this respect, by evaluating the subsets of circulating T-lymphocytes, by the cutaneous hypersensitivity reactions to purified protein derivatives of common antigens (*Candida*, tetanus, *Mycobacterium tuberculosis*, *Trichophyton*, *Streptococcus*, diphtheria, *Proteus*) and by the *in vitro* responses of lymphocytes to stimulation with mitogens. In our group of elderly subjects cellular immunity was evaluated by a cutaneous hypersensitivity test (Multitest I.M.C. Merieux Institute), by subsets of lymphocytes (T3, T4, T8, T4/T8, NK) measured by the immunofluorescence technique, and by HLA-DR. Immunity was not found to be significantly impaired and was not influenced by a 3-week supplementation with 110 mg t.i.d. zinc sulphate orally (Figures 29.5–29.7). Since, as suggested by Chandra[21], large amounts of zinc supplementation may suppress (instead of stimulate) immunity, we used a small dosage, i.e. 100 mg zinc sulphate t.i.d. A moderate dietary zinc

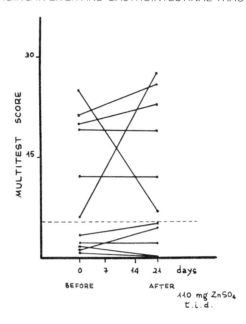

Figure 29.5   Zinc and immunity in the elderly: multitest score

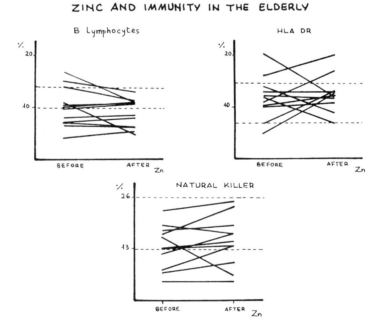

Figure 29.6   Zinc and immunity in the elderly: B lymphocytes, HLA-DR and natural killer cells. Zinc dose as in Figure 29.5

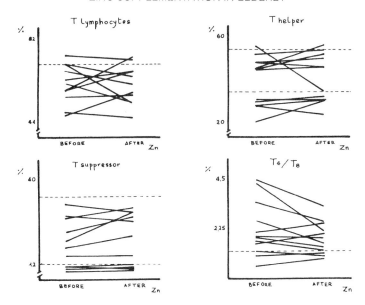

Figure 29.7   Zinc and immunity in the elderly: T lymphocytes, T helper cells, T suppressor cells and the T_4:T_8 ratio. Zinc dosage as in Figure 29.5

supplementation (comparable to the dose we used) was shown to increase the plasma levels of thymic hormone and to increase the absolute number of T-lymphocytes with a concomitant reduction of recurrent infections[21].

CONCLUSIONS

In conclusion we cannot definitively support the hypothesis that a zinc deficiency exists in the healthy elderly population living at home and eating a self-chosen diet. Serum zinc is reduced, but is not statistically different from young adults. Tissue and urinary zinc are normal. Only zinc absorption is significantly impaired. Even if it is impossible to exclude a marginal zinc deficiency, at least in our subjects, no consequences of zinc deficiency were demonstrated by evaluating the nutritional status (within the normal limits) or the immunological indices, that were not significantly impaired. Zinc supplementation did not modify the immunological parameters, even when these were clearly impaired in some subjects.

Thus, in our experience, zinc status is not impaired in the healthy elderly population and there is no reason to justify zinc supplementation.

References

1. Pories, W. I., Henlel, J. H., Rob, C. G. and Strain, W. H. (1967). Acceleration of healing with zinc sulphate. *Ann. Surg.*, **165**, 432–6

2. Prasad, A. S. (1983). The role of zinc in gastrointestinal and liver disease. *Clinics in Gastroenterology*. pp. 713–41. (Eastbourne: W. B. Saunders)

3. Bales, C. W., Steinman, L. C., Freeland-Graves, J. H., Stone, J. M. and Young, R. K. (1986). The effect of age on plasma zinc uptake and taste acuity. *Am. J. Clin. Nutr.*, **44**, 664–9

4. Sandstead, H. H., Henriksen, Z. K., Greger, J. L., Prasad, A. S. and Good, R. A. (1982). Zinc nutriture in the elderly in relation to taste acuity, immune response, and wound healing. *Am. J. Clin. Nutr.*, **36**, 1046–59

5. Hallbook, T. and Lanner, E. (1972). Serum-zinc and healing of venous leg ulcers. *Lancet*, **2**, 780–2

6. Duchateau, J., Delepesse, G., Vrijens, R. and Collet, H. (1981). Beneficial effects of oral zinc supplementation on the immune response of old people. *Am. J. Med.*, **70**, 1001–4

7. Sturniolo, G. C., Gurrieri, G., Mastropaolo, G., Martin, A., Corsano, A., Fagiolo, U. and Naccarato, R. (1983). Effects of zinc treatment of peripheral T-cell subsets in Crohn's disease. *Ital. J. Gastroenterol.*, **15**, 220

8. Greger, J. L. and Geissler, A. H. (1978). Effect of zinc supplementation on taste acuity on the aged. *Am. J. Clin. Nutr.*, **31**, 633–7

9. Abdulla, M. (1986). Inorganic Chemical Elements in Prepared Meals in Sweden. (Department of Clinical Chemistry, University of Lund)

10. Burke, D. M., De Micco, F. J., Taper, L. J. and Ritchey, S. J. (1981). Copper and zinc utilization in elderly adults. *J. Gastroenterol.*, **36**, 558–63

11. Wilson, C. W. M. and Myskow, L. (1985). Reduced serum zinc levels and oral zinc supplementation in geriatric patients. *Int. J. Vit. Nutr.*, **55**, 331–6

12. Busher, G. L., Lockwood, I. J., Cochrane, H. R., Delves, H. T. and Hali, M. R. P. (1982). Serum zinc in old age. *J. Clin. Exp. Geriatr.*, **4**(3), 249–56

13. Fickel, J. J., Freeland-Graves, J. H. and Roby, M. J. (1986). Zinc tolerance test in zinc deficient and zinc supplemented diets. *Am. J. Clin. Nutr.*, **43**, 47–58

14. Valberg, L. F., Flanagan, P. R., Brennan, J. and Chamberlein, M. J. (1985). Does the oral zinc tolerance test measure zinc absorption? *Am. J. Clin. Nutr.*, **41**, 37–42

15. Bunker, V. W., Hindl, L. J., Lawson, M. S. and Clayton, B. E. (1984). Assessment of zinc and copper status of healthy elderly people using metabolic balance studies and measurement of leucocyte concentrations. *Am. J. Clin. Nutr.*, **40**, 1096–102

16. Molokhia, M., Sturniolo, G. C., Shields, R. and Turnberg, L. A. (1980). A simple method for measuring zinc absorption in man using a short-lived isotope (^{69}Zn). *Am. J. Clin, Nutr.*, **33**, 881–6

17. Zinc and polymorphonuclear leukocyte functions. *Nutrition Reviews 1977*, **35**, 266–68

18. Flynn, A. (1985). *In vitro* levels of copper, magnesium and zinc required for mitogen stimulated T-lymphocyte proliferation. *Nutr. Res.*, **5**, 487–95

19. Fernandes, G., Madhavan, N., Kazunori, O., Toshio, T., Floyd, R. and Good, R. A. (1978). Impairment of all-mediated immunity function by dietary zinc deficiency in mice. *Immunology*, **1**, 457–61

20. Fabris, N., Mocchegiani, E., Amadio, L., Zannotti, M., Licastro, F. and Franceschi, C. (1984). Thymic hormone deficiency in normal ageing and Down's syndrome: is there a primary failure of the thymus? *Lancet*, **1**, 983–6

21. Chandra, R. K. (1984). Excessive intake of zinc impairs immune responses. *J. Am. Med. Assoc.*, **252**, 1443–6

30
The aging pancreas

L. GULLO

Judging by the size of the literature published on age-related changes in the exocrine pancreas, it would seem that the interest of investigators in this subject has had a biphasic trend over time: from about 1945 to 1960–65 interest was fairly high, after which it declined until about 1980, picking up again in recent years in accordance with the general re-awakening of interest in the elderly and in their physiology and diseases. This means that most of the data available on pancreatic changes in the elderly come from studies carried out many years ago, when the means for studying the pancreas were few and rather imprecise. In this chapter, the human pancreas will be mainly dealt with, and specifically, the following questions:

1. Does the exocrine pancreas undergo changes in structure as a result of aging?
2. Does the exocrine pancreas undergo changes in function as a result of aging?
3. If such changes occur, can they impair the digestive capacity of the elderly person and thereby alter nutritional status?

As is well known, the pancreas plays a crucial role in the digestion of food. In this respect, it should be remembered that this organ has a functional characteristic which ensures long-term protection of its role in food assimilation even in pathological states of the gland: normally, enzyme secretion in response to food ingestion is much greater than the actual digestive requirements. In fact, only about 10% of the enzymes secreted into the duodenal lumen are needed for normal digestion[1]. This means that when the structure of the gland is damaged, maldigestion and malabsorption occur only if functional impairment exceeds 90% with respect to normal, i.e. when the pancreas is practically destroyed. One could therefore assume that if the pancreas undergoes structural and functional changes as a result of age, these changes may have clinical significance only if they are severe.

STRUCTURAL CHANGES

The information on this topic is fragmentary and insufficient. Although some investigators[2] have reported a decrease in weight and size of the gland with aging, others[3] have not. Both peripancreatic and intrapancreatic fat has been reported to increase with aging[4,5], but the degree of this change is not defined. The increase in fat has been believed to be one of the factors contributing to the increased echogenicity of the elderly pancreas at ultrasound examination[6]. Changes in the ductal system have been a little better defined. A post-mortem study[7] of the pancreatic ductal system in a large number of subjects older than 60 years has shown that definite changes in pancreatic duct morphology occur with increasing age. The most important of these are: (1) a progressive increase, of about 8% per decade, of the caliber of the main pancreatic duct along its whole length (the dilated duct retains its uniform tapering appearance with smooth margins, in contrast to the changes associated with chronic pancreatitis or pancreatic cancer); and, (2) dilatation of interlobular and intralobular ducts and small cyst formation. It is worth mentioning that histologic examination has shown intact lobular structure and ducts in cases with ductal dilatation. The authors of this study did not offer any explanation of the mechanisms responsible for the dilatation of the pancreatic ducts with aging. The present author is not aware of any studies *in vivo* of the pancreatic ductal system in the elderly which can confirm or refute these post-mortem observations. It is clear, in any case, that these changes should be taken into consideration in assessing endoscopic retrograde pancreatograms in elderly patients.

From a histologic viewpoint, the changes most often described are fibrosis, fat infiltration, degenerative changes of the acinar cells, arteriolosclerosis, and lesions of the interlobular and intralobular ducts consisting of proliferation and squamous metaplasia of the epithelium, and cystic dilatation[2,5,8-10]. Many of these lesions, however, are not specific, since they may occur at any age.

Two questions arise in interpreting these data: (1) were the observed lesions caused by the basic aging process or by superimposed disease and/or malnutrition ? (most studies were carried out on patients who died in the hospital, who were affected by a variety of systemic diseases and whose nutritional status was unknown); and, (2) if the changes described were indeed caused by aging, what were their degree and extent? At present, we do not have sufficient information to answer these questions adequately. The answer to the first question raised at the beginning of this chapter cannot therefore be precise and definitive. It is probable that a certain degree of fibrosis will develop with aging (most likely as a result of vascular impairment and ischaemia), together with some dilatation of the ductal system. However, fibrosis should be slight and not associated with significant loss of exocrine parenchyma[9,10].

Before concluding this topic, the recent work of Nagai *et al.*[11] who reported a rather high frequency of pancreatic lithiasis found incidentally at autopsy in elderly patients (22 of 418 cases, or 5.3%) should be mentioned. Similar findings were reported in a study published in 1941 by Ludin and Scheidegger[12]. In the Nagai study, the incidence of pancreatic stones increased in proportion to age after 70 years (0% in those younger than 69 years, 4.2% in those in their 70s, 7.7% in patients in their 80s, and 16.7% in those in their 90s). The stones had a gross appearance and chemical composition similar to those found in younger patients with chronic calcific pancreatitis, but it is of interest that the clinical and pathological features were quite different. In fact, pancreatic lithiasis in the aged was rarely associated with pain or other symptoms or with a history of alcoholism, which is the usual cause of this pathological condition. Moreover, parenchymal atrophy and fibrosis were usually limited to the areas upstream from the sites of ductal lesions. These differences could raise the question if, rather than a painless idiopathic chronic pancreatitis, pancreatic lithiasis may not be, at least in some cases, a natural manifestation of aging. Clearly, further studies are necessary in order to clarify this point.

FUNCTIONAL CHANGES

Relatively few studies have examined exocrine pancreatic function in the elderly, and results have been conflicting: some investigators have found no substantial modification of pancreatic function, whereas others have found a reduction[13-17]. Subject selection and methodological differences may probably explain these discrepancies. Moreover, since most of these studies have been carried out in hospitalized patients, it is difficult to establish whether the functional changes observed by some investigators were owing to aging or to superimposed disease and/or malnutrition. In this regard, it is important to mention that even mild degrees of malnutrition may significantly impair exocrine pancreatic function[18]. In an attempt to better define age-related pancreatic functional changes, we recently studied[19] exocrine pancreatic function in a group of aged persons by means of duodenal intubation. Our first concern was to choose individuals without any past or present disease and with a normal nutritional status. We studied 15 subjects between 61 and 68 years of age, 10 subjects between 71 and 78 years of age, and 30 younger controls. The pancreas was stimulated by a 90-min intravenous infusion of maximal doses of secretin and caerulein and the outputs of bicarbonate, trypsin, chymotrypsin, and lipase were measured[20]. The results showed that the pancreatic secretory capacity of bicarbonate and enzymes (Figure 30.1) in almost all the elderly subjects was not significantly different from that of the younger individuals. Pancreatic outputs below the control range were observed in only three elderly persons, but the reduction was slight. In this study, we examined relatively few individuals, and their age did not exceed 78 years. With the aim of extending the assessment of pancreatic function to a wider group of elderly persons and, above all, to those older than the previous group, we recently carried out a second investigation[21]. Pancreatic function was assessed by means of the pancreolauryl test, which is one of the most recent tubeless pancreatic function tests[22,23]. This test requires oral administration of fluorescein dilaurate, a synthetic ester which is specifically hydrolyzed by pancreatic arylesterases into lauric acid and free water-soluble

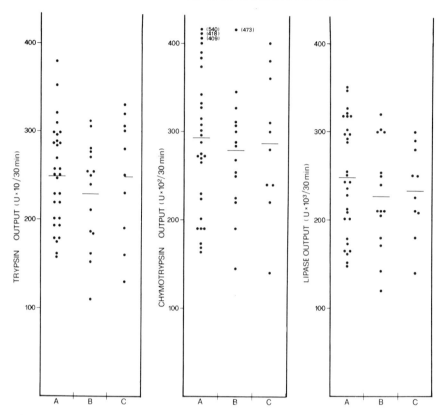

Figure 30.1 Individual values for trypsin, chymotrypsin, and lipase output in (A) young controls, (B) individuals 61–68 years of age, and (C) those 71–78 years of age. The values indicate pancreatic secretory responses during the final 30 min of a 90-min i.v. infusion of maximal doses of secretin and caerulein. The horizontal lines represent the mean. [From Gullo, L. *et al.* (1983). *Gerontology*, **29**, 407–11]

fluorescein. This is absorbed in the small intestine, partly conjugated in the liver, and excreted in the urine. To evaluate individual absorption, conjugation, and excretion, the test is repeated 2 days later using free fluorescein only. The urinary recovery rate of both days is expressed as a ratio and taken as an index of pancreatic function. It is a reliable test of pancreatic digestive capacity, which is easy to perform, and has a high sensitivity and negative predictive value[22,23]. We have examined 60 healthy elderly persons, 25 men and 35 women, with normal nutritional status, and with no history of disease: 8 were 66–70 years of age, 31 were 71–80 years of age, and 21 were 81–90 years of age. The test proved strictly normal in all 60 subjects studied (Figure 30.2). No significant differences were observed between those under 75 years and those over 75 years. These results confirm and extend the results of our previous study and clearly show that the pancreatic digestive capacity is not affected at all by the age of the individual. Since the sensitivity of the pancreolauryl test in the detection of mild pancreatic insufficiency is not

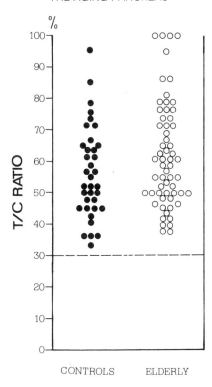

Figure 30.2 Individual results of the fluorescein dilaurate test in young controls and in elderly persons. The broken horizontal line represents the lower normal value. [From Gullo, L. *et al.* (1986) *J. Am. Geriatrics Soc.*, **34**, 790–2]

high[22,23], it cannot be excluded, on the basis of this study, that a slight impairment of pancreatic function may occur in some aged persons.

The answer then to the second question is that exocrine pancreatic function is not significantly affected by age. If a decline occurs in pancreatic secretory capacity in some individuals, it is slight.

The third of the initial questions is of practical interest: can nutritional status be impaired as a result of age-related pancreatic changes? It is clear from the data discussed that the answer is 'no'. Maldigestion and malabsorption occur only when pancreatic function is reduced by more than 90% of normal[1]. Thus, even if in some individuals a slight pancreatic insufficiency develops with age, the enzymes secreted into the duodenum after a meal are still more than sufficient to ensure normal digestion.

Up to this point, only human studies have been consulted. Now some reference to animal studies should be made. A relatively high number of studies have examined the influence of aging on exocrine pancreatic secretion of the rat, and the results have been controversial. Only some of the more recent studies can be mentioned. Khalil *et al*[24] assessed the pancreatic response to increasing doses of secretin and cholecystokinin-8 in Sprague–

Dawley rats and found that the responsiveness of the pancreas to these hormones was depressed in aged rats. In a similar study done with Fischer rats, Miyasaka et al.[25] found that basal pancreatic secretion and bicarbonate stimulated by secretin were not affected by aging. The pancreatic enzyme response to low doses of cholecystokinin-8 also did not differ for young and old rats, but there was a significant attenuated response to the higher doses of cholecystokinin-8 in old rats. Greenberg et al.[26] examined the response of pancreatic growth and enzyme content to prolonged (7 days) administration of secretin and caerulein in Fischer rats, and found that these hormones induced significant pancreatic growth and stimulation of pancreatic enzyme content in both young and adult rats. However, adult pancreas responded less well than young pancreas to these trophic hormones. They concluded that although basal pancreatic output and enzyme secretion may not be affected by the aging process, aging pancreas shows a sub-optimal adaptive response to hormonal stimuli. Finally, Wang et al.[27] analysed the activity of different lipolytic enzymes in young, adult, and senescent Fischer rats. They found that cholesterol esterase and pancreatic lipase activity did not show any consistent change with age. Pancreatic carboxylesterase, on the other hand, was lower in adult and old animals, probably because of a decline of the physiological importance of this enzyme after weaning.

Therefore, these recent experimental studies also seem to indicate that exocrine pancreatic function does not undergo significant modifications with aging. In fact, some reduction of function was demonstrated, but only after pancreatic stimulation by very high doses of hormones or after very prolonged administration of hormones, i.e., under particular, and probably non-physiological, conditions.

In conclusion, the available information indicates that the human exocrine pancreas does not undergo substantial changes in structure and function with advancing age. Further studies aimed at assessing more specifically the influence of aging on structure and function in the acinar cell at the intracellular level should result in a better understanding of the aging pancreas.

References

1. Di Magno, E. P., Go, V. L. W. and Summerskill, W. H. J. (1973). Relations between pancreatic enzyme outputs and malabsorption in severe pancreatic insufficiency. N. Engl, J. Med., **288**, 813–15
2. Andrew, W. (1952). Cellular Changes with Age. (Springfield, Ill.: Charles C. Thomas)
3. Calloway, N. O., Foley, C. F. and Lagerbloom, P. (1965). Uncertainties in geriatric data. II. Organ size. J. Am. Geriatrics Soc., **13**, 20–30
4. Geokas, M. C. and Haverback, B. J. (1969). The aging gastrointestinal tract. Am. J. Surg., **117**, 881–92
5. Andrew, W. (1944). Senile changes in the pancreas of Wistar Institute rats and of man with a special regard to the similarity of locule and cavity formation. Am. J. Anat., **74**, 97–127
6. Worthen, N. J. and Beabeau, D. (1982). Normal pancreatic echogenicity: relation to age and body fat. Am. J. Roent., **139**, 1095–8
7. Kreel, L. and Sandin, B. (1973). Changes in pancreatic morphology associated with aging. Gut, **14**, 962–70
8. Houcke, E., Houcke, M. and Leblois, J. (1964). Le pancréas du vieillard. Etude histologique. Presse Méd., **72**, 1887–92

9. Morgan, Z. R. and Feldman, M. (1957). The liver, biliary tract and pancreas in the aged: an anatomic and laboratory evaluation. *J. Am. Geriatrics Soc.*, **5**, 59–65

10. Pitchumoni, C. S., Glasser, M., Saran, R. M., Panchacharam, P. and Thelmo, W. (1984). Pancreatic fibrosis in chronic alcoholics and nonalcoholics without clinical pancreatitis. *Am. J. Gastroenterol.*, **79**, 382–8

11. Nagai, H. and Ohtsubo, K. (1984). Pancreatic lithiasis in the aged. Its clinicopathology and pathogenesis. *Gastroenterology.*, **86**, 331–8

12. Ludin, M. and Scheidegger, S. (1941). Ueber pankreaskonkremente. Rontgenologisch–pathologisch–anatomische Untersuchungen. *Klin. Wochenschr.*, **20**, 690–4

13. Rosenberg, I. R., Friedland, N., Janowitz, H. D. and Dreiling, D. A. (1966). The effect of age and sex upon human pancreatic secretion of fluid and bicarbonate. *Gastroenterology*, **50**, 191–4

14. Fikry, M. E. (1968). Exocrine pancreatic functions in the aged. *Am. J. Geriatrics Soc.*, **16**, 463–8

15. Bartos, V. and Groh, J. (1969). The effect of repeated stimulation of the pancreas on the pancreatic secretion in young and aged men. *Geront. Clin.*, **11**, 56–62

16. Laugier, R. and Sarles, H. (1984). Pancreatic function and diseases. In Hellemans, J. and Vantrappen, G. (eds.) *Gastrointestinal Tract Disorders in the Elderly*. pp. 243–51. (Edinburgh: Churchill Livingstone)

17. Dreiling, D. A., Triebling, A. T. and Koller, M. (1985). The effect of age on human exocrine pancreatic secretion. *Mount Sinai J. Med.*, **52**, 336–9

18. Barbezat, G. O. and Hansen, J. D. L. (1968). The exocrine pancreas and protein calorie malnutrition. *Paediatrics*, **42**, 77–88

19. Gullo, L., Priori, P., Daniele, C., Ventrucci, M., Gasbarrini, G. and Labò, G. (1983). Exocrine pancreatic function in the elderly. *Gerontology*, **29**, 407–11

20. Gullo, L., Costa, P. L., Fontana, G., and Labò, G. (1976). Investigation of exocrine pancreatic function by continuous infusion of caerulein and secretion in normal subjects and in chronic pancreatitis. *Digestion*, **14**, 97–107

21. Gullo, L. Ventrucci, M., Naldoni, P. and Pezzilli, R. (1986). Aging and exocrine pancreatic function. *J. Am. Geriatrics Soc.*, **34**, 790–2

22. Lankisch, P. G., Schreiber, A. and Otto, J. (1983). Pancreolauryl test. Evaluation of a tubeless pancreatic function test in comparison with other indirect and direct tests for exocrine pancreatic function. *Dig. Dis. Sci.*, **28**, 490–3

23. Ventrucci, M., Gullo, L., Daniele, C., Priori, P. and Labò, G. (1983). Pancreolauryl test for pancreatic exocrine insufficiency. *Am. J. Gastroenterol.*, **78**, 806–9

24. Khalil, T., Fujimura, M., Townsend, C. M., Greeley, G. H. and Thompson, J. C. (1984). Effect of aging on pancreatic secretion in rats. *Am. J. Surg.*, **149**, 120–5

25. Miyasaka, K. and Kitani, K. (1986). The effect of age on pancreatic exocrine function in the conscious rat. *Gastroenterology*, **90**, 1554. (Abstract)

26. Greenberg, R. E., Dominguez, A., Washington, A. and Holt, P. R. (1986). Impaired response of aging rat pancreas to cerulein-secretin stimulation. *Gastroenterology*, **90**, 1438. (Abstract)

27. Wang, C. S. Floyd, R. A. and Kloer, H. U. (1986). Effect of aging on pancreatic lipolytic enzymes. *Pancreas*, **1**, 438–42

31
Gastrointestinal motility and aging

W. PELEMANS

Our knowledge of the changes in gastrointestinal motility owing to aging in the absence of overt pathology is rather limited. Only a handful of studies have been done on this topic. Parts of the gut that are more easily accessible to motility studies have been explored by priority. Aging in the colon is discussed in another contribution; so this review will concentrate on the motility changes of the proximal gastrointestinal tract and of the oesophagus in particular.

OESOPHAGUS

The pharyngo-oesophageal transition zone

At the pharyngo-oesophageal junction the upper oesophageal sphincter (UES) protects the entrance of the gastrointestinal tract. With adequate manometric techniques a high-pressure zone of about 4 cm can be demonstrated at this level. The resting pressure profile of this sphincter is characterized by a radial and axial asymmetry[1]. On deglutition the upper oesophageal sphincter first relaxes; the subsequent contraction is a part of the peristalsis which travels from the nasopharynx to the oesophagus. Microtransducers are needed for accurate manometric recording of these fast and high peristaltic contractions[2].

Comparing the maximal resting pressure in the UES in different age groups we found a progressive decline in pressure (Figure 31.1). In the four radial orientations a significant reduction in pressure is found between the age of 20 and 80.

The relaxations of the UES on deglutition have the same duration in different age groups (Table 31.1). However, 9% of the swallows are not accompanied with relaxations in old people. The amplitude of the contractions in the pharynx and in the proximal part of the high-pressure zone is not different in different age groups. However, with accurate manometric techniques a lower contractile force is documented in the distal part of the high pressure zone and in the proximal oesophagus in 80-year-old subjects[3].

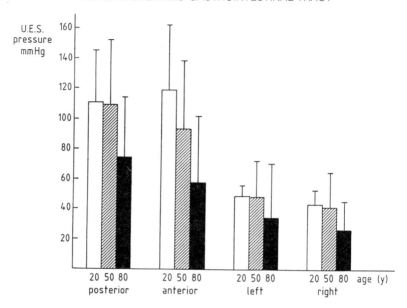

Figure 31.1 Maximal UES pressure ($\pm$ S.D.) in different age groups

Table 31.1 Relaxation in the UES in different age groups

	Age		
	20 years	*50 years*	*80 years*
Number of swallows	142	106	100
No relaxation	1%	4%	9%
Duration	0.9 ± 0.29 sec	0.81 ± 0.27 sec	0.81 ± 0.25 sec

Oesophageal motility

Oesophageal motility can be studied with radiological, manometric and electromyographic techniques. Manometry is most popular. To record faithfully the pressure changes in the oesophagus catheters perfused by means of a low compliant system, or a catheter assembly containing small intraluminal transducers have to be used[4,5].

The gastro-oesophageal junction is characterized by a high-pressure zone 2–4 cm in length. Using current low-compliance manometric systems the normal pressure range is 10–30 mmHg. Pressure recorded within this sphincter varies to some degree according to the orientation of the recording orifice. Pressures from left and left posterior orientations are higher than those recorded from other orientations in the sphincter[6]. When the subject swallows, the lower oesophageal sphincter relaxes. Measuring the pressure by means of a perfused catheter system in normal subjects, relaxations lasting 8–9 sec are found[7]. This relaxation occurs before the peristaltic contraction of the oesophageal body arrives at the level of the lower oesophageal sphincter and is followed by a sphincteric contraction in peristaltic sequence with that of the oesophageal body.

In the oesophagus deglutition causes a peristaltic contraction. In the distal oesophagus these contractions have a mean pressure of 81 ± 30 mmHg (mean ± 1 S.D.)[8]. The speed of progression of these peristaltic contractions depends on the level of the oesophagus and is much slower than in the pharynx.

A few oesophageal manometric studies have been done in the elderly[9–13]. However the selection criteria with regard to pathology and medication and the age of the patients are very divergent in these studies. Moreover, the manometric techniques used by some workers have been criticized afterwards. Manometric studies without perfusion of the catheter assembly with a low compliance system may give unreliable results. Finally no clear distinction is made between wet and dry swallows; these factors also may influence the motility pattern in the oesophagus[14].

A very critical review would therefore reject many existing data on the change in oesophageal motility in elderly people. Nevertheless some general and descriptive findings on the changes in oesophageal motility in elderly people can be given.

(1) Normal primary peristaltic contractions become less frequent with increasing age. The peristaltic progression remains normal in the proximal 4–6 cm, the striated muscle part of the oesophagus. More distally the progression gets disturbed in elderly people and the peristaltic contractions are often replaced by simultaneous activity. In addition, there is a gradual rise in the number of tertiary and repetitive contractions according to age[10]. A lower incidence of peristaltic contractions in old age was also noted in the study of Csendes et al.[13], Khan et al.[12] and Soergel et al.[9]. However in the study of Hollis and Castell[11] this trend was not observed.

(2) A decrease in amplitude of the contractions in the distal oesophagus can be demonstrated with adequate manometric techniques. According to the work of Hollis and Castell[11] these changes are only detectable after the age of 80. In this age group the pressure of the oesophageal contraction falls to less than 50% of the control values.

(3) The pressure response to a second swallow is influenced by the precedent deglutition when two swallows take place in rapid succession. The contraction induced by a second swallow, after an interval of 10 sec, generates a pressure in the oesophagus of lower amplitude. Only $\pm 80\%$ of these contractions have a normal peristaltic progression. It takes at least 18 sec before a second swallow generates a contraction with a normalized amplitude and progression in elderly people. In young subjects there is already some recuperation 12 sec after the first swallow[7].

(4) A lower incidence of normal relaxations in the lower oesophageal sphincter is found in elderly people[10,12]. However, the studies of Csendes et

al.[13] and Hollis and Castell[11] could not confirm the lower incidence of relaxations of the lower oesophageal sphincter in elderly people. Manometric studies with perfused catheters indicate that the resting pressure of this sphincter is not influenced by age[12,13]. There are no studies that have measured lower sphincter tone over long time periods in older subjects.

GASTRIC AND SMALL INTESTINAL MOTILITY

Available methods to study gastric motility include radiography, manometry, electromyographic recording and gastric emptying studies. No radiological manometric or myoelectric studies have recently been done in elderly subjects.

There are four recent studies of gastric emptying times in the elderly. Kupfer et al.[15] measured gastric volume by means of real time ultrasound. Horowitz et al.[16], Moore et al.[17] and Evans et al.[18] assessed gastric emptying rates by radioisotopic methods in young and old subjects. However the selections of the elderly subjects who have participated is quite different.

Studies with isotope techniques suggest that the emptying of liquids by the stomach could be slower in older subjects[16,17] especially in the recumbent position[18]. However, Kupfer et al.[15] measured gastric emptying of liquid by means of ultrasound. The initial rate of gastric emptying was significantly higher in elderly patients than in young controls. The two groups' gastric emptying rates after 5 min were not significantly different.

The data on solid emptying by the stomach are also equivocal. Horowitz et al.[16] measured a significantly slower emptying rate in older subjects. However Moore et al.[17] found no significant difference in solid food emptying.

Small bowel motility function in human subjects can be quantified very roughly by measuring the transit time. Small intestinal transit time of barium from the stomach to the caecum was the same in young adults and elderly subjects without gastrointestinal disease[19]. Kupfer et al.[15] measured the transit by means of the hydrogen breath test. Small bowel transit in 15 elderly patients was not significantly different from that found in 15 younger volunteers.

However, the foregut has a more complex pattern of motility. During fasting there is a cyclical activity called migrating motor complex. It can be divided into three phases. Phase 1 is a quiescent period, phase 2 is characterized by intermittent contractions that increase in frequency until phase 3 occurs when there are intense uninterrupted phasic pressure changes at the maximum frequency for that locus. After phase 3 the foregut becomes quiescent again and enters a new phase 1. This cyclical pattern continues until the subject eats. After feeding the migrating motor complex is replaced by frequent intermittent contractions (fed pattern). The fed pattern of motility usually lasts for hours after feeding and then the fasting pattern returns.

The variations in patterns of the human interdigestive motility from oesophagus to colon have been recently documented[20]. Half the interdigestive cycles involved the oesophagus, approximately one-third began in the gastroduodenal region, and the remainder commenced more distally. Fewer than half the migrating motor complexes were recognizable beyond the midpoint of the small bowel, and $< 10\%$ reached the distal ileum.

There are only a few studies that concentrate upon the interdigestive or digestive motility pattern in older subjects. Bortolotti et al.[21] found an absence of phase 3 activity in the gastroduodenal area in 10 elderly subjects without gastrointestinal diseases. In most cases phase 3 activity was replaced by an intense 'minute rhythm' activity. Anuras and Sutherland[22] did not find any changes in the three phases of the migrating motor complex in healthy elderly subjects at the level of the proximal jejunum. However, after a meal the intestinal motility was significantly lower in the elderly subjects than in the group of young adults. Kellow et al.[20] noted the following significant variations in the migrating motor complex owing to age: the cycle length between migrating motor complexes in the proximal jejunum tended to increase with age. Furthermore, a significantly higher proportion of migrating motor complexes involved the oesophagus in subjects aged $\geqslant 35$ years old as compared to subjects < 35 years old.

CONCLUSION

This contribution reviews the existing data on the motility changes in the proximal gastrointestinal tract in aging. It clearly demonstrates our limited knowledge in this field. Moreover, it is not always evident that the described changes are the expression of aging. Known or unknown pathology and medication may also interfere with gastrointestinal function and motility. Therefore, much work has still to be done before we will understand the 'normal' gastrointestinal motility in healthy elderly subjects.

References

1. Winans, C. S. (1972). The pharyngoesophageal closure mechanism: a manometric study. *Gastroenterology*, **63**, 768–77
2. Orlowski, J., Dodds, W. J., Linehan, J. H., Dent, J., Hogan, W. J. and Arndorfer, R. C. (1982). Requirements for accurate manometric recordings of pharyngeal and esophageal peristaltic pressure waves. *Invest. Radiol.*, **17**, 567–72
3. Pelemans, W. (1983). *Functie van de Faryngo-esofagale Overgangszone en Dysfunctie bij Bejaarden*. (Leuven: Acco)
4. Dodds, W. J., Stef, J. J. and Hogan, W. J. (1976). Factors determining pressure measurement accuracy by intraluminal esophageal manometry. *Gastroenterology*, **70**, 117–23
5. Arndorfer, R. C., Steff, J. J., Dodds, W. J., Linehan, J. H. and Hogan, W. J. (1977). Improved infusion system for intraluminal esophageal manometry. *Gastroenterology*, **73**, 23–7
6. Winans, C. S. (1977). Manometric asymmetry of the lower esophageal high pressure zone. *Dig. Dis.*, **22**, 348–54
7. Hellemans, J. and Vantrappen, G. (1974). Physiology. In Vantrappen, G. and Hellemans, J. (ed.) *Diseases of the Esophagus*. pp. 40–102. (Berlin-Heidelberg-New York: Springer-Verlag)
8. Benjamin, S. B., Gerhardt, D. C. and Castell, D. O. (1979). High amplitude peristaltic esophageal contractions associated with chest pain and/or dysphagia. *Gastroenterology*, **77**, 418–83
9. Soergel, K. H., Zboralske, F. F. and Amberg, J. R. (1964). Presbyesophagus: esophageal motility in nonagenarians. *J. Clin. Invest.*, **43**, 1472

10. Hellemans, J. (1970). Invloed van de Leeftijd op de Motorische Funktie van de Slokdarm. Thesis. (Tielt: Lannoo)

11. Hollis, J. B. and Castell, D. O. (1974). Esophageal function in elderly men. A new look at 'Presbyesophagus'. *Ann. Intern. Med.*, **80**, 371–4

12. Khan, T. A., Shragge, B. W., Crispin, J. S. and Lind, J. F. (1977). Esophageal motility in the elderly. *Dig. Dis.*, **22**, 1049–54

13. Csendes, A., Guiraldes, E., Bancalari, A., Braghetto, I. and Ayala, M. (1978). Relation of gastroesophageal sphincter pressure and esophageal contractile waves to age in man. *Scand. J. Gastroenterol.*, **13**, 443–7

14. Janisch, H. D. and Eckardt, V. F. (1983). Wet swallows stimulate abnormal contractions in patients with oesophageal motility disorders. *Z. Gastroenterol.*, **21**, 574–9

15. Kupfer, R. M., Heppell, M., Haggith, J. W. and Bateman, D. N. (1985). Gastric emptying and small bowel transit rate in the elderly. *J. Am. Geriatr. Soc.*, **33**, 340–3

16. Horowitz, M., Maddern, G. J., Chatterton, B. E., Collins, P. J, Harding, P. E. and Shearman, D. J. C. (1984). Changes in gastric emptying rates with age. *Clin. Sci.*, **67**, 213–18

17. Moore, J. G., Tweedy, C., Christian, P. E. and Datz, F. L. (1983). Effect of age on gastric emptying of liquid–solid meals in man. *Dig. Dis. Sci.*, **28**, 340–4

18. Evans, M. A., Triggs, E. J., Cheune, M., Broe, G. A. and Creasey, H. (1981). Gastric emptying rate in the elderly: Implications for drug therapy. *J. Am. Geriatr. Soc.*, **29**, 201–5

19. Kim, S. K. (1968). Small intestine transit time in the normal small bowel study. *Am. J. Roentgenol. Radium Ther. Nucl. Med.*, **104**, 522–5

20. Kellow, J. E., Borody, T. J., Phillips, S. F., Tucker, R. L. and Haddad, A. C. (1986). Human interdigestive motility: variations in patterns from esophagus to colon. *Gastroenterolgy*, **91**, 386–95

21. Bortolotti, M., Frada, G., Barbagallosangiorgi, J. R. and Abo, G. (1984). Interdigestive gastroduodenal motor activity in the elderly. *Gut*, **25**, A1320. (Abstract)

22. Anuras, S. and Sutherland, J. (1984). Small intestinal manometry in healthy elderly subjects. *J. Am. Geriatr. Soc.*, **32**, 581–3

32
Aging and the colon

N. W. READ

INTRODUCTION

Ageing is associated with a reduction in blood supply to organs, loss of neurons and nervous control, loss of muscle bulk and replacement of muscle by fibrous tissue. Such changes could result in quite gross alterations in colonic function. Nevertheless, two large studies have shown that there is no significant difference in bowel habit in elderly subjects compared with the young[1,2]. Stool output is also not significantly different in elderly subjects and there is also no significant difference in whole gut transit time in old people compared with young controls[3]. Nevertheless, more elderly than young people take laxatives[1] and greater proportions of elderly than young patients suffer from faecal impaction, faecal incontinence and diverticular disease. Ischaemic colitis is also largely considered a disease of the elderly and carcinoma of the colon is, of course, more common in older people.

ANORECTAL STUDIES IN HEALTHY SUBJECTS

Anorectal manometry[4] has shown that healthy elderly subjects have lower anal pressures compared with young normal subjects, but have higher rectal pressures during balloon distension (Table 32.1). The reduction in anal pressures that occurs with aging is greater in women than men and may be due in part to age-related reduction in muscle contractility and bulk and in part to progressive neuropathic damage to the external anal sphincter as indicated by electrophysiological evidence of pudendal neuropathy in elderly women[5]. Damage to the muscle and/or nerve supply to the levatores ani, sustained during childbirth[6] is thought to result in abnormal descent of the perineum as the subject increases her intra-abdominal pressure. This stretches the pudendal nerve below its attachment to the ischial spine, causing damage to the nerve and weakness of the external anal sphincter. In support of this hypothesis, elderly women have a significantly greater degree of perineal descent than young women both at rest and on straining[4], whereas the

Table 32.1 Ano-rectal function in young and old subjects (expressed as mean ± S.E.M.)

Test	Male			Female			Total (male + female)		
	Young	Old	p	Young	Old	p	Young	Old	p
1. Anal pressures (cmH₂O)									
Mean highest basal	100±5	73±7	<0.01	103±8	57±4	$p<0.001$	102±5	65±4	$p<0.001$
Mean highest squeeze	284±20	214±23	<0.05	217±16	132±9	$p<0.001$	247±14	171±15	$p<0.001$
2. Anal response to rectal distension									
Rectal volume required to cause anal relaxation (ml)	23±3	29±8	NS	21±2	23±4	NS	22±2	26±4	NS
Rectal volume required to cause sustained anal relaxation (ml)	74±9	48±9	NS	60±7	39±7	$p<0.05$	69±6	42±5	$p<0.05$
3. Rectal pressures and volumes (cmH₂O)									
*Distending volume (ml)**									
50	15.7±2.3	18.3±2.8	NS	11.9±0.8	25.1±2.6	$p<0.01$	13.4±1.0	21.4±2.1	$p<0.01$
100	20.6±3.0	22.0±3.4	NS	16.6±1.2	28.1±3.1	$p<0.01$	18.1±1.4	24.9±2.3	$p<0.05$
150	27.2±4.2	31.0±3.8	NS	20.5±1.7	32.6±3.4	$p<0.01$	23.1±2.0	31.8±2.5	$p<0.01$
Maximum tolerable volume (ml)	265±20	209±19	NS	297±19	250±17	NS	283±14	225±13	$p<0.01$
Maximum tolerable pressure (cm H₂O)	46±6	35±4	NS	38±4	47±4	NS	41±4	41±3	NS
4. Radiographic measurements									
Ano-rectal angle (degrees)									
At rest	91±1	95±4	NS	88±3	90±3	NS	89±2	92±2	NS
Straining	105±8	111±5	NS	115±7	98±4	$p<0.05$	112±5	104±4	NS
*Distance of ano-rectal angle from pubococcygeal line (cm)***									
At rest	+0.1±0.1	−0.2±0.4	NS	0±0.3	−1.5±0.3	$p<0.01$	0±0.2	−0.8±0.3	NS
Straining	−1.8±0.4	−1.6±0.6	NS	−1.6±0.3	−3.6±0.4	$p<0.01$	−1.7±0.2	−2.6±0.4	NS

* Values are given only for distending volumes up to 150 ml since some patients could not tolerate distension above that volume

** Positive values denote distances above and negative values below the pubococcygeal line

position of the ano-rectal angle in relation to the pubococcygeal line is similar in elderly compared with young men.

The increase in rectal pressure during balloon distension may reflect the generalized loss of tissue elasticity that occurs with age or it may occur as a result of rectal ischaemia and fibrosis[7]. Changes in rectal pressure in the elderly were associated with a more sensitive recto-anal inhibitory reflex (lower volumes were required to completely inhibit the anal sphincter tone) and also with increases in rectal sensitivity (less rectal distension was required to elicit a desire to defecate in the elderly). Our previous studies[8] have shown that incontinence to rectally infused saline occurs when the rectal pressure is greater than the anal pressure. The combination of low anal pressure and high rectal pressures upon rectal distension and the observation that it takes lower rectal volumes to cause sustained relaxation of the anal sphincter could all predispose to incontinence in the elderly.

Perineal descent and a weak sphincter are thought to encourage the rectal mucosa to prolapse and plug the anal canal, obstructing defaecation[9,10]. Our studies showed that a lower proportion of elderly subjects than young subjects could pass either a cylindrical balloon containing 50 ml of air or a plastic sphere 1.8 cm in diameter within 20 sec though this difference disappeared when the time limit extended to 5 min. The elderly may therefore strain for longer periods than the young while attempting to pass a stool possibly causing further damage to the innervation of the pelvic floor[11]. The observation that elderly women that did not find it more difficult to expel a simulated stool than elderly men even though they had significantly more perineal descent suggests the degree of perineal descent is not necessarily related to impaired defaecation in the elderly.

FAECAL IMPACTION

Faecal impaction affects a considerable proportion of elderly patients, who are referred for admission to geriatric hospitals. To give an impression of the extent of the problem, we found that 192 out of 460 (42%) patients admitted in one year (1982) to two acute geriatric wards in Tickhill Road Hospital in Doncaster, had faecal impaction. In another study, faecal impaction was the main reason for admission in 18% acutely ill and 27% chronically ill patients[12].

Faecal impaction is often regarded as a behavioural problem, a failure to respond to the sensation of a stool in the rectum[13–15] until this becomes so large it cannot be passed. Factors such as the decline in mental function and confusion leading to neglect of personal hygiene[16–20], immobility, inadequate toilet facilities and physical weakness[15] may all play an important role in the pathogenesis of faecal impaction. The increased use of laxatives may exacerbate the problem by causing damage to the myenteric plexus[21]. Some investigators have suggested that physiological rather than psychological factors may play an important role. These include absence of the gastro-colonic response[22], increased re-absorption of fluid from the colon[13,15], decreased rectal sensitivity[23], loss of rectal tone and contractility[15,23], elevated

Table 32.2 Results of ano-rectal radiology in patients with faecal impaction and elderly controls (results are expressed as mean ± S.E.M.)

	Impacted patients	Elderly controls	Statistical significance
Age (years)	83 ± 1	78 ± 1	NS
Sex (M:F)	13:12	11:9	
Ano-rectal angle (degrees)			
Resting	119 ± 3	92 ± 3	$p < 0.001$
Squeezing	113 ± 4	93 ± 3	$p < 0.001$
Straining	130 ± 4	106 ± 3	$p < 0.001$
Anal canal length (cm)	3.2 ± 0.2	2.5 ± 0.3	NS
Rectal width (cm)	6.1 ± 0.4	5.1 ± 0.3	NS
Perineal descent (cm)*			
Resting	− 1.2 ± 0.2	− 1.1 ± 0.3	NS
Squeezing	− 0.8 ± 0.2	− 0.9 ± 0.6	NS
Straining	− 2.9 ± 0.3	− 2.6 ± 0.4	NS

* Negative sign indicates descent below the pubococcygeal line
The degree of statistical significance between groups was assessed by Student's paired t test (NS = not significant, $p > 0.05$)

colonic pH[24], and intake of anticholinergic and other constipating medications[25]. Since few attempts have been made to investigate ano-rectal or colonic function in impacted patients there is no consensus regarding the pathogenesis of the condition.

We conducted tests of ano-rectal function in a total of 55 elderly patients with faecal impaction: 28 females, aged between 69 and 95 years (mean ± S.E.M. = 81 ± 1 year) and 27 males, aged between 70 and 89 years (79 ± 1 year)[26]. All the patients had hard masses of faeces filling the rectum on admission and all had a previous history of problems with defecation, including hard stools, infrequent bowel movements and straining at stool, necessitating regular use of laxatives and/or enemas.

Tests were also carried out on a control group of 36 elderly patients (18 female; age range, 68–87; mean, 78 ± 1 year; and 18 male; age range, 66–87; mean, 77 ± 1 year) who had no history of ano-rectal disorders or difficulties of defecation. All of these patients were ambulant, and none was mentally confused or disturbed.

Our results showed that the range of clinical diagnoses related to the rectal or anal canal were similar in patients with impacted faeces and control subjects[26]. However, all except one of the patients with impacted faeces had prominent haemorrhoids. None of the control group had haemorrhoids or any other local conditions involving the anal canal ($p < 0.001$). The presence of haemorrhoids in patients with faecal impaction may suggest that instead of ignoring the cause of defecation, these patients may have been straining to pass their motions[27]. In a recent study we have argued that the anal cushions have solid-like properties resembling erectile tissue[28], and under 'resting' conditions, they plug the anal canal and help to preserve continence. However, it is evident that if solid plug of vascular tissue does not become flaccid during defecation, then the anal cushions could obstruct the passage of the stool and contribute to constipation.

Not surprisingly, a higher proportion of impacted patients than elderly patients were ingesting irritant laxatives prior to admission[26]. In many cases, laxatives had been taken for many years and could have contributed to impaction by damaging the myenteric plexus[21]. In addition, a greater proportion of impacted patients were taking analgesics containing dextropropoxyphene compared with elderly controls. Dextropropoxyphene induces analgesia by interacting with opiate receptors and could in theory contribute to faecal impaction. However, dextropropoxyphene only causes constipation in a small proportion of patients taking it[29] and is a less-potent constipating agent than other opiate-like agents such as codeine[30].

Manometric results showed that sphincter pressures in 'impacted patients' were no different from elderly controls. Moreover, in all except one patient, internal sphincter tone was normally relaxed by rectal distension, though in some patients basal pressures were so low that relaxation could not be demonstrated. Thus, unlike constipation in children and young adults[31-34] faecal impaction in the majority of elderly patients was not related to a hypertonic anal canal, or impairment or sphincter relaxation upon rectal distension.

In contrast with many younger patients with constipation[35] most elderly patients who had been admitted with faecal impaction could pass simulated stools, consisting of balloons filled with water, from the rectum, although a lower percentage of impacted patients compared with controls could defecate a small solid sphere[26]. Thus, patients with a tendency to faecal impaction should have no difficulty in passing normal sized stools from the rectum, as long as they can recognize their presence in the rectum. However, rectal sensation is blunted in impacted patients. We found that the rectum of impacted patients needed to be distended with much larger volumes compared with elderly controls before sensations of fullness, pain or desire to defecate were perceived[26] (Figure 32.1). A similar blunting of rectal sensation has been observed in children with megarectum and adults with megacolon[31,36-38], though the majority of young adults with slow transit constipation show a selective blunting of the sensation of a desire to defecate but no change in the threshold for sensation of pain or the perception of the presence of a balloon in the rectum[39]. Higher distending volumes were also required to elicit rectal contractions in impacted patients; and in some no rectal contractions were generated at all[26]. Similarly, the rectal volumes which induced anal relaxations were higher in impacted patients. All of these features would facilitate the accumulation of faeces in the rectum.

The disturbances in rectal sensation, found in impacted patients were associated with low steady-state rectal pressures upon distension compared with values recorded in elderly controls[26]. In some patients with faecal impaction, the rectum could be distended with volumes as high as 500 ml before rectal pressures increased.

The responses to rectal distension suggest that faecal impaction may result from neuropathic impairment of rectal function which not only affects rectal sensation, but also blunts the mechanisms responsible for maintaining rectal

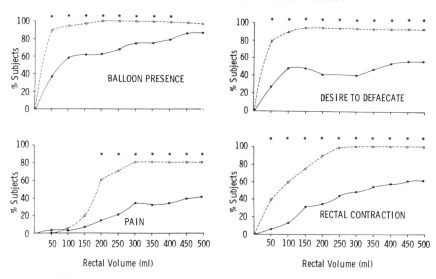

Figure 32.1 Diagrams showing the percentages of patients admitted with fecael impaction (●—●) and elderly controls (o---o) who had experienced sensations of the presence of a balloon, pain and the desire to defecate and who demonstrated rectal contractions during distension of a rectal balloon with increasing volumes of air. *indicates points that are significantly different ($p < 0.05$)

tone and initiating rectal contractions and anal relaxations. It is possible that prolonged presence of a faecal mass in the rectum leads to blunting of sensation and reflex activity; the rectal wall is said to assume a normal size and tone 5 or 6 weeks after faecal masses have been removed from the rectum[22]. Several studies have shown that ganglion cells in the colonic wall are abnormal in patients with constipation[40,41] though it is not certain whether this is a primary abnormality in the nerve supply to the rectum or whether it is secondary to prolonged laxative intake[21]. A hypotonic rectum which is relatively insensitive to rectal distension in association with an altered though intact recto-anal inhibitory reflex is also typical of patients who have damaged the sacral cord[42-44]. The observation that anal and perianal sensation is also impaired in impacted patients could also be explained by spinal-cord damage. Similar somatic changes could also be caused by damage to the pudendal nerve caused by prolonged straining at stool[9-11], although we did not find that perineal descent was any greater in impacted patients compared with controls.

FAECAL INCONTINENCE

Although the weak anal sphincter, the more sensitive recto-anal inhibitory reflex and the decreased rectal compliance found in elderly subjects could predispose to faecal incontinence[4], most cases of incontinence in the elderly are related to faecal impaction. This 'spurious or overflow' incontinence is often explained by suggesting that the faecal mass stretches the anal sphinc-ter[45] or causes a reflex reduction in internal sphincter tone[46].

Our results[47] showed that the anal pressures in the rectum containing impacted faeces were no lower than in the disimpacted rectum, indicating that the anal canal was not stretched and the anal tone was not inhibited by the chronic faecal distension of the rectum. In fact, distension of the rectum elicited a normal recto-anal inhibitory reflex even in the presence of the impacted faeces.

Normal subjects may be able to prevent to leakage of faeces because they can perceive the levels of rectal distension which would normally cause relaxation of the internal anal sphincter and consciously contract the external anal sphincter to prevent incontinence. When we distended the rectum of patients with faecal impaction, we found that rectal sensation was blunted and external sphincter contraction only occurred in 53% patients (compared with 80% elderly controls) and at higher distending volumes than in

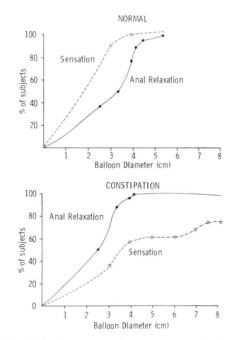

Figure 32.2 The relationship between the cumulative percentage of patients who could perceive a balloon distended with increasing volumes of air in the rectum and the percentage of patients, in whom the distension caused anal inhibition, in both faecally impacted patients and elderly controls

controls[47]. Thus patients with faecal impaction were unable to detect an increase in rectal volume that would cause anal relaxation and were therefore unable to contract the external anal sphincter to present incontinence that could ensue. To add to these difficulties, anal sphincter relaxation occurred at lower levels of rectal distension than in normal volunteers[47]. A similar impairment of rectal sensation has been invoked to explain incontinence in diabetics, patients with meningomyelocoele and children with encopresis[48-51]. Such patients often do not have adequate external sphincter responses to rectal distension[48,51-53].

The risk of incontinence is further exacerbated in patients with faecal impaction by the impairment of anal sensation. Thus, patients with faecal impaction may have no warning that leakage is about to take place and are unable to prevent leakage by conscious contraction of the external sphincter and puborectalis.

References

1. Connell, A. M., Hilton, C., Irwin, G. Lennard-Jones, J. E. and Misiewicz, J. J. (1965). Variations in bowel habit in two population samples. *Br. Med. J.*, **2**, 1095–9
2. Milne, J. S. and Williamson, J. (1972). Bowel habit in older people. *Gerontologica Clinica*, **14**, 55–60
3. Cann, P. A. (1985). A Study of the Gastrointestinal Transit of a Physiological Meal in Relation to Symptoms and Response to Treatment with Patients with the Irritable Bowel Syndrome. MD thesis, University of Leeds.
4. Bannister, J. J., Abouzekry, L. and Read, N. W. (1987). Effect of aging on anorectal function. *Gut*, **28**, 353–7
5. Bartolo, D. C. C., Jarrett, J. A. and Read, N. W. (1983). The use of conventional electromyography to assess external sphincter neuropathy in man. *J. Neurol. Neurosurg. Psych.*, **46**, 1115–18
6. Snooks, S. A., Setchell, L. M., Swash, M. and Henry, M. M. (1984). Injury to innervation of pelvic floor sphincter musculature in childbirth. *Lancet*, **2**, 546–50
7. Devroede, G., Vobecky, E., Masse, S. *et al.* (1982). Ischaemic faecal incontinence in rectal angina. *Gastroenterology*, **83**, 970–80
8. Read, N. W., Haynes, W. G. and Bartolo, D. C. C. (1983). The use of anorectal manometry during rectal infusion of saline to investigation sphincter function in continent patients. *Gastroenterology*, **85**, 105–13
9. Parks, A. G., Porter, N. A. and Hardcastle, J. D. (1966). The syndrome of the descending perineum. *Proc. R. Soc. Med.*, **59**, 477–82
10. Hardcastle, J. D. (1969). The descending perineum syndrome. *Practitioner*, **203**, 612–20
11. Snooks, J. S., Barnes, G. R. H., Swash, M. and Henry, M. M. (1985). Damage to the innervation of the pelvic floor musculature in constipation. *Gastroenterology*, **89**, 977–81
12. Geboes, K. and Bossaert, H. (1977). Gastrointestinal disorders in old age. *Age Ageing*, **6**, 197–200
13. Exton-Smith, A. N. (1973). Constipation in geriatrics. In Jones, F. A. and Godding, E. W. (eds.) *Management of Constipation*. pp. 156–75. (London: Blackwell Scientific Publications)
14. Fabris, F. and Robino, A. (1971). Diarrhoea and constipation in the aged. *Giorio Gerantol.*, **19**, 200–19
15. Banks, S. and Marks, I. N. (1977). The aetiology, diagnosis and treatment of constipation and diarrhoea in geriatric patients. *South African Med. J.*, **51**, 409–14
16. Ehrentheil, O. F. and Wells, E. P. (1955). Megacolon in psychotic patients: A clinical entity. *Gastroenterology*, **29**, 285–90
17. Johnston, I. D. and Gibson, J. B. (1960). Megacolon and volvulus in psychotics. *Br. J. Surg.*, **47**, 394–5
18. Watkins, G. A. and Oliver, G. A. (1965). Giant megacolon in the insane: Further observations in patients treated with subtotal colectomy. *Gastroenterology.*, **48**, 718–27
19. Gurll, N. and Steer, M. (1975). Diagnostic and therapeutic considerations for faecal impaction. *Dis. Colon Rectum*, **18**, 507–11
20. Brocklehurst, J. C. and Khan, M. Y. (1969). A study of faecal stasis in old age and the use of Dorbanex in its prevention. *Geront. Clin. (Basel)*, **11**, 293–300

21. Smith, B. (1968). Effect of irritant purgatives on the myenteric plexus in man and the mouse. *Gut*, **9**, 139–43
22. Stratton, J. W. and MacKeigan, J. M. (1982). Treating constipation. *Am. Fam. Physician*, **25**, 139–42
23. Newman, H. F. and Freeman, J. (1974). Physiologic factors affecting defecation sensation. *J. Am. Geriat. Soc.*, **22**, 553–4
24. Calloway, N. O. (1964). A clinical investigation of fecal pH in geriatric constipation. Corrective Therapy. *J. Am. Ger. Soc.*, **12**, 368–71
25. Read, N. W. (1983). Drug induced constipation. *Mims Magazine*, January, pp. 19–21
26. Read, N. W., Abouzekry, L., Read, M. G., Howell, P., Ottewell, D. and Donnelly, T. C. (1985). Anorectal function in elderly patients with fecal impaction. *Gastroenterology*, **89**, 959–66
27. Thompson, W. H. F. (1975): The nature of haemorrhoids. *Brit. J. Surg.*, **62**, 542–52
28. Gibbons, G. P., Trowbridge, E. A. Bannister, J. J. and Read, N. W. (1986). The role of the anal cushions in maintaining continence. *Lancet*, **1**, 886–7
29. Farrell, J., Brown, A. W. and Sturrock, R. D. (1979). The use and abuse of Distalgesic. *Br. Med. J.*, **1**, (No. 6173), 1284
30. Wang, R. I. H. (1980). Another look at the therapeutic value of propoxyphene. *J. Med. Therapeutics*, **1**, 14–16
31. Meunier, P., Marechal, J. M. and de Beaujeu, M. J. (1979). Rectoanal pressures and rectal sensitivity studies in chronic childhood constipation. *Gastroenterology*, **77**, 330–6
32. Martelli, H., Devroede, G., Ahran, P. and Dugay, C. (1978). Mechanism of idiopathic constipation; outlet obstruction. *Gastroenterology*, **75**, 623–31
33. Meunier, P. (1984). Physiological study of the lower digestive tract in primary constipation. In Roman, C. (ed.) *Gastrointestinal Motility*. pp. 469–75. (Lancaster: MTP Press)
34. Behar, J. and Biancani, P. (1984). Rectal function in patients with idiopathic chronic constipation. In Roman, C. (ed.) *Gastrointestinal Motility*. pp. 459–66. (Lancaster: MTP Press)
35. Barnes, P. R. N. and Lennard-Jones, J. (1984). Patients with constipation of different types have difficulty in expelling a balloon from the rectum. *Gut*, **25**, A526–7
36. Porter, N. H. Megacolon – a physiological study. *Proc. R. Soc. Med.*, **54**, 1043–7
37. Callaghan, R. P. and Nixon, H. H. Megarectum – physiological observations. *Arch. Dis. Child.*, **39**, 153–7
38. Nixon, H. H. (1967). Megarectum in the older child. *Proc. R. Soc. Med.*, **60**, 801–3
39. Bannister, J. J., Timms, J. M., Barfield, L. and Read, N. W. (1986). Physiological studies in young women with chronic constipation. *Int. J. Colorectal Dis.*, **1**, 175–82
40. Krishnamurthy, S., Schuffler, M. D., Pope, C. C. and Rohrmann, C. A. Severe idiopathic constipation is caused by distinct abnormality of the colonic myenteric plexus. In Roman, C. (ed.) *Gastrointestinal Motility*. pp. 467–8. (Lancaster: MTP Press)
41. Preston, D. M., Butter., M. G., Smith, B. and Lennard-Jones, J. E. (1983). Neuropathology of slow transit constipation. *Gut*, **25**, A997
42. Freckner, B. and Ihre, T. (1976). Influence of autonomic nerves on the internal anal sphincter in man. *Gut*, **17**, 306–12
43. Meunier, P. and Mollard, P. (1977). Control of the internal anal sphincter (manometric study with human subjects). *Pflügers Arch.*, **370**, 233–9
44. White, J. C., Verlot, M. G. and Ehrentheil, O. (1940). Neurogenic disturbances of the colon and their investigation by the colonmetrogram. *Am. Surg.*, **112**, 1042–57
45. Exton-Smith, A. N. (1973). Constipation in geriatrics. In Jones, F. A. and Godding, E. W. (eds.) *Management of Constipation*. (pp. 156–75). (London: Blackwell)
46. Schuster, M. M., Hendrix, T. R. and Mendeloff, A. I. (1963). The internal sphincter response. *J. Clin. Invest.*, **42**, 1966–207
47. Read, N. W and Abouzekry, L. (1986). Why do patients with faecal impaction have faecal incontinence? *Gut*, **27**, 283–7
48. Wald, A. and Tunuguntla, A. K. (1984). Anorectal sensation dysfunction in fecal incontinence and diabetes mellitus. *N. Engl. J. Med.*, **310**, 1282–7
49. Wald, A. (1983). Biofeedback for neurogenic faecal incontinence: rectal sensation is a determinant of outcome. *J. Paediatr. Gastroenterol Nutr.*, **2**, 302–6
50. Molnar, D., Taitz, L. S., Unwin, O. M. and Wales, J. K. H. (1983). Anorectal manometry results in defecation disorders. *Arch. Dis. Child.*, **58**, 257–61

51. Meunier, P., Mollard, P. and Marechal, J-M. (1976). Physiology of megarectum: the association of megarectum with encopresis. *Gut*, **17**, 224–7

52. Wald, A. (1981). Biofeedback therapy for faecal incontinence. *Ann. Intern. Med.*, **95**, 146–9

53. Cerulli, M. A., Nikoomanesh, P. and Schuster, M. M. (1979). Progress in biofeedback conditioning for faecal incontinence. *Gastroenterology.*, **76**, 742–6

Section 6
Clinical Application

33
Nutritional needs of the elderly

I. H. ROSENBERG

In the past two decades the nutritional status of the elderly population in many countries has received increasing scientific attention. The average age of citizens in most industrial nations is rising and thus the percentage of the total population represented by older and even very old individuals is increasing. It is most important therefore to assess the validity of the data assessing the nutritional status of the elderly[1]. Such studies often produce conflicting observations. In the U.S. National Health and Nutrition Examination Survey (HANES) of 1979, approximately one-half of those over age 65 had vitamin A intakes less than two-thirds of the Recommended Dietary Allowance[2]. Nevertheless, only 0.3% of this population had low blood levels of vitamin A[1]. Similar data and discrepancies between dietary intake and the biochemical indices of vitamin nutriture have been observed for other vitamins in HANES and again in the recent comprehensive survey of non-institutional elderly females in Boston conducted by the Human Nutrition Research Center on Aging[3] (Table 33.1). A large review of available infor-

Table 33.1 Boston Nutrition Status Survey – Percentage of female subjects receiving less than two-thirds of RDAs from diet

Nutrient	60–69 years	70–79 years	80+ years
Vitamin A	8	7	11
Vitamin D	65	60	68
Ascorbic acid	6	3	7
Thiamin	5	5	4
Riboflavin	3	3	2
Niacin	1	2	1
Folic acid	70	74	69
Vitamin B_6	70	75	74
Vitamin B_{12}	32	30	30
Iron	2	5	3
Calcium	35	38	29
Zinc	65	69	64

mation on nutritional status of the elderly found limited clinical evidence of nutritional deficiency despite low intakes as judged by available norms[4].

Certain questions arise in the face of these observations. The first can be simply put: Are the diets of the healthy elderly in nations such as the United States and other industrialized nations inadequate? Or do the diets fail to meet recommended norms which are themselves too high? We could further examine the validity of the values for officially released Recommended Dietary Allowances generically and question the applicability of these recommendations to the population with which we are concerned here, the elderly. It will not be the purpose in this chapter to examine the assumptions and methods that give rise to Recommended Dietary Allowances in general. That topic has been eloquently discussed in the recent past and one can be confident that such discussions will continue, perhaps indefinitely. We can, however, examine the particular problem of the applicability of general recommended dietary allowances to the elderly and explore the question of what is known and needs to be known about changing nutritional requirements in that population. Such information must, after all, determine the final recommendation for their dietary intake.

Continuing to take the American case as our study example, we observe that the Recommended Dietary Allowances which are promulgated under the auspices of the National Academy of Sciences and Food and Nutrition Board were most recently published in 1980[5]. In those recommendations, consideration of changing nutritional allowances for the elderly was highly limited. For example, the age breakdown was such that recommendations for most nutrients were presented for the adult population up to the age of 50 and for those 51 and over. No concessions were made at that time to consider the different requirements for the true elderly, sometimes identified as 75 and over, except in the case of calories. In those recommendations, which are widely used not only in the U.S. but also in other countries, the only micronutrients for which there were recommended changes in intake for those over age 51 were thiamin and riboflavin, where the recommended amounts decreased in recognition of the decreasing calorie intake for the elderly population, and decreased in the recommendation for iron intake for older women reflecting the lower iron requirement after menopause.

The concern for nutrition in the elderly population is increasing and that concern has had an impact on the revisions currently under consideration for the Recommended Dietary Allowances (RDAs). Various drafts of these newer allowances have appeared and although there is at present no official release of the latest version of the RDAs, it is of interest to note that current drafts now add categories of age groups from 50 to 69.9 (which are now distinguished from the younger adults as 'mature adults' and the population of 70 and above, which will be called 'older adults'). We see an extension of the concept of decreasing dietary recommendations for mature and older adults as shown in Table 33.2. The decrease in lean body mass with progression into elderly life results in an estimated decrease in basal metabolic rate of 2% per decade[5]. In addition, there are the lower requirements for a decrease in total activity amounting to 200 kcal/day for men and women between 51 and 75, 500 kcal for men and 400 fewer for women over 75. As

Table 33.2 Recommended Dietary Allowances for Energy[5]

Age (years)	Males	Females
23–50	2700	2000
51–75	2400	1800
76+	2050	1600

shown in Table 33.3, lower energy intakes translate into declining needs for those vitamins whose requirements are largely determined by energy intake, thiamin and riboflavin. Although recommended protein intakes might also decline with age when expressed as a function of declining body mass, recent data on protein requirements in the elderly suggest a possible increased allowance[14]. One change under consideration is an increase in the calcium recommendation for adult women from 800 mg/day to 1000 mg/day to take into account the concern that failure to meet dietary calcium requirements may be a factor in the well-documented loss of bone mass and mineral content which occurs most strikingly in post-menopausal women.

Table 33.3 Recommended Dietary Intakes 1987. Nutrients for which recommended values are different for the elderly

Nutrients	Men			Women		
	25–50	50–69.9	70+	25–50	50–69.9	70+
Protein (g)	66	64	?	38	34	?
Thiamin (mg)	1.4	1.3	1.1	1.1	1.1	0.9
Riboflavin (mg)	1.6	1.4	1.3	1.3	1.3	1.2
Folacin (μg)	240	230	220	190	190	190
Iron (mg)	10	10	10	15	10	10
Vitamin A (μg)	700	700	700	600	600	600
Vitamin C (μg)	40	40	40	30	30	30

But what do we know of requirements for all the other nutrients which are not directly linked to declining energy intake, activity, lean mass, and/or skeletal mass? Newer recommendations for several other nutrients suggest lower allowances for the adult population. This is true of vitamin A[6], vitamin C[7], and folic acid[8]. Controversy has arisen around some of these newer suggestions and no attempt is made to reproduce the arguments on both sides but rather address the question of whether these lower recommendations can and should apply to the elderly population. First, in the case of vitamin A, there is now increasing evidence that the circulating vitamin A levels in the elderly tend to be higher than in younger adults[9]. This phenomenon is best explained by some loss of capacity in the elderly to clear plasma retinol along with a tendency to store increased amounts of retinol in the form of esters. It would seem therefore prudent to lower the recommended allowance for vitamin A slightly in respect to the elderly whether or not that change is made for younger adults based on observed changes in utilization noted above. The case of vitamin C is somewhat more complicated and the final decisions will depend upon which criteria are used to judge optimal vitamin C nutriture. Prevailing attention currently is directed to set dietary intake so as to produce body stores which would be available to meet all requirements for vitamin C over various periods of deprivation. That method of determining vitamin C requirements and allowances will continue to be challenged by those who will argue that increasing amounts of vitamin C in the diet may counteract specific processes that lead to degenerative conditions of aging. One such example is the recent extrapolation from animal studies that there is a dose–response between vitamin C intake and protection from the destructive effects of UV radiation on the lens of the eye leading to central cataract[10]. As research on the relationship between anti-oxidant vitamins like vitamin C and specific degenerative processes continues, we can expect to hear continued arguments for recommendations which take into account the interaction of nutrients, the environment and the process.

In the third example, that of folic acid or folacin the newer recommendations are to bring down the recommended intake for adults to a level of 3 μg/kg, which is rounded to 240, 230, and 220 mg for adults, mature, and older men, and 190 mg for the average adult female. These are substantially below the previous recommendations but are now much more in keeping with increasing data from both Canada and the U.S. on the amounts of intake required to meet allowances. These new recommendations are also much more consistent with modern information about the bioavailability of complex folates from food even though that latter subject continues to need a good deal more study. These lower recommendations for folate for adults raise a number of interesting questions in respect to their application to the elderly. Should the 3 μg/kg figure be extrapolated from adults to mature adults to older adults on the basis of their declining body mass so that the folate allowances for mature adults are lower and those for older adults still lower than those for younger adults? Or should some of the considerations about folate utilization in the elderly be brought to bear on these decisions? Among those considerations are the suggestions about the efficiency of absorption of folate in the elderly population. The general data would seem to indicate that the elderly absorb folic acid about as well as younger adults[11], although the information of the efficiency of absorption of food folates is still incomplete. Another potentially confounding factor, which has not been adequately addressed in most surveys, is the issue of the declining ability to produce gastric acid in the elderly population so that 30% of individuals over 70 will have a demonstrable defect in gastric acid production as described by Russell et al.[12,13]. This could have an effect, at least in a subset of the elderly population with hypochlorhydria, on the efficiency of absorption of folic acid which is highly dependent upon the ability of the stomach to acidify the pH in the proximal intestine[12]. However as Russell has indicated, surveys have not shown lower levels of circulating folate in the elderly and thus the hypochlorhydria factor may be offset by other differences in the physiology of the elderly including the increased synthesis of bacterial folate in the face of increased intestinal populations of such bacteria in the elderly[13].

The efficiency with which these nutrients are utilized in elderly individuals has been minimally explored. Russell and co-workers have performed short-term studies of vitamin A disposition in the elderly[9] but overall efficiency of utilization over periods of time has not really been explored for vitamin A or for the other nutrients under consideration. Such studies are now increasingly within technical reach, particularly with the use of labelled substances including stable isotopes. These newer techniques offer the possibility of doing studies at minimal risk and will become an essential addition to our research armamentarium. The information obtained on nutrient turnover and utilization will be essential to our progress on establishing nutritional requirements and allowances for the older population.

Given the increase in absolute and relative numbers of the elderly population in our countries, it would be a mistake to dismiss the problem of nutrition in the elderly as a conceptual one of setting nutritional allowances and standards, important as that may be. There still are socioeconomic problems which do put the elderly at special risk as do problems of mobility, dentition, etc. These issues demand sensitive and aggressive attention by progressive and compassionate societies, but the goals of programs will be best served by a set of standards which most realistically defines the nutritional needs of elderly individuals and populations. The quest for better standards continues to be a major challenge in gerontology and nutrition.

References

1. Bowman, B. B. and Rosenberg, I. H. (1982). Assessment of nutritional status of the elderly. *Am. J. Clin. Nutr.*, **35**, 1142–51
2. Department of Health, Education and Welfare. (1974). Preliminary Findings of the First Health and Nutrition Examination Survey, United States. 1071–72. Dietary intake and biochemical findings. DHEW Publication No. (HRA) 74–1219–1. (Washington, DC: U.S. Government Office)
3. McGandy, R. B., Russell, R. M., Hartz, S. C., Jacob, R. A., Tannenbaum, S., Peters, M. S., Sahyoun, N. and Otradovec, C. L. (1986). Nutritional status survey of healthy non-institutionalized elderly: energy and nutrient intakes from three-day diet records and nutrient supplements. *Nutr. Res.*, **6**, 785–98
4. Young, E. A. and Rivlin, R. S. (1982). Symposium on Evidence Relating Selected Vitamin Minerals to Health and Disease in the Elderly Population in the United States. *Am. J. Clin. Nutr.*, **36** (suppl.), 977–1086
5. National Academy of Sciences. National Research Council. (1980). *Recommended Dietary Allowances*. 8th revised edn. (Washington, DC: National Academy of Sciences)
6. Olson, J. A. (1987). Recommended Dietary Intakes (RDI) of vitamin A in humans. *Am. J. Clin. Nutr.*, **45**, 704–16
7. Olson, J. A. and Hodges, R. E. (1987). Recommended Dietary Intakes (RDI) of vitamin C in humans. *Am. J. Clin. Nutr.*, **45**, 693–703
8. Herbert, V. (1987). Recommended Dietary Intakes (RDI) of folate in humans. *Am. J. Clin. Nutr.*, **45**, 661–70
9. Krasinski, S. D., Russell, R. M. and Schaefer, E. J. (1987). Delayed plasma clearance of chylomicron-retinyl esters in the elderly. *Gastroenterology*. (In press)
10. Blondin, J. and Taylor, A. (1987). Measures of leucine aminopeptides can be used to anticipate UV-induced age-related damage to lens proteins; ascorbate can delay this damage. *Mech. Ageing Develop.* (In press)
11. Rosenberg, I. H., Bowman, B. B., Cooper, B. A., Halsted, C. H. and Lindenbaum, J. (1982). Folate nutrition in the elderly. In Rivlin, R. S. and Young, E. A. (eds.) Symposium on Evidence Relating Selected Vitamins and Minerals to Health and Disease in the Elderly Population in the United States. *Am. J. Clin. Nutr.*, **36** (suppl.), 1060–6

12. Russell, R. M., Dhar, G. J., Dutta, S. K. and Rosenberg, I. H. (1979). Influence of intra-luminal pH on folate absorption: Studies in control subjects and in patients with pancreatic insufficiency. *J. Lab. Clin. Med.,* **93** (3), 428–36
13. Russell, R. M., Krasinski, S. D., Samloff, I. M., Jacob, R. A., Hartz, S. C. and Brovender, S. R. (1986). Folic acid malabsorption in atrophic gastritis: compensation by bacterial folate synthesis. *Gastroenterology,* **91** (6), 1476–82
14. Gersovitz, M., Motil, K., Munro, H. N., Scrimshaw, N. S. and Young, V. R. (1982). Human protein requirements: Assessment of the dietary adequacy of the current Recommended Daily Allowances for dietary protein in elderly men and women. *Am. J. Clin. Nutr.,* **35,** 6–14

34
Age-related changes in retinoid status and some parameters of retinoid metabolism

H. F. J. HENDRIKS, W. S. BLANER, A. BROUWER, D. S. GOODMAN and D. L. KNOOK

INTRODUCTION

Numerous disorders occur during the aging process, which are associated with alterations in regulatory processes[1,2] and affect cell proliferation[3] and, under extreme conditions, with intercellular communication and cell function[4]. Retinoids (vitamin A) are required for the regulation of reproduction, development and normal growth of higher animals. They are also required for the maintenance of mucus secretion and of differentiated epithelia in adult life. The maintenance of retinoid homeostasis, which is complex and highly regulated, is essential in this respect. The liver plays a central role in retinoid homeostasis by regulating serum retinol levels and by storing the majority of the body retinoids[5].

Naturally-occurring retinoids are taken up in the mucosal cells of the intestine[6], converted into retinyl esters and then secreted into the lymph as chylomicron constituents[7]. The chylomicra are metabolized to chylomicron remnants during their circulation in the blood[8]. Chylomicron remnants still contain the majority of the retinyl esters[9] and are rapidly taken up by the liver parenchymal cells[10]. The plasma half-life of these chylomicron remnants is in the order of minutes[11,12].

Subsequently, the chylomicron remnant retinoids are metabolized in the liver. In the liver, both the parenchymal and the fat-storing cells play essential roles in retinoid metabolism. Uptake and processing of retinoids occurs in the liver parenchymal cells, whereas the fat-storing cells are involved in the storage of retinoids[13,14]. The parenchymal cells take up retinyl esters primarily as chylomicron remnant constituents[15,16]. After uptake, retinyl esters are hydrolyzed by retinyl palmitate hydrolase (RPH) to yield retinol[17-19]. After the hydrolysis of retinyl esters, a part of the retinol generated is bound to the retinol-binding protein (RBP). The retinol–RBP is secreted into the circulation and complexed to transthyretin (TTR)[20]. Another part of the retinol, as well as its metabolite retinoic acid, is bound to intracellular binding proteins, viz. the cellular retinol-binding protein (CRBP) and the cellular retinoic acid-binding protein (CRABP). It was previously shown that parenchymal cells contain high concentrations of CRBP, RBP and RPH activity, while fat-storing cells contain high concentrations of CRBP and RPH activity, but very little RBP[14]. These data indicate that fat-storing cells do not only store retinyl esters, but are also important in retinoid metabolism.

It was previously shown that the retinoid content of rat liver increases with age[13]. In the present study, retinoid contents of a number of tissues and organs were determined to investigate the age-related changes in retinoid status. Age-related changes in retinoid uptake and transport were investigated by determining the half-lives of [³H]retinoid chylomicra and [³H]retinoid chylomicron remnants and the plasma retinol levels. Furthermore, the levels of retinoids, RBP, CRBP, CRABP and RPH activity were determined in total liver homogenates and in the four main liver cell types, i.e. parenchymal, endothelial, Kupffer and fat-storing cells isolated from young and old rats.

MATERIALS AND METHODS

Animals

Female BN/BiRij rats aged 3, 6, 30, and 36 months, weighing 150 ± 10 g ($n = 5$), 159 ± 13 g, ($n = 10$), 215 ± 21 g ($n = 4$), and 205 ± 10 g ($n = 10$), respectively, were used. Life-span characteristics of this rat strain include a 50% survival of 32 months and a maximum life-span of approximately 41 months. The age-associated pathology of this rat strain has been described previously[3]. All rats were fed standard laboratory chow (Diet AM II, Hope Farms, Woerden, The Netherlands) *ad libitum*. This diet contained (per kilogram) 5.5 mg retinyl acetate and approximately 1.5 mg mixed carotenoids derived from alfalfa and dried grasses. These specific pathogen-free derived rats were maintained under 'clean conventional' conditions[21].

Preparation of [³H]retinoid chylomicra and [³H]retinoid chylomicron remnants

The intestinal lymphatic trunk of 3-month-old rats was cannulated as described by Drevon[22]. Rats were given about 1 mCi [³H]retinol in 1 ml of Intralipid 20% (Vitrum AB, Stockholm, Sweden) through duodenal tubing and lymph was collected overnight in EDTA at a final concentration of 1 mM. Chylomicra were isolated from the lymph as described previously[13] and resuspended in 0.9% NaCl containing 1 mM EDTA.

Chylomicron remnants were prepared from the isolated chylomicra using 3-month-old, overnight fasted, functionally hepatectomized rats[23]. Chylomicron remnants were recovered with the serum from the animal. The serum was stored at 4°C and injected the next day.

Plasma disappearance of [³H]retinoid chylomicra and [³H]retinoid chylomicron remnants

Half-lives of both [³H]retinoid chylomicra and [³H]retinoid chylomicron remnants were determined in 6-month-old and in 36-month-old rats on two consecutive days. Rats were fed *ad libitum* prior to the first experiment, and fasted prior to the second experiment.

Young (6-month-old) and old (36-month-old) rats received a dose of 2–5 μCi [³H]retinoids. Blood samples were taken from the tail vein and were collected into heparinized glass capillaries, centrifuged, and the radioactivity present in 20-μl plasma samples was determined. In general, 5 samples were taken during the first 5 min and another 5 at longer time intervals up to about 20 min after the injection. Half-lives were calculated for each individual animal using the elimination phase of the plasma disappearance curve.

Organ distribution studies

Endogenous retinoid distribution was determined in 6-month-old and 30-month-old rats. Under ether narcosis, the portal vein was cannulated, a blood sample was taken, and the liver was perfused with Gey's balanced salt solution to rinse out the blood. Subsequently, the following organs were taken out: liver, kidneys, peri-renal fat, adrenal glands, spleen, lungs, small intestines, skeletal muscle, sub-mandibulary lymph nodes, eyes and brains. The organs were cleaned, weighed and stored at $-70°C$ until analysis.

Cell isolation procedures

From one individual animal either liver parenchymal cells or sinusoidal cells were isolated.

Parenchymal cells

Parenchymal cells were isolated[24] at 37°C by a first perfusion with perfusion medium[25] lacking Ca^{2+} and collagenase, followed by a perfusion and an incubation with perfusion medium containing Ca^{2+} and collagenase[13]. Parenchymal cells were further purified by centrifugal elutriation in a JE-6 elutriator rotor using a Sanderson chamber (Beckman Instruments, Palo Alto, CA). At a rotor speed of 1350 r.p.m., parenchymal cells were elutriated between 32 and 41 ml of perfusion medium per minute.

Kupffer, endothelial and fat-storing cells

Non-parenchymal cell suspensions were prepared by perfusion and incubation of the liver with pronase and collagenase as described previously[26]. From this non-parenchymal cell suspension fat-storing cells were purified using a discontinuous two-layer Nycodenz gradient[13,14]. Endothelial and Kupffer cells were further purified by centrifugal elutriation. At a rotor speed of 3250 r.p.m., endothelial cells were elutriated at a flow of 41 ml and Kupffer cells at a flow of 58 ml of Gey's balanced salt solution per min.

The yield and purity of all cell preparations were determined by light and electron microscopy[14]. The purity of the cell fractions was 99%, 90%, 80%, and 40–70%, for parenchymal, endothelial, Kupffer, and fat-storing cell fractions, respectively.

HPLC method

Retinoids, including retinol, retinyl oleate, retinyl palmitate, and retinyl stearate were analysed by high-performance liquid chromatography as described previously[13] using retinyl acetate as an internal standard.

Assays for RBP, CRBP, CRABP and RPH activity

RBP, CRBP, and CRABP were measured by specific radioimmunoassays[27,28]. RPH activities were determined using a sensitive microassay which measures the formation of [1-^{14}C]palmitate from retinyl[1-^{14}C]palmitate[29].

Statistical analysis

Elimination half-lives as determined in the experimental groups were compared by a two-tailed Mann–Whitney U test[30]. All regression lines were acceptable at the 5% level of probability.

Student's t test was used for the statistical evaluation of the other data.

RESULTS

[^{3}H]Retinoid chylomicra and [^{3}H]retinoid chylomicron remnants half-lives

Half-lives of [^{3}H]retinoid chylomicra and chylomicron remnants were determined in 6- and 36-month-old rats given food *ad libitum* overnight. Half-lives of these particles were also determined in young and old rats after an overnight fasting period. Half-lives of [^{3}H]retinoid chylomicron remnants were significantly shorter than those of [^{3}H]retinoid chylomicra. The results of this experiment indicate that the half-life of [^{3}H]retinoid chylomicra in young rats did not differ significantly from that in old rats (Table 34.1).

After an overnight fasting period, half-lives of [^{3}H]retinoid chylomicron remnants observed in old rats were significantly ($p < 0.05$) shorter than those observed in young rats (Table 34.2).

Table 34.1 Half-lives of [³H]retinoid chylomicra and [³H]retinoid chylomicron remnants in 6-month-old and 36-month-old female BN/BiRij rats*

	6-month-old**		36-month-old**	
	n	$t_{\frac{1}{2}}$ (min)	n	$t_{\frac{1}{2}}$ (min)
[³H]retinoid chylomicra	4	10.3 ± 1.5	4	10.2 ± 1.7
[³H]retinoid chylomicron remnants	4	4.8 ± 3.2	3	3.2 ± 0.4

* Values are expressed as the mean ± S.D.
** No significant differences existed between 6- and 36-month-old animals

Table 34.2 Half-lives of [³H]retinoid chylomicron remnants in 6-month-old and 36-month-old fasted female BN/BiRij rats*

	6-month-old		36-month-old	
	n	$t_{\frac{1}{2}}$ (min)	n	$t_{\frac{1}{2}}$ (min)
[³H]retinoid chylomicron remnants	4	4.3 ± 0.7	4	2.7 ± 0.7**

* Values are expressed as the mean ± S.D.
** Value differs significantly ($p < 0.05$) from 6-month-old value

Organ distribution studies

The endogenous retinoid contents of several organs and tissues of young (6-month-old) and old (30-month-old) rats were determined. Retinoid content of the liver was highest of all organs and tissues tested. Liver retinoid content increased significantly ($p < 0.01$) from 876 ± 110 in 6-month-old rats to 1584 ± 636 μg retinol equivalents/g wet weight in 30-month-old rats. Of the other organs and tissues tested, the retinoid content of the eyes only decreased significantly ($p < 0.01$) from 1.0 ± 0.3 in 6-month-old to 0.2 ± 0.2 μg retinol equivalents/g wet weight in 30-month-old rats. No age-related changes were observed in the plasma retinol levels or in the other organs and tissues tested (data not shown).

Distribution of retinoids and retinoid-related parameters in rat liver

The concentrations of retinoids, RBP, CRBP, CRABP, and RPH activities were determined in liver homogenates and isolated liver cell types, viz. parenchymal, Kupffer, endothelial and fat-storing cells from 6-month-old rats and 36-month-old rats (Table 34.3)

Liver fat-storing cells contained high concentrations of retinoids (Table 34.3). Low retinoid concentrations were present in the other cell types. This confirms our earlier finding that fat-storing cells are the main retinoid storage sites in rat liver[13]. A significant ($p < 0.05$) age-related increase in the retinoid

Table 34.3 Contents of total retinoids, some retinoid binding proteins and RPH activity in isolated liver cell types and total liver from female 6-month-old and 36-month-old BN/BiRij rats*

Fraction	Retinoids	(n)	RBP	(n)	CRBP	(n)	CRABP	(n)	RPH	(n)
1. 6-Month-old rats										
Fat-storing cells	33.6± 4.5	(5)	7.1± 1.8	(5)	223 ±53	(5)	86.3±47.9	(9)	1187±400	(5)
Endothelial cells	0.7± 0.1	(5)	1.8± 0.2	(5)	5.8± 2.2	(5)	2.7± 1.7	(3)	80± 33	(6)
Kupffer cells	0.6± 0.1	(5)	3.4± 0.6	(5)	10.8± 1.6	(5)	0.5± 0.5	(3)	112± 56	(5)
Parenchymal cells	1.0± 0.1	(6)	110 ±31	(6)	195 ±59	(5)	4.4± 1.3	(5)	4408±728	(5)
Total liver**	876 ±45	(6)	23.7± 3.1	(6)	117 ± 3	(5)	1.1± 0.1	(6)	55± 2	(6)
2. 36-Month-old rats										
Fat-storing cells	78.1± 15.1†	(5)	3.5± 0.7	(5)	301 ±118	(5)	26.7±14.2	(9)	997±215	(5)
Endothelial cells	1.5± 0.2†	(5)	3.1± 0.3	(5)	8.7± 1.3	(5)	2.6± 0.7	(3)	30± 14	(6)
Kupffer cells	1.2± 0.4	(5)	6.5± 1.6†	(5)	10.7± 2.8	(5)	8.8± 2.9	(5)	145± 27	(5)
Parenchymal cells	4.1± 1.1	(6)	148 ±26	(5)	523 ±111†	(5)	3.8± 1.4	(6)	4875±428	(6)
Total liver**	1141±290	(6)	27.6± 2.7	(6)	108 ± 14	(6)	1.6± 0.2	(6)	65± 2†	(2)

* Values are given as the mean ±S.E.M. Retinoids are expressed as μg retinol equivalents per 10^6 cells or as μg retinol equivalents per gram wet weight **. RBP, CRBP and CRABP are expressed as ng per 10^6 cells or as μg per gram wet weight ** and RPH activity is expressed as pmol free fatty acid formed per hour per 10^6 cells or as pmol per minute per mg protein **. † Value differs significantly from 6-month-old value ($p < 0.05$). n = the number of experiments performed.

content of liver homogenates and of the fat-storing cell fractions was observed. In all other cell fractions a small increase in retinoid content was also observed. It was calculated that fat-storing cells in both young and old rats contained more than 70% of the retinoids stored in the liver.

RPH activity was detected in high concentrations in both parenchymal cells and fat-storing cells. An age-related increase in the liver RPH activity was observed. This small increase is only based on two observations. The cellular distribution of this parameter was not changed with age.

RBP was present mainly in liver parenchymal cells. Low, but detectable levels of this serum protein were found in all non-parenchymal cell types tested. No age-related change could be observed in the cellular distribution of this binding protein.

CRBP was detected in high concentrations in both fat-storing cells and parenchymal cells and in low concentrations in endothelial cells and Kupffer cells. A significant age-related increase was observed in the CRBP content of the parenchymal cell fractions. This increase was significant ($p < 0.05$) both when the data were expressed per 10^6 cells and when expressed per mg cell protein. No such age-related increase, however, could be observed in the liver homogenates of the two age groups tested.

CRABP was present in low concentrations in the liver homogenates and cell preparations tested. Relatively high concentrations of CRABP were detected in fat-storing cell fractions. A similar cellular distribution of CRABP was observed for both 6-month-old and 36-month-old rats.

DISCUSSION

In this study several parameters of retinoid metabolism as a function of age were investigated. The elimination half-life of [³H]retinoid chylomicron remnants was significantly shorter in old fasted rats as compared to young fasted rats. These results were obtained using [³H]retinoid chylomicron remnants prepared in 3-month-old rats. The shortening of the elimination half-life might be the result of alterations in lipoprotein particles combined with a changed receptor affinity. Lipoprotein particles and lipoprotein receptors should be further characterized to obtain more insight into the mechanisms underlying the observed phenomena.

The results presented in this study show that both liver fat-storing cells and parenchymal cells play an important role in retinoid metabolism. Both cell types contain the enzyme RPH, which hydrolyses retinyl esters. The retinyl esters hydrolyzed in the parenchymal cells might represent the retinyl esters taken up as chylomicron remnant constituents, while the esters in the fat-storing cells might represent the retinyl esters stored in the fat-storing cell lipid droplets[24]. The CRBP present in the two cell types is possibly important in the intracellular transport of retinol.

These studies also indicate that retinoid stores in the laboratory rat kept on a normal diet increase with age. The increase in retinoid stores is only observed in the liver. Retinoid stores are specifically located in the fat-storing cells. Therefore, the increase in liver retinoid content with age is primarily due to an increase in fat-storing cell retinoid content. This change does not seem to affect the handling of the vitamin in the liver, since levels of binding proteins and enzyme activities are not significantly changed with age in the different liver cell types and liver homogenates. Furthermore, plasma retinol levels are not changed with age indicating that retinoid homeostasis is maintained in the old rat.

Acknowledgements

This work was in part supported by the foundation for Medical Research and Health Research (MEDIGON), which is subsidized by the Netherlands Organization for Advancement of Pure Research (ZWO).

References

1. Popper, H. (1986). Aging and the liver. In Popper, H. and Schaffner, F. (eds.) *Progress in Liver Disease*. Vol. 8, pp. 673–89. (New York: Grune and Stratton)
2. Kitani, K. (ed.) (1978). *Liver and Aging*. (Amsterdam: North-Holland, Elsevier Biomedical Press)
3. Burek, J. D. (1978). Pathology of Aging Rats. Thesis. (Cleveland, Ohio: CRC Press)
4. Brouwer, A., Horan, M. A., Barelds, R. J. and Knook, D. L. (1986). Cellular aging of the reticuloendothelial system. *Arch. Gerontol. Geriatr.*, **5**, 317–24
5. Goodman, D. S. and Blaner, W. S. (1984). Biosynthesis, absorption, and hepatic metabolism of retinol. In Sporn, M. B., Roberts, A. B. and Goodman, D. S. (eds.) *The Retinoids*. pp. 1–39. (New York: Academic Press)
6. Hollander, D. (1981). Intestinal absorption of vitamin A, E, D, K. *J. Clin. Invest.*, **97**, 449–62
7. Goodman, D. S., Blomstrand, R., Werner, B., Huang, H. S. and Shiratori, T. (1966). The intestinal absorption and metabolism of vitamin A and β-carotene in man. *J. Clin. Invest.*, **45**, 1615–23
8. Green, P. H. R. and Glickman, R. M. (1981). Intestinal lipoprotein metabolism. *J. Lipid Res.*, **22**, 1153–73
9. Hazzard, W. R. and Bierman, E. L. (1978). Delayed clearance of chylomicron remnants following vitamin-A-containing oral fat loads in broad β-disease (type III hyperlipoproteinemia). *Metab. Clin. Exp.*, **25**, 777–801
10. Shelburne, F., Hanks, J., Meyers, W. and Quarfordt, S. (1980). Effect of apoproteins on
11. Redgrave, T. G. (1970). Formation of cholesteryl ester-rich particulate lipid during metabolism of chylomicrons. *J. Clin. Invest.*, **49**, 465–71
12. Norum, K. R., Berg, T., Helgerud, P. and Drevon, C. A. (1983). Transport of cholesterol. *Physiol. Rev.*, **63**, 1343–419
13. Hendriks, H. F. J., Verhoofstad, W. A. M. M., Brouwer, A., de Leeuw, A. M. and Knook, D. L. (1985). Perisinusoidal fat-storing cells are the main vitamin A storage sites in rat liver. *Exp. Cell Res.*, **160**, 138–49
14. Blaner, W. S., Hendriks, H. F. J., Brouwer, A., de Leeuw, A. M., Knook, D. L. and Goodman, D. S. (1985). Retinoid, retinoid-binding proteins, and retinyl palmitate hydrolase distributions in different types of rat liver cells. *J. Lipid Res.*, **26**, 1241–51
15. Nilsson, A. (1977). Effects of antimicrotubular agents and cycloheximide on the metabolism of cholesteryl esters by hepatocyte suspensions. *Biochem. J.*, **162**, 367–77
16. Blomhoff, R., Helgerud, P., Rasmussen, M., Berg, T. and Norum, K. R. (1982). *In vivo* uptake of chylomicron [³H]retinyl ester by rat liver: Evidence for retinol transfer from parenchymal to nonparenchymal cells. *Proc. Natl. Acad. Sci. USA*, **79**, 7326–30
17. Harrison, E. H., Smith, J. E. and Goodman, D. S. (1979). Unusual properties of retinyl palmitate hydrolase activity in rat liver. *J. Lipid Res.*, **20**, 760–71

18. Prystowsky, J. H., Smith, J. E. and Goodman, D. S. (1981). Retinyl palmitate hydrolase activity in normal rat liver. *J. Biol. Chem.*, **256,** 4498–503

19. Blaner, W. S., Prystowsky, J. H., Smith, J. E. and Goodman, D. S. (1984). Rat liver retinyl palmitate hydrolase activity: Relationship to cholesteryl oleate and triolein hydrolase activities. *Biochim. Biophys. Acta,* **794,** 419–27

20. Navab, M., Smith, J. E. and Goodman, D. S. (1971). Rat plasma prealbumin. Metabolic studies on effects of vitamin A status and on tissue distribution. *J. Biol. Chem.,* **252,** 5107–14

21. Hollander, C. F. (1976). Current experience using the laboratory rat in aging studies. *Lab. Animal Sci.,* **26,** 320–8

22. Drevon, Ch.A. (1978). Cholesteryl ester metabolism in fat- and cholesterol/fat-fed guinea pigs. *Atherosclerosis,* **30,** 123–36

23. Redgrave, T. G. (1970). Formation of cholesteryl ester-rich particulate lipid during metabolism of chylomicrons. *J. Clin. Invest.,* **49,** 465–71

24. Hendriks, H. F. J., Brekelmans, P. J. A. M., Buytenhek, R., Brouwer, A., de Leeuw, A. M. and Knook, D. L. (1987). Liver parenchymal cells differ from the fat-storing cells in their lipid composition. *Lipids,* **22,** 266–73

25. Brouwer, A., Barelds, R. J. and Knook, D. L. (1984). Centrifugal separations of mammalian cells. In Rickwood, D. (ed.) *Centrifugation, a Practical Approach.* pp. 183–218. (Oxford and Washington: IRL Press)

26. Knook, D. L., Blansjaar, N. and Sleyster, E. Ch. (1977). Isolation and characterization of Kupffer and endothelial cells from the rat liver. *Exp. Cell Res.,* **109,** 317–29

27. Smith, J. E., Deen, D. D., Jr., Sklan, D. and Goodman, D. S. (1980). Colchicine inhibition of retinol binding protein secretion by rat liver. *J. Lipid Res.,* **21,** 229–37

28. Adachi, N., Smith, J. E., Sklan, D. and Goodman, D. S. (1981). Radioimmunoassay studies of the tissue distribution and subcellular localization of cellular retinol-binding protein in rats. *J. Biol. Chem.,* **256,** 9471–6

29. Prystowsky, J. H., Smith, J. E. and Goodman, D. S. (1984). Retinyl palmitate hydrolase activity in normal rat liver. *J. Biol. Chem.,* **256,** 4498–503

30. Hollander, M. and Wolfe, D. A. (1973). *Nonparametrical Statistical Methods.* (New York: J. Wiley)

35
Parenchymal liver disease in the elderly

O. F. W. JAMES

By now well-rehearsed demographic changes in the population are leading to a higher and higher proportion of elderly and very elderly patients in hospitals and consulting rooms. With these demographic changes an increasing awareness is occurring of the importance of diagnosis and management of liver disease in elderly individuals. Thus it has become more important to ask ourselves how we translate the half-understood alterations in morphology and function of the liver into statements about the susceptibility of the aged human liver to damage and disease. At a simple clinical level we should ask three questions:

1. Are the elderly more susceptible to liver damage or disease?
2. Is liver disease different in the elderly?
3. Are the principles of treatment and management altered in any way?

In an attempt to answer these questions, and provide a background on which we can begin to answer them, data are presented here, largely from our own unit, on several parenchymal liver diseases in elderly subjects – these data should be regarded as background information upon which subsequent prospective clinical studies can be intelligently based, particularly as little hard data currently exist although frequent *ex cathedra* statements have been made about the clinical features of liver disease in older individuals.

DRUG-INDUCED LIVER DISEASE

There is an almost universal impression that adverse drug reactions (ADRs) in general are much more common in elderly subjects and that hepatic ADRs are no exception to this rule. In order to critically examine this question Woodhouse[1], Mortimer and Wiholm recently have examined all hepatic ADRs reported to the Swedish Adverse Drug Reactions Advisory Committee from 1980 to 1984. Reporting of ADRs is arguably more thorough in Sweden than in any other major country. In addition prescribing information is monitored by the National Corporation of Swedish Pharmacies and from these data the percentage prescriptions for any individual drug given to patients over age 65 may be calculated[1]. The total reported hepatic ADRs were 807 of which 234 (29%) were in individuals over age 65. In Sweden 17% of the population is over age 65; superficially therefore there was a marked excess in the proportion of hepatic ADRs occurring in over 65 year olds compared to that expected purely on the basis of the proportion of persons in this age group. From the monitoring of prescribing data however it is possible to show that about 30% of prescriptions are given to individuals over age 65. By obtaining prescribing data for the individual drugs most commonly implicated in hepatic ADRs Woodhouse *et al.* were able to derive a ratio: (% Reports > 65 years):(% Prescriptions > 65 years). In this way a true reflection as to whether elderly individuals were truly more susceptible to developing ADRs to individual drugs could be obtained. A high ratio indicated increased susceptibility in the elderly, a ratio of 1 being that which would be expected in the population as a whole, a ratio substantially below

Table 35.1 Hepatic ADR and the effect of age, corrected for age-related prescribing variables

Drug	% Reports >65 years	% Prescriptions >65 years	Ratio % Reports >65 years to % Prescriptions >65 years
Zimelidine	24%	24%	1.00
Co-trimoxazole	40%	34%	1.18
Cimetidine	32%	27%	1.18
Sulindac	50%	37%	1.32
Carbamazipine	18%	17%	1.05
Nitrofurantoin	43%	30%	1.43
Chlorpromazine	20%	32%	0.63
Hydralazine	37%	55%	0.67
Phenytoin	12%	23%	0.52
Naproxen	37%	37%	1.00
Piroxicam	20%	44%	0.45
Overall	30%	32%	0.94

1 indicating reduced susceptibility to a particular ADR in the elderly. It will be seen from Table 35.1 that for the 11 most frequently reported hepatic ADRs there was no marked increase in susceptibility (no ratio > 1.5) for any drug although there was a suggestion that a higher proportion of elderly individuals receiving nitrofurantoin over age 65 might be susceptible to an hepatic ADR (ratio 1.43).

It will be seen that the mean ratio of (% Reports > 65:% Prescriptions > 65) is only 0.94 indicating no increased susceptibility whatever to the development of hepatic ADRs in this Swedish population. It is suggested that the impression that the elderly are more susceptible to hepatic ADRs has been given because of the substantially greater number of drugs which they receive.

Woodhouse *et al.* also examined the possibility that ADRs were less commonly reported in the elderly thus biasing the sample, from the pattern of ADRs recorded and from other data available in Sweden they concluded that this was most unlikely.

There remains the possibility that while the elderly may not be more likely to develop hepatic ADRs in general there may be specific, possibly not common ADRs, to which they are more susceptible or, more likely, if certain ADRs do develop they may be more severe in elderly subjects. Because of the general lack of data corrected for age-related prescribing variables it is extremely difficult to examine the first possibility [2-4]. In relation to the second possibility it does seem however in the cases of halothane and benoxaprofen that if an elderly individual develops an hepatic ADR then this is liable to be more severe. In the case of halothane, Neuberger and Williams[5] reviewed the age distribution of patients admitted to the King's College Hospital Liver Failure Unit with halothane-associated fulminant hepatic failure and compared this to data on the distribution of patients undergoing anaesthesia in general and individuals admitted with viral fulminant hepatic failure. Among 48 patients with halothane-associated fulminant hepatic failure the median age was 57 years with a considerable shift towards an older age group among individuals with halothane-associated FHF compared to the generality of individuals undergoing anaesthetic (the majority receiving halothane). In the case of the non-steroidal anti-inflammatory drug benoxaprofen, unpublished data from the UK DHSS suggests that while the mean age of individuals receiving the drug was about 59 years the mean age of those sustaining ADRs was about 66 and in individuals with severe or fatal ADRs (almost always hepatic) the mean age was 75. Of the 9 patients described by Taggart and Alderdice[6] and Goudie et al.[7] with fatal hepatic failure associated with benoxaprofen, 6 were over age 80, the remainder over age 70.

At present one should probably conclude on the still insubstantial evidence available that the liver does not grow more likely to develop drug-related disease as age progresses; possibly, if damage does develop it is more likely to be severe and this is perhaps not surprising.

CAUSES OF CIRRHOSIS

It is among the causes of cirrhosis that demographic changes and increasing clinical awareness are combining most closely to sharpen the realisation that liver disease is a major problem in old age.

Alcoholic liver disease

Although it is now 8 years since Garagliano et al.[8] showed that among White males in Baltimore the peak decade for presentation of cirrhosis was the 70s there has been very little data presented specifically on the clinical and histological features of alcoholic liver disease (ALD) and its prognosis in respect of advancing age. We have therefore carried out a retrospective analysis of all patients in whom a diagnosis of ALD had been made on our medical/geriatric unit from August 1977 through July 1985[9]. The diagnosis of ALD was based on history, clinical examination, liver blood tests, blood film, random blood and urine ethanol examinations together with compatible or diagnostic liver histology. Other conventional serological examinations for patients with liver disease were also carried out. A full alcohol consumption history was taken with corroborating data from relatives and/or health-care workers. Patients received standard treatment for ALD and its complications; they were strongly urged to abstain from alcohol consumption following discharge; many received further support on leaving hospital. A minimum follow-up of 1 year, maximum 8 years was available on all subjects in July 1986.

Results

208 were identified with a firmly established diagnosis of ALD. 149 of these presented up to age 59 years, 45 presented for the first time age 60–69 years,

Table 35.2 Main symptoms at presentation ranked in order of frequency (percentages in parentheses) for each age group males and females combined

Ranking of frequency	Age groups (years)					
	20–59 (n = 149)		60–69 (n = 45)		≥70 (n = 14)	
Anorexia	1	(40%)	1	(36%)	1	(33%)
Nausea/vomiting	2	(23%)	6	(16%)	6	(17%)
Abdominal pain	3	(21%)	7	(13%)	6	(17%)
Weight loss	3	(21%)	3	(20%)	6	(17%)
NSS* + abnormal LFTs**	5	(20%)	8	(9%)		
Ankle swelling	6	(13%)	2	(22%)	3	(21%)
Jaundice	7	(13%)	8	(9%)	3	(21%)
Tremor/shakes	8	(12%)	11	(8%)		
Haematemesis/melaena	9	(12%)	4	(18%)		
Abdominal swelling	10	(10%)	4	(18%)	3	(21%)
Diarrhoea	11	(8%)	8	(9%)		
Dizziness/falls			12	(7%)	2	(29%)

* NSS = non-specific symptoms; ** LFT = liver function tests

12 presented over the age of 70. Thus 57 of 206 patients (28%) were over age 60 at presentation. Presenting symptoms were as shown in Table 35.2, presenting signs as in Table 35.3. It is worth noting that the very elderly presented with a rather higher proportion of symptoms suggestive of severe liver disease – ankle swelling, jaundice, abdominal swelling – than the youngest group. Similarly while 20% of the young ALD patients presented with essentially mild or absent symptoms but with abnormal liver blood tests found on insurance screening, this became progressively rarer with increasing age.

Table 35.3 Main clinical signs at presentation ranked in order of frequency (percentages in parentheses) for each age group males and females combined

Ranking of frequency	Age groups (years)		
	20–59 (n = 149)	60–69 (n = 45)	≥ 70 (n = 14)
Hepatomegaly	1 (54%)	1 (53%)	1 (50%)
Spider naevi	2 (38%)	2 (27%)	3 (29%)
Palmar erythema	3 (30%)	3 (24%)	5 (21%)
Jaundice	4 (22%)	6 (11%)	3 (29%)
Ascites	5 (17%)	5 (20%)	2 (36%)
Oedema	7 (11%)	4 (22%)	5 (21%)
Gynaecomastia	7 (11%)	8 (8%)	7 (14%)
Neuropathy/myopathy	9 (8%)	6 (11%)	7 (14%)
Splenomegaly	6 (15%)	8 (8%)	7 (14%)

Liver histology

Liver histology was available on 199 patients (96%) either within 3 months of presentation or at post-mortem (if this was within 6 months of presentation). In the remaining 4% patients' histology could not be obtained because of poor coagulation. The histological classification is presented in Table 35.4.

Table 35.4 Dominant histological features at presentation or at post-mortem (if within 6 months of presentation) by sex and age (years). The classification is by the most severe lesions seen; individuals with, for example, alcoholic hepatitis together with steatosis are classified as having hepatitis, not steatosis. All individuals over age 70 in whom histology was obtained had cirrhosis at presentation

Sex/age	Unknown	Steatosis	Fibrosis	Hepatitis	Cirrhosis
Men, 20–59 (n = 112)	5%	26%	8%	7%	55%
Women, 20–59 (n = 37)	—	28%	5%	17%	50%
Men, 60–69 (n = 29)	7%	19%	7%	15%	52%
Women, 60–69 (n = 16)	6%	42%	6%	16%	30%
Men, ≥ 70 (n = 7)	—	—	—	—	100%
Women, ≥ 70 (n = 7)	14%	—	—	—	86%

Estimated alcohol consumption

There appeared little evidence that the more elderly individuals were either consuming significantly less alcohol just prior to presentation and diagnosis or that any of the elderly subjects were 'new' drinkers – almost all patients were long-term heavy alcohol abusers although a few of the elderly had clearly progressively reduced consumption in retirement.

Mortality

A minimum 1-year follow-up (maximum 8 years) was obtained in 198 patients (8 subjects lost to follow-up have been excluded from analysis). Minimum 3-

Table 35.5 Alcoholic liver disease mortality at 1 and 3 years

Age	1 year (n = 198)		3 years (n = 128)	
	n	mortality (%)	n	mortality (%)
20–59	145	5	92	24
60–69	41	22 ⎫	25	40 ⎫
		⎬ 34%		⎬ 53%
⩾ 70 +	12	75 ⎭	11	91 ⎭

year follow-up was available in 128 patients. The mortality figures are shown in Table 35.5. Mortality at both 1 and 3 years was significantly ($P < 0.05$) greater in subjects over age 60 than those below. Among the 37 men who died 12 had primary liver cancer (PLC), of those presenting under age 60, 4 out of 21 had serological evidence of previous infection with the hepatitis B virus. Of the 16 men dying with ALD over age 60, 8 (50%) died with PLC, among these 5 of the 7 men dying over age 70 had PLC.

Conclusions

It seems that alcoholic liver disease is by no means uncommon with increasing age. The symptoms, histological findings and mortality data suggest that, particularly in the very elderly, ALD presents 'further along the line' than in younger individuals. The reasons for this are not clear but in a separate community study of the prevalence of possible alcoholism and alcohol consumption in our local community as many as 13% of the elderly could be classed as heavy drinkers. It seems possible that there may be some selection in referral patterns both by the patients themselves and by their referring family physician so that older individuals with relatively mild symptoms or complaints associated with possible alcoholic liver disease are not presented to hospital[10]. Further evaluation is clearly needed.

PRIMARY BILIARY CIRRHOSIS (PBC)

With the recognition that the anti-mitochondrial antibody (AMA) is a sensitive and rather specific marker for the presence of PBC together with the ·increased use of biochemical and serological screening, there is an understanding that the clinical spectrum of the disease is wider than had hitherto been appreciated. The mean age at diagnosis is now about 55 to 60 years and many patients are asymptomatic of liver disease at the time of detection. We have therefore carried out a study of the presentation and prognosis of patients age 65 years or more at the time of diagnosis in comparison with the features seen in younger patients[11].

Patients and methods

We examined 121 consecutive patients seen in the clinic between 1974 and 1983 in whom a diagnosis of PBC was made on the basis of either:

1. AMA titre >1 in 20, abnormal cholestatic liver blood tests together with diagnostic or compatible liver histology or
2. Positive AMA titre >1 in 40 together with diagnostic liver histology even in the absence of cholestatic liver blood tests.

Patients were grouped as follows:

Group 1 had no symptoms at the time of presentation which could be related to liver disease.
Group 2 had symptoms of liver disease.
Group 3 patients presented with symptoms of portal hypertension or hepatic failure.

Results

121 patients with PBC were studied of whom 35 (29%) were >65 years at presentation of detection. Those aged ⩾65 will be referred to as the old group. There were 12 men (10% of the total), 5 in the old group. All symptoms which could conceivably be related to liver disease were recorded as were clinical signs of liver disease. No single sign or symptom was significantly commoner in either age group, however the total number of signs and symptoms recorded per patient was significantly less in the older than the younger group ($P < 0.05$). Thus although the pattern of clinical findings was the same in both age groups more features were detected in younger patients. 31% of the older group were asymptomatic at detection, 20% of the younger. Asymptomatic patients had a higher mean age at presentation than symptomatic (60 vs. 56 years); this was not statistically significant. Similarly the biochemical and other serological findings were compared between groups; there was no difference in titres of AMA nor in levels of serum immunoglobulins between old and young, and while marked abnormalities in bilirubin, serum alkaline phosphatase and serum albumin were each more common in the younger rather than the older age group in no instance did this reach statistical significance. There was no difference between the histology at the time of first liver biopsy between groups – 40% of the younger, 37% of the older patients had cirrhosis.

Follow-up

The patients were followed-up for a mean 55 months with a minimum follow-up of 2 years (no difference between young and old groups). After follow-up a higher proportion of young patients was symptomatic of liver disease or had symptoms of liver failure or portal hypertension ($P < 0.05$); almost exactly the same proportion of patients in each group (ca. 10%) had died of liver disease although 14% over 65-year-olds had died of liver unrelated causes in a mean follow-up of almost 5 years (compared with 3 in the under 65-year-old group). There was no difference in total deaths in the old group and that predicted for an age and sex matched control population. The prognostic importance of serum bilirubin led us to examine the progression of serum bilirubin: during the follow-up period the mean change in bilirubin was $+55$ mmol/litre in young, $+8$ mmol/litre in the old patients ($P < 0.001$).

Since other usually autoimmune conditions are thought to be possibly associated with PBC these were examined in the two groups. There was no difference in the occurrence of autoimmune thyroid disease, rheumatoid arthritis or Sjögren's syndrome between the two groups.

Conclusions

Although Christensen et al.[12] and Roll et al.[13] have both suggested that increased age carries an adverse prognostic implication in PBC patients, when age-adjusted mortality was taken into account there was no increase in mortality in the study of Christensen. Our own study did not support the concept that age was an independent adverse prognostic variable for PBC. Indeed while there was no suggestion that PBC presenting in an older age group differed substantially from 'classical' disease there was some suggestion that the spectrum of the disease was shifted, at least in a proportion of individuals, towards a more mild clinical course. There was a higher proportion of asymptomatic patients in the older group, the clinical features were rather less marked in older patients and the progression of bilirubin was less. This slightly more 'benign' course of the disease may balance the possible lack of compensatory mechanisms in the ageing liver thus leading to a net lack of alteration in overall mortality. One would certainly draw attention to the fact that this disease is far from rare in elderly females.

α_1-ANTITRYPSIN DEFICIENCY

Both increasing use of full serological testing in patients with suspected liver disease and improved sophistication of histological techniques has substantially reduced the proportion of individuals now thought to have 'cryptogenic' cirrhosis. Nonetheless there remains a substantial proportion, perhaps 20%, of individuals where no clinical or haematological evidence as to the cause of the liver disease is available; this may be particularly true in the elderly and indeed led earlier generations to speculate as to whether a condition known as 'senile cirrhosis' exists[14]. Recently, a number of case reports of elderly individuals presenting with previously unsuspected cryp-togenic cirrhosis have been described in whom a histological diagnosis of α_1-antitrypsin deficiency has been made[15,16]. The advent of a specific immu-noperoxidase technique for detection of α_1-antitrypsin granules within the liver has supplemented the classical method of identification of periodic acid Schiff-positive diastase-resistant intracytoplasmic inclusion granules within liver cells in the identification of α_1-antitrypsin deficiency.

We have identified 55 individuals presenting with cryptogenic cirrhosis over age 65 at the time of liver biopsy or post-mortem histology in the 6 years from 1981 to 1986. In all cases autoantibody screen, full screening for HBsAg, anti-HBs, anti-HBc and serum ferritin estimations were all negative: fur-thermore there was no suggestion in any individual, from clinical history or examination of biochemical data, of alcohol as a cause of the liver disease. All such biopsies were routinely stained with an immunoperoxidase specific for α_1-antitrypsin: 9 were found to have strongly positive hepatocyte staining together with PAS-positive diastase-resistant intracytoplasmic granules; 3 of these were found at post-mortem examination in patients not suspected in life of having liver disease. A further 3 >65-year-olds had 'cryptogenic' chronic active hepatitis not amounting to cirrhosis. The 6 cirrhotics identified before death together with the 3 found to have histological chronic active hepatitis were all phenotypically PiMZ heterozygous for the α_1-antitrypsin gene. These data suggest that a not insubstantial proportion of elderly indi-viduals with cirrhosis may be individuals presenting very late in life with the first manifestation of previously occult α_1-antitrypsin deficiency. We are investigating this possibility further.

COMPLICATIONS OF LIVER DISEASE

It is one's impression that the serious complications of liver disease are less actively and invasively treated in elderly individuals than in younger ones. While this might sometimes be owing to a laudable desire on the part of physicians not to 'strive officiously to keep alive' one suspects that it is more because elderly patients are held to have a worse prognosis from these complications and a poorer quality of life than their younger colleagues with a similar severity of disease. In order to test these questions we have begun to examine the results of treatment of severe complications of liver disease among our own patients, drawn from a wide age spectrum and with a 'non-ageist' approach to treatment.

Acute variceal haemorrhage

As a first attempt to evaluate the above question the preliminary results of a retrospective study of outcome of acute variceal haemorrhage are presented. During the 5-year period from 1982 to 1986, 92 patients made a first pres-entation with acute upper gastrointestinal haemorrhage endoscopically proven to be from oesphageal varices. These 92 patients required 131 emergency admissions to hospital during this period. 37 patients were over age 60 on first presentation, these required 54 admissions. The Childs grading for severity of liver disease was comparable in the 2 groups.

In the total patient group haemorrhage was controlled in 112 (85%) of all 131 admissions, discharge achieved in 98 (75%). Among the 54 admissions in over 60-year-olds, haemorrhage was controlled in 46 (85%), discharge achieved in 38 (70%). It seems therefore that for acute haemorrhage the outcome is no different in older subjects; however further analysis of prognosis, quality of life and length of hospital stay per admission is required before firm conclusions may be drawn from this data.

Primary Hepatocellular Cancer (HCC)

While HCC is the major malignant scourge of the Far East and Sub-Saharan Africa and while in these areas it is a disease of young people, the picture is quite different in Western communities. Here HCC does not appear to be so closely linked with the hepatitis B virus (HBV) – rather it is associated with cirrhosis whatever the cause and probably with the length of time for which an individual has had cirrhosis. The other major association is of course male sex. It is becoming increasingly clear that hepatocellular cancer is on the increase and where associated with cirrhosis in Western countries is a disease of advancing age. Melia et al.[17] in a specialized liver unit in London found 45% cirrhotic patients with HCC presented over age 60, among our own patients 38 out of 46 patients (82%) presenting with HCC in a cirrhotic liver in a British community were over age 60 at presentation, almost half of these were over 70. We have recently drawn attention to the fact that a substantial proportion of these elderly male cirrhotics with HCCs had experience in World War II in the Far East or Sub-Saharan Africa. While this is only conjecture at this stage I would suggest that such factors as HBV infection in adult life, environmental exposure to potential carcinogens, alcoholic liver disease and such connected factors as war experience in Vietnam and intravenous drug abuse may well lead to a very considerable rise in the incidence of HCC in coming years among the elderly after a suitable 'lag' time.

There is little to suggest that HCC in the elderly cirrhotic Western male is in any significant way different from that seen in his younger Eastern counterpart in terms of presentation and prognosis.

Conclusions

One would conclude by saying that the elderly are probably not more susceptible to liver disease than when they were younger although the accumulation of possibly damaging insults to the liver over a life time may increasingly lead us to see chronic liver disease presenting in older individuals. Preliminary data suggest that the clinical features and prognosis of such liver disease are not strikingly different in the elderly and that complications arising from liver disease in an older person should be treated as for a younger individual; any features which might adversely affect recovery in such an elderly individual might not result from 'faults' within the liver – rather from other organ systems. If anything the study of the diseased liver suggests that liver cells are among the most hardy and resistant to the effects of ageing in the human organism.

References

1. Woodhouse, K. W., Mortimer, O. and Wiholm, B. E. (1986). In Kitani, K. (ed.) *Hepatic Adverse Drug Reactions: The Effect of Age in Liver and Aging – 1986*. pp. 75–80. (Amsterdam: Elsevier)
2. James, O. F. W. (1985). Drugs and the ageing liver. *Eur. J. Hepatol.*, **1**, 431–5
3. Weber, J. C. P. and Griffin, J. P. (1986). Prescriptions, adverse reactions, and the elderly. *Lancet*, **1**, 1220
4. Pickles, H. (1986). Prescriptions, adverse reactions, and the elderly. *Lancet*, **2**, 40–1
5. Neuberger, J. and Williams, R. (1984). Halothane anaesthesia and liver damage. *Br. Med. J.*, **289**, 1136–9
6. Taggart, H. Mc. A. and Alderdice, J. M. (1982). Fatal cholestatic jaundice in elderly persons taking benoxaprofen. *Br. Med. J.*, **284**, 1372
7. Goudie, B. M., Birnie, G. F., Watkinson, G. *et al.* (1982). Jaundice associated with the use of benoxaprofen. *Lancet*, **1**, 959–61
8. Garagliano, C. F., Lilienfeld, A. M. and Mendeloff, A. I. (1979). Incidence rates of liver cirrhosis and related diseases in Baltimore and selected areas of the United States. *J. Chron. Dis.*, **32**, 543–54
9. Potter, J. F. and James, O. F. W. (1988). The clinical features and prognosis of alcoholic liver disease in respect of advancing age. *Gerontology* (In press)
10. Bridgewater, R., Leigh, S., James, O. F. W. and Potter, J. F. (1988). Alcohol consumption and alcohol dependence in the elderly in an urban community. *Brit. Med. J.* (In press)
11. Lehmann, A. B., Bassendine, M. F. and James, O. F. W. (1985). Is primary biliary cirrhosis a different disease in the elderly? *Gerontology*, **31**, 186–94
12. Christensen, E., Crowe, J., Doniach, D. *et al.* (1980). Clinical pattern and course of the disease in primary biliary cirrhosis based on an analysis of 236 patients. *Gastroenterology*, **78**, 236–46
13. Roll, J., Boyer, J. L., Barry, D. *et al.* (1983). The prognostic importance of clinical and histological features in asymptomatic and primary biliary cirrhosis. *N. Engl. J. Med.*, **308**, 1–7
14. Ludwig, J. and Baggenstoss, A. H. (1970). Cirrhosis of the aged and senile cirrhosis – are there two conditions? *J. Gerontol.*, **25**, 244–8
15. Roggli, V. L., Hausner, R. J. and Askew, J. B. (1981). Alpha-1-antitrypsin globules in hepatocytes of elderly persons with liver disease. *Am. J. Clin. Pathol.*, **75**, 538–42
16. Battle, W. M., Maltaranzzo, A., Selhat, G. F. *et al.* (1982). Alpha-1-antitrypsin deficiency – A cause of cryptogenic liver disease in the elderly. *J. Clin. Gastroenterol.*, **4**, 269–73
17. Melia, W. M., Wilkinson, M. L., Portmann, B. C. *et al.* (1984). Hepatocellular carcinoma in Great Britain; influence of age, sex, HBsAg status and aetiology of underlying cirrhosis. *Q. J. Med.*, **53**, 391–400
18. Cobden, I., Bassendine, M. F. and James, O. F. W. (1986). Hepatocellular carcinoma in North-East England: Importance of hepatitis B infection and ex-tropical military service. *Q. J. Med.*, **60**, 855–63

36
Vaccination in old age

F. DEINHARDT and W. JILG

INTRODUCTION

Infectious diseases are important in producing morbidity in the elderly, and are a leading cause of death amongst those older than 65 years. Thus, prevention is of particular importance in this group and should be achievable by vaccination.

The available evidence suggests that vaccination in old age should be considered differently. The aged do not respond as well to vaccination, the number of non-responders is higher than in the young, and some of those who do respond have impaired responses. The major underlying reason is a loss of immunological ability, either due to diseases such as diabetes and renal failure or associated with poor nutrition (for example, vitamin deficiencies), changes in hormone levels, and immunosuppression owing to treatment with anti-inflammatory drugs or radiation. However, even normal, healthy individuals may respond less well to antigenic stimuli in advanced years, and this is important in establishing vaccination strategies for older age groups.

Our understanding of the mechanisms underlying the immunological responses that relate to vaccination has increased considerably (B and T cell recognition, the definition of various lymphocyte classes, particularly in the T cells, the dynamics of antibody responses, etc.). Despite this increase in knowledge, we are still faced with difficulties in vaccinating the elderly because immune capacity declines with age, and although some of this age-related decline is attributable to qualitative changes in immune cells, the specific changes and their relationship to vaccination responses are still largely undefined. In normal aging, delayed-type hypersensitivity reactivity declines, tumours and allografts survive longer, and antibody responses to foreign antigens decline[1], and these reduced immune functions significantly affect survival, as seen in an age-matched control study[2]. Nevertheless, healthy old people can produce good (i.e. adequate) antibody responses[3], for example to pneumococcal vaccines. In this chapter, we discuss briefly vaccination against influenza, pneumococcal pneumonia, and tetanus, and consider hepatitis B vaccination in the elderly in more detail. Strategies to ensure that vaccination responses are adequate for protection also are considered.

EVALUATION OF VACCINATION RESPONSES

The efficacy of response to vaccination is measured from the proportion of vaccinees responding to the vaccine (seroconversion) and/or the proportion of the vaccinees that develop protective levels of antibodies. Clinical response is judged by the reduction on a population-wide basis in hospitalization rates, length of disease, mortality and morbidity.

VACCINATION OF THE ELDERLY

Influenza

Analysis of influenza pandemics and of outbreaks of influenza between pandemics shows that the highest death rates occur in the elderly[4], that closed populations (such as in residential homes) have increased mortality in outbreaks of influenza A and B[5], and that underlying chronic diseases further increase mortality rates[6].

Influenza vaccines have been shown to elicit antibody responses in the chronically ill and elderly[7,8], and vaccine efficacy has been demonstrated in a controlled retrospective study by reduction in hospitalization and mortality. Barker and Mullooly[9] studied a non-institutionalized population of persons 65 years of age or older, and compared the reduction in pneumonia- and influenza-associated hospitalizations and mortality during two major influenza epidemics in persons vaccinated in the summer and autumn preceding the epidemics and in non-vaccinated individuals of comparable age and with similar underlying chronic conditions. One epidemic with a major antigenic shift showed no benefit of vaccination whereas in the other a reasonable cross-reactivity existed between the vaccine and epidemic virus strain: hospitalization was reduced by 72% and mortality by 87%, results that were comparable to those obtained in young, healthy adults. Other studies have indicated that influenza vaccines are less effective in elderly patients with chronic diseases than in younger patients[10], and some failures to respond may be owing to poor antigenicity or ineffective responses associated with deficient numbers and percentages of IgD-bearing peripheral blood lymphocytes[11].

Annual influenza vaccination is recommended in several countries, particularly for individuals over 65 years of age, but implementation and compliance with this policy have not been high. Lower responses potentially could be offset by two booster vaccinations but in face of the inadequate, initial acceptance of influenza vaccination this seems to be only a counsel of perfection.

Pneumococcal vaccine

Pneumococcal infections occur most frequently in patients with chronic pulmonary, cardiac or renal diseases, and are a leading cause of morbidity and mortality. Randomized, double-blind trials of pneumococcal vaccines have been conducted in such high-risk patients above 55 years (mean age 61 years old)[12] but did not prevent pneumonia or bronchitis in contrast to studies in younger subjects such as military recruits. One non-randomized study in institutionalized elderly also failed to demonstrate any major effect in reducing cases of pneumonia or pneumococcal pneumonia[13]. It is possible that other serotypes should be used but vaccinees who had infections neither made nor maintained serum antibody concentrations that were likely to be protective. Most probably inadequate immune responses explain such failures of vaccination[12], so that vaccines with greater immunogenicity may be necessary to protect the elderly.

Tetanus toxoid immunisation

In one small study, serum titres of total and IgG antibodies were significantly lower in 10 elderly individuals (65–84 years old) than in 12 subjects 25–34 years old after primary and booster immunisations with tetanus toxoid; IgG antibody against tetanus toxoid decreased more rapidly in the older vaccinees[14]. This and similar studies suggest that IgG synthesis and T-cell helper activity may be impaired in the elderly, but 'age-related immuno-depression is multifactorial'[14] and the underlying mechanisms need further study. Whatever the cause, elderly persons who are immunized against tetanus appear to be protected against disease. Low antibody levels in the elderly population could be readily corrected by a modified vaccination program that considers these impaired responses.

Hepatitis B

In contrast to the immune responses of elderly individuals to vaccines against influenza and tetanus and the pneumococcal vaccines, which usually represent recall stimulation after previous exposure to these antigens, immunization against hepatitis B (HB) presents the opportunity of studying the initial responses of older age groups to vaccination.

HB vaccines derived from plasma of hepatitis B virus (HBV) carriers or containing recombinant HBsAg produced in yeast cells have been shown to be safe, effective and free of serious side reactions in many volunteer studies. This vaccine usually is administered in 3 or 4 doses at 0, 1 and 6 months or at 0, 1, 2 and 12 months. More recent studies in young vaccinees with one hepatitis vaccine (H-B-Vax Merck, Sharp and Dohme) administered at months 0, 1 and 12 gave better responses to the third inoculation than subjects who received the third dose at 6 months[15]. Seroconversion rates of more than 95% were observed in vaccinated healthy young adult volunteers (18–25 years old) but seroconversion rates dropped to about 80–90% when general populations were vaccinated. Improper storage of vaccines (freezing) or inoculation into fat tissue (intragluteal) instead of intramuscular (deltoid) inoculation could be responsible for some vaccine failures. However, the age of the vaccinees also played a role: the rate of seroconversion and the antibody

Table 36.1 Immune response to hepatitis B vaccine in different age groups

Age (years)	n	Sex (f/m)	Positive (%)	anti-HBs >10 IU/l GMT (%)	GMT (IU/l) +
10–19	21	15/6	100	100	820
20–29	62	43/19	97	95	481
30–39	46	30/16	98	89	565
40–49	40	29/21	96	92	538
50–59	17	15/2	·71	65	34

+ of *all* vaccinees

titres declined with increase in the age of the vaccinated individuals. A summary of the result of vaccination of individuals of various ages in one of our studies is given in Table 36.1.

In a study that included much older vaccinees, Steketee and his co-workers studied the immune responses in 444 haemodialysis patients and 128 staff members of dialysis units[16]. The seroconversion rate in the staff ranged from 96% in the age group below 34 to 71% in those of 45 years and older. Overall, only 208 (47%) of the hemodialysis patients seroconverted (these patients have impaired immune systems), and the response appeared to be age dependent so that seroconversion rates declined from 86% in patients below 30 to 32% in those over 70 years.

The risk of HBV infection in residential institutions, such as homes for the aged, may be increased[17] and the consequences may be severe. The incidence of the symptomatic HBsAg carrier rate is higher than in the young and asymptomatic carriers often are positive for HBeAg. These increased risks may be greater for the elderly from higher socioeconomic backgrounds who have a low prevalence of anti-HBs and become exposed to HBV for the first time in old age. Clearly, vaccination against HBV should be considered for these high risk groups, but the impaired cellular and humoral immunity observed in the elderly[1], which may contribute to the development of carrier states (while possibly also explaining the milder courses of diseases in some patients), means that usual vaccination strategies may have to be modified.

In another study, 70 seronegative individuals in good general health between the ages of 61 to 96 years living in a 'chronic care facility' were vaccinated with three 5 μg doses of an HBsAg alum vaccine (Hevac-B, Pasteur) at one-month intervals[18]. In young adults, this vaccine induced anti-HBs in 96% of vaccinees but only seroconversion rates of 69.2% to 33.3% were observed in older age groups (Table 36.2).

DISCUSSION

In general, responses to vaccination in older individuals are less than optimal, and vaccination strategies should take this into account by increasing vaccine immunogenicity or modifying vaccination schedules. A public health focus should reach the elderly for vaccination, emphasizing particularly for influ-

Table 36.2 Seroconversion after 3 doses of 5 μg Hevac-B*

Age (years)	n	Seroconversion (%)
61–70	13	69.2
71–80	16	43.7
81–90	38	39.5
91–96	3	33.3

* Ref. 16

enza vaccination; raising the level of vaccination, particularly for those in residential institutions or in chronic care facilities, would seem to require no more than a determined effort on the part of national and local public health authorities to achieve success. However, a study of long-term immunogenicity of HB vaccine in homosexual men indicated that boosters or revaccinations are not very effective in initially poor or non-responders; antibody levels usually only reached moderate levels after a booster series, and became undetectable after 18 months, so that the attack rate for viral hepatitis was similar to that before vaccination[20] so some other approach seems to be needed for HB vaccination of the elderly.

Another approach for accentuating the immune response in older individuals is the use of immunomodulators or adjuvants, which either augment antigenic immunogenicity or potentiate antibody production. A placebo-controlled study with a glycoprotein from *Klebsiella* (RU 41 740) showed a significant increase in levels of antibodies to two of three inactivated influenza virus strains in people over 65 years old whose haemagglutination-inhibiting titres before vaccination were low[19]. Such a combination of adjuvant therapy with vaccination seems worth testing with vaccines other than influenza in elderly persons with immunological impairment.

To offset the lower responses in the elderly, higher vaccine doses and more frequent vaccinations with booster doses about 12 months after the primary course of vaccination should be tried. In addition, future vaccine formulations containing the pre S1 and/or pre S2 gene products of HBV in addition to HBsAg (major polypeptide p-24) may prove more immunogenic in immunocompromised individuals such as haemodialysis patients and also the elderly.

References

1. Makinodan, T. and Kay, M. (1980). Age influence on the immune system. In Kunkel, H. and Dixon, F. (eds.). *Adv. Immunology*, pp. 287–330. (New York: Academic Press)
2. Roberts-Thomson, I., Youngchaiyud, U., Whittingham, S. and Mackay, I. (1974). Ageing, immune response, and mortality. *Lancet*, **2**, 368–70
3. Schwartz, J. S. (1982). Pneumococcal vaccine: clinical efficacy and effectiveness. *Ann. Intern. Med.*, **96**, 208–20
4. Alling, D., Blackwelder, W. and Stuart-Harris, C. (1981). A study of excess mortality during influenza epidemics in the United States, 1968–1976. *Am. J. Epidemiol.*, **113**, 30–43

5. Goodman, R., Orenstein, W., Munro, T., Smith, S. and Sikes, R. (1982). Impact of influenza A in a nursing home. *J. Am. Med. Assoc.*, **247**, 1451–3

6. Barker, W. and Mullooly, J. (1982). Pneumonia and influenza deaths during epidemics. *Arch. Intern. Med.*, **142**, 85–9

7. Douglas, R. G., Bentley, D. and Brandriss, M. (1977). Responses of elderly and chronically ill subjects to bivalent influenza A/New Jersey/8/76 (HswlNI)-A/Victoria/3/75 (H3N2) vaccines. *J. Infect. Dis.*, **136** (suppl.), S526–32

8. Feery, B., Evered, M. and Morrison, E. (1976). Antibody responses to influenza virus sub-unit vaccine in the aged. *Med. J. Austr.*, 540–2

9. Barker, W. and Mullooly, J. (1980). Influenza vaccination of elderly persons. Reduction in pneumonia and influenza hospitalizations and deaths. *J. Am. Med. Assoc.*, **244**, 2547–9

10. Outbreaks of influenza among nursing home residents – Connecticut, United States. (1985). *Morbidity and Mortality Weekly Report*, **34**, 478–82

11. Phair, J., Kauffman, C., Bjornson, A., Adams, L. and Linnemann, C. (1978). Failure to respond to influenza vaccine in the aged: correlation with B-cell number and function. *J. Lab. Clin. Med.*, **92**, 822–8

12. Simberkoff, M., Cross, A., Al-Ibrahim, M., Baltch, A., Geiseler, P., Nadler, J., Richmond, A., Smith, R., Schiffman, G., Shepard, D. and Van Eeckhout, J. (1986). Efficacy of pneumococcal vaccine in high-risk patients. *N. Engl. J. Med.*, **315**, 1318–27

13. Bentley, D., Ha, K., Mamot, K., Moon, D., Moore, L., Poletto, P. and Springett, A. (1981). Pneumococcal vaccine in the institutionalized elderly: design of a nonrandomized trial and preliminary results. *Rev. Infect. Dis.*, **3** (suppl.), S71–81

14. Kishimoto, S., Tomino, S., Mitsuya, H., Fujiwara, H. and Tsuda, H. (1980). Age-related decline in the *in vitro* and *in vivo* synthesis of anti-tetanus toxoid antibody in humans. *J. Immunol.*, **125**, 2347–52

15. Jilg, W., Schmidt, M. and Deinhardt, F. Immune responses to late booster doses of hepatitis B vaccine. (1985). *J. Med. Virol.*, **17**, 249–54

16. Steketee, R., Ziarnik, M. and Davis, J. (1988). Seroresponse to hepatitis B vaccine in patients and staff of renal dialysis centers, Wisconsin. *Am. J. Epidemiol.* (In press)

17. Chiaramonte, M., Floreani, A. and Naccarato, R. (1982). Hepatitis B virus infection in homes for the aged. *J. Med. Virol.*, **9**, 247–55

18. Denis, F., Mounier, M., Hessel, L., Michel, J. P., Gualde, N., Dubois, F., Barin, F. and Goudeau, A. (1984). Hepatitis-B vaccination in the elderly. *J. Infect. Dis.*, **149**, 1019

19. Profeta, M. L., Guidi, G., Meroni, P. L., Palmieri, R., Palladino, G., Cantone, V. and Zanussi, C. (1987). Influenza vaccination with adjuvant RU41740 in the elderly. *Lancet*, **1**, 973

20. Hadler, S., Francis, D., Maynard, J., Thompson, S., Judson, F., Echenberg, D., Ostrow, D., O'Malley, P., Penley, K., Altman, N., Braff, E., Shipman, G., Coleman, P. and Mandel, E. (1986). Long-term immunogenicity and efficacy of hepatitis B vaccine in homosexual men. *N. Engl. J. Med.*, **315**, 209–14

Summary – Gastrointestinal tract

P. R. HOLT

In his introductory remarks, Dr Popper described this conference on aging of the liver and the gastrointestinal tract as unusual or atypical. Most of the previous Falk conferences have dealt with a single physiologic or biochemical problem, or a small number of conditions affecting a particular organ or details of a new or current therapy.

In contrast, this conference has been inhomogeneous, not only because it involved the liver and the gastrointestinal tract, as exemplified by these two summaries, but also because the audience has comprised gerontologists, clinical gastroenterologists, experimental hepatologists and viscologists. Thus, it was impossible to ensure the cohesion that has been achieved in some of the other Falk conferences, but I believe the purpose of this conference was somewhat different. Certainly, many participants have said 'I heard a lot of new facts that have given me serendipitous ideas and leads for my own bench or clinical research'. In that stimulating sense, this conference has been a tremendous success.

What I should like to do in this summary is to describe the state of some of the data about the gastrointestinal tract and aging a decade or so ago, to extract the main messages from this conference and, finally, to describe areas which I believe will or should be studied intensively in the next 5–10 years. Since the gut absorbs, grows, moves, differentiates and secretes fluid and peptides, we can consider all of these processes.

In the late 1970s, the current belief was that in the aging gastrointestinal tract 'something must be wrong'. The stomach secreted less acid, in the small intestine the villus architecture was altered sufficiently to reduce villus surface area which would be expected to be accompanied by a lower small intestinal mucosal enzyme content, intestinal absorption was assumed to be reduced – the best example being after administration of a test dose of xylose – cell replication and intestinal cell turnover in the gut must be decreased, secretion from auxiliary organs such as the pancreas was reduced and the motility of the oesophagus, stomach and colon was deranged. On the other hand, from a clinical point of view, if malnutrition occurred in the elderly, this was due to a reduction in caloric intake and not to altered intestinal nutrient absorption. Thus, the current prejudice suggested that, although many physiologic processes in the gastrointestinal tract were deranged as a consequence of aging, these were not clinically important. What have we learned in some of these areas?

The observations of Sharp, Ecknauer and our own group, in rodents, and Corazza (who, unfortunately, could not present his studies at this meeting), in man, clearly show that, in the absence of intestinal disease and malnutrition, small bowel villus architecture and villus surface area is normal. Wright, at this meeting, re-emphasized that the vincristine metaphase arrest technique is the best method of determining proliferative rates in the bowel. Studies from his group showed that proliferation was reduced to a major extent in the early developmental period followed by a small but constant decline in proliferation thereafter. In addition, his data showed that, despite an increase in intestinal mass, water absorption was maintained at normal rates except when calculated per unit mass of tissue, suggesting that the older small intestine was relatively inefficient in this absorptive process. However, until we can actually quantitate the number of absorbing cells and then use this number as a denominator for study of absorption rates in animals of differing ages, it is premature to accept his conclusion that the aging rat has lower rates of water absorption. Although all investigators appear to agree that cell proliferation in the small intestine of aging rodents is altered as a function of age, we should hold in abeyance a final decision about what changes occur since the studies of some investigators have implied increased intestinal proliferation in aging rodents.

Both Brasitus and Thomson, in work presented here and elsewhere, have shown that membrane fluidity (and membrane composition) of the gut can readily be altered by diet, specifically in the content of cholesterol and of saturated and unsaturated lipids or by pharmacologic measures such as administration of the bile salt binding resin, cholestyramine. Their studies and those of others have shown that microvillus membranes are very susceptible to experimental manipulation but intestinal basolateral membranes generally are resistant. They emphasized that it is essential to use the optimal methodology which includes ensuring the harvest of pure membranes, the use of several different molecular probes and parallel studies of membrane composition. Some compositional changes occur very rapidly, an example being changes in the basolateral membrane within 30 to 60 min following the administration of 1,25-hydroxycholecalciferol. It should also be remembered that membrane fluidity and composition may be affected by cellular events; for example, structural membrane cholesterol may be altered more by changes in *de novo* synthesis than by cholesterol feeding, and phospholipid and fatty acid composition affected by the activity of cellular lipophilic enzymes. Furthermore, the studies of Thomson and his group have demonstrated that functional membrane changes such as altered fluxes and changes in enzyme activity, induced by feeding different diets, may be maintained for several weeks after the experimental diet is withdrawn. These effects cannot possibly occur as a result of generalizable alteration in the gut membranes but, rather, result in changes in microdomains of the membranes.

What have we learned about changes in membrane composition and fluidity in advanced age?

Few studies of this kind have been performed. Brasitus described studies of rat microvillus membrane fluidity using several probes which demonstrated major compositional and fluidity changes in the early postnatal period after weaning but none between 4 and 27 months. Compositional and fluidity changes with age in hepatic intracellular membranes have been described by several investigators. However, the gastrointestinal tract has been investigated insufficiently to exclude the possibility that membrane factors alter enzyme activity and transport processes.

Studies of gut enzymes in rodents of different ages have begun to elucidate possible age-related changes in cellular differentiation of enzymes and in enterocyte macromolecular synthesis and turnover. The preliminary results of our own group, which has studied changes in enterocyte enzymes with age, are in accord with the experiments described by David Gershon, suggesting that the aging process may be accompanied in part by minimal changes in protein composition.

Studies of intestinal absorption in aging animals in order to define age-dependent changes are in their infancy. However, the work of Esposito on glucose absorption, presented at this meeting, and that of others imply that one can detect a fall in V_{max} without changes in K_m in older animals, suggesting insufficient or inadequately functioning glucose transporters. Now that the structure of glucose transporters has been elucidated and cDNA probes are available, more data on the molecular mechanisms for changes in glucose transport (and that of other active transport molecules) in enterocytes may be forthcoming.

Dr Ambrecht elegantly described the present state of knowledge of the cellular basis for calcium absorption. Even though experimental gerontologists may argue whether the intestinal absorption of sugars or fats is increased or decreased or whether changes in their absorption is important, all agree that calcium absorption is impaired and this contributes to the osteopenia of old age. At a cellular level, calcium flux falls dramatically with age during the early development of rodents. Calcium uptake and transport is dependent upon calcium binding protein, calcium binding complex (whose function is presently unclear) and the specific mechanisms for pumping calcium out of intestinal cells at the basolateral membrane. Two different systems have been described and it is generally felt that both are ATP dependent and crucially responsive to 1,25-hydroxycholecalciferol. Administration of this hormone involves transcription of mucosal calcium binding protein and perhaps a rapid change in lateral membrane fluidity. Dr Ambrecht presented his observations suggesting that the steady state levels of mRNA for calcium binding protein fall dramatically with age, accompanied by a reduction in 1,25-hydroxycholecalciferol responsiveness. Thus, it is possible, though not completely proven, that some of the changes in calcium absorption, and particularly the adaptation of the intestine to a low calcium diet that has been found in older organisms and in man, may be due to this cellular defect.

Turning to changes in receptor-dependent mechanisms in the gastrointestinal tract, Dr Abrass beautifully illustrated that both the normal receptor-associated system and post-receptor mechanisms may be altered during the process of aging. At the present time, a sparse amount of information that applies to the gastrointestinal tract, including the enteric nervous system, is available. Data for the effect of aging in other systems do not permit a definition of generalizable changes that may occur as a function of advanced age.

James Thompson, at the very last minute, was able to introduce data from his laboratory, suggesting that gallbladder contraction is diminished in some older individuals associated with a reduced sensitivity to exogenous CCK. In his studies, CCK basal and postprandial levels were increased in the old. Furthermore, experiments in the aging guinea pig gallbladder have shown a reduction in K_m for the CCK receptor. These preliminary observations have emphasized to this conference the importance of studies of gastrointestinal peptides for the understanding of potential changes in gastrointestinal function and suggested that elevated hormone levels may be found in aging. Presently, it is difficult to determine what is the cart and what is the horse; that is, whether increased peptide levels may downregulate the receptor or whether such increased levels may be adaptive responses to altered cellular receptor mechanisms.

Turning to the clinical presentations at this conference, there appears to be a consensus that there are no major deficits in intestinal absorption in healthy normal man, but there may well be a reduction in absorptive reserve or absorptive capacity. One must introduce some caveats in this overall opinion since we do not know what happens in the very old, most studies having been performed in elderly well individuals in their seventies. We also do not know whether absorptive function may decrease more in older individuals during the stress of major illnesses, treatment of neoplasms with alkylating agents etc. We do not know very much about the effects of aging on drug absorption. One question that was raised during this conference, by the studies of both Hollander and Russell, was whether excessive accumulation of vitamin A might occur in the elderly who are taking vitamin supplements since some evidence suggests that vitamin A absorption may be increased when compared to young controls. The studies of Russell introduced the intriguing question whether hypochlorhydria in the elderly may lead to special problems, related to the absorption of micronutrients, such as food-bound vitamin B_{12} or folate, or whether such hypochlorhydria results in intestinal bacterial overgrowth syndrome. The potential nutritional impact of hypochlorhydria has not been evaluated to the present time.

Turning to age-related changes in the pancreas, it is well recognized that the pancreas is an organ with enormous capacity for protein synthesis, produces very well defined proteins, is an organ whose function is modulated by hormones, diets and other extraneous agents, has a special mechanism for enzyme product transport, the elucidation of which resulted in the award of a Nobel prize in Medicine, and also that much is known of pancreatic intracellular messengers that follow hormonal and cholinergic stimuli. Furthermore, pancreatic acinar cell culture systems are available. Thus, it is an unusual useful organ for the study of the cellular biology of aging. However, very few studies have been performed to date. The observations of Gullo strongly indicate that pancreatic digestion is maintained in the elderly although there is much scatter in the data from his laboratory and others. It is unclear at the present time whether some individuals may not lose pancreatic acinar function in advanced age. Pancreatic carcinoma is the commonest pancreatic disease in the elderly but, to date, no work has been done on pancreatic ductal cell aging.

Studies of changes in gastrointestinal motility perfectly illustrate the difficulties in determining whether phenomena that occur in elderly animals or humans are the consequence of age-related diseases or physiologic aging. To date, studies of motility changes usually have been descriptive of abnormal states. For example, in the pharynx, abnormal striated muscle function in the initiation of swallowing has been shown to be present. Pelemans told us that the changes that are seen in the esophagus are akin to those of excess vagal stimulation. Anorectal studies, described by Nicholas Read in this symposium, have begun to analyze changes that occur in the distal colon and rectum of elderly humans. It is of importance that such clinical research has started with the very common clinical problem of 'why do elderly individuals frequently have fecal impaction?' The data that Dr Read presented indicates that the rectum is relatively non-pliant and resistant and that sensory changes occur which imply that neuropathic disease is centered in the lower spinal reflexes. If this is the case, such changes may be susceptible to modulation by sensory hyperstimulation or by biofeedback.

We must try, as much as possible, as Schneider asked, to determine what phenomena in the elderly are related to degeneration in advanced age and what are adaptive responses to aging? What are physiologic changes and what are the consequences of disease?

Now for questions that I believe we must answer by further research in the future:

1. Are intestinal homeostatic control mechanisms for metabolic processes and enzyme content impaired and, specifically, is there evidence for impaired adaptation of the enterocyte to rapid changes?
2. How is proliferation of gut cells affected by the aging process? May gut cell proliferation be deranged and be a contributor to the frequency of cancer of the gastrointestinal tract in the old?
3. We must continue to clarify changes in the lipid composition and viscosity of intestinal membranes and specifically develop methods to determine changes that may occur in membrane microdomains since such domains may be susceptible to experimental manipulation.
4. Can the calcium malabsorption of the elderly be improved by changing the sensitivity or responsiveness of the enterocyte to normal adaptive stimuli?
5. We must study the barrier function of the gut, including gut permeability (the barrier to macromolecules), which some data suggest may be increased, including the immune barrier, and specifically the gut-associated lymphoid tissue and IgA production, and including the barrier function that is produced by enterocyte detoxification capacity.
6. Research on motility or dysmotility in the elderly crucially is needed since we must find ways of evaluating swallowing difficulties more carefully and to define which can be treated at the gastrointestinal level

381

and we must clarify further the physiology and pathophysiology of the colon, rectum and anus in the hope of ameliorating the frequency of impaction and incontinence.

7. Gastrointestinal peptides and tissue responsiveness and receptors, numbers and affinity and post-receptor mechanisms all must be studied.

8. From a clinical point of view, we must be able to more carefully evaluate absorptive capacity for different nutrients, determine whether bacterial overgrowth syndrome is a frequent problem in the elderly and may lead to malnutrition and understand better such phenomena as atrophic gastritis and the association of this disorder with the production of carcinoma.

If we learn to understand only a small fraction of these problems, we will have made major strides in this field. Aging presents a model for studies of organ physiology so that, in the process, we probably will shed light on other gastrointestinal changes that occur throughout the life span.

Summary – Hepatologic problems in aging

H. POPPER

To supplement Peter Holt's excellent summary on the multiple gastrointestinal problems of aging, I am to review the relation of the liver to aging. This should start with the expression of the common prejudice that liver function deteriorates in older age. That means the organ should not only become older but should also senesce or wither. For emphasis my remarks are restricted to the transition from maturity to aging and omit the development to maturity, despite its biologic importance.

We might assume senescence of the liver from the here well-presented theories of aging which I would divide simply into a genetic one with 6.7% of the genome possibly involved in aging and the response to the myriad of environmental influences of which the effect of toxic or activated oxygen species is only one example. We heard of a global molecular biologic change and that protein synthesis is somewhat diminished in 37 out of 38 examined proteins. The synthesis of some specific proteins, such as the α_{2u}-urinary globulin in male rats, is convincingly reduced as reflected in a diminution of its mRNA. Omitting names of all the excellent speakers, first academic problems and then practical questions will be discussed, closing with a list of the new concepts which had been developed.

The academic problems start with a consideration of the liver's relation to the organism. By virtue of its position between the gastrointestinal tract and the rest of the body, it serves as a guardian, as already emphasized by the ancients. It handles material in the food by metabolism, de-toxification, and storage. Many compounds undergo oxidation or reduction resulting in metabolites representing or bound to toxic oxygen species. They are, in turn, controlled by the anti-oxidant capacity of the liver exerted by glutathione dismutases and other enzymes as well as by binding compounds which include vitamins E and C. The liver is a main blood depot and is furthermore endowed with many other constitutive functions, but it is also the target of extended regulation by mediators which are either produced in or are acting on the liver.

The question arises to what degree constitutive or regulatory processes of the liver are altered in aging. As already mentioned, the metabolism of the macromolecules may be changed which includes the well-established sequence from DNA to RNA to proteins of which some, in turn, act on DNA as we now increasingly appreciate; ligands taken up by receptors in plasma membrane, cytosol and even nuclei become enhancers of DNA, including its promoters. In this cycle the transcription to RNA and the translation to proteins are at this time better established than the protein action on DNA. Aging changes seem to involve prominently reduced catabolism of mRNA with a characteristic poly-A tail. This accounts particularly for increased albumin mRNA. But also total DNA has been found increased in the hepatocytes in aging. Since transcription appears normal, the increase in albumin mRNA suggests a reduction of its catabolism. However, since the plasma albumin level is normal, elimination appears raised, probably by enhanced fluid phase endocytosis. These observations would indicate that aging reduces the catabolism of RNA and enhances the clearance of its product from the plasma. Moreover, the fidelity of the translation of RNA appears reduced.

This leads to the second problem, namely the probable alteration of proteins or enzymes, recently also demonstrated by determination of their breakdown products by specific monoclonal antibodies. This supplements the abnormalities of enzymes previously shown by discrepancies between their immunologically determined amounts and their relatively reduced catalytic potencies, seemingly a result of modified three-dimensional structure. This introduces the concept of 'junk macromolecule' proteins and also RNA and possible DNA. These junk proteins call for a compensation since they may increase susceptibility to stress. Part of this compensation may represent increased synthesis of macromolecules or recruitment of additional cells into the synthetic process.

Lipids are increased in amount. Cholesterol formation is enhanced with at least two significant consequences. One is an increase in biliary cholesterol content coupled with lower bile acid concentration, the latter possibly from decreased bile acid synthesis. The result is a bile with raised cholesterol saturation and a tendency to gallstone formation. Secondly, the raised cholesterol in the phospholipid membranes reduces their fluidity. The activity of the enzymes localized in such membranes, for instance the microsomal cytochrome P-450 system, depends on the constitution of the surrounding phospholipid membrane; reduced fluidity tends to decrease enzyme activity. Two further lipid-related aspects include alteration of the carrier protein, apolipoprotein A, which plays a major role in the hepatic lipid uptake, and finally the increase of vitamin A in the liver localized in both the interstitial fat-storing cells (lipocytes) and the hepatocytes with the former important in storage and the latter in vitamin A metabolism and its distribution in the body. Storage of excess vitamin A in fat droplets in the lipocytes increases their volume, particularly in their perinuclear main body. This might hypothetically reduce the cells' fibroblastic potential, probably temporarily, and, by reduction of their star-like extensions, decrease their ability to modulate the hepatic microcirculation.

Turning to morphologic observations on the liver, one is the increased lipofuscin reflected in its brown color and in the accumulation of lysosomes representing material accumulated during the life of the hepatocytes. It also is junk protein which the body cannot dispose of by digestion or excretion. But lipofuscin does not influence hepatic function and thus its accumulation represents a mere cosmetic feature as does the increased occurrence of functionally insignificant, benign tumors and cysts. The second observation is the great variability in the size of the hepatocytes, the presence of microhepatocytes and macrohepatocytes. Similar variations involve some hepatocellular organelles, such as the mitochondria. This also includes the nuclei which show focal polyploidy. In addition to the lysosomes, glycogen is increased, possibly as a result of alteration in the pentose phosphate shunt, while the peroxisomes are reduced. To what degree this variability represents compensation for the junk macromolecules remains to be established. The third feature is an apparent smaller size of the liver, particularly in male rats, but so far not established in man. Even more questionable are changes in the stroma of the liver in which increased focal fibrosis has been claimed, probably from reduced collagen metabolism as exists in cirrhosis, but no firm data are available.

The next academic problem concerns the significance of functional constitutive defects of the hepatocytes. While some data exist, their overall functional significance is indeed questionable. Hepatic blood flow is apparently reduced, seemingly between 8 and 10%. This cannot be of great functional significance since the blood flow to the liver far exceeds its demands. Modern Doppler circulation studies on the aged have not been reported; moreover, portal venous flow is regulated in the mesenteric vessels. Some reduction of the hepatic blood flow may simply reflect reduced cardiac output. Bile flow is apparently normal. Whether there is reduced constitutive uptake by the hepatocytes remains to be proven; intrahepatocellular transport, at least of some substance, is impaired. A new observation is aging changes of intermediate filaments, some cytokeratins and also tubulin which influences the transport of ligands, with or without receptors, in the liver. This supplements previous observations on the movement of IgA through the rat hepatocytes.

In contrast to the hepatocytes, the sinusoidal cells exhibit well-documented functional changes, more the Kupffer cells than the endothelial cells. The major defect involves the uptake of particular substances. Some may be subtle changes recognized by small test doses, but a lack of compensation to stress is better appreciated with large doses.

In conclusion, there is a questionable and probably variable, but not global, impairment of hepatocellular function in contrast to a global disturbance of endocytosis by sinusoidal cells, particularly of phagocytosis by Kupffer cells.

Turning from the constitutive functions to regulation or adaptive abilities of the liver, the proliferative potential of the hepatocytes deserves consideration. It is important to stress that in the absence of liver injury, the hepatocytes have a long lifespan with only few mitoses during their entire life, seemingly about three, since the lifespan of the hepatocytes depends on the organism's lifespan or, better its maximal lifespan potential which, in humans, is at least 30 times longer than in the widely examined rodent models, such as mice. Thus mitosis is very rare in the human liver and increased DNA synthesis without mitosis accounts for the nuclear polyploidy which is frequently seen in aging hepatocytes as an expression of junk protein impaired cell division. It deserves further emphasis that metabolic rate, oxygen production by at least one variant of cytochrome P-450, and the amount of oxidizable material are also related to body size and therefore are much lower in man compared to the laboratory rodents. Another important point is that in the liver the signal transduction via receptors, second messengers, and phosphokinases serves far more regulatory processes than differentiation and proliferation than in most other organs. In general, the mitogenic growth factors act in the liver rather on regulation than on differentiation or proliferation. Moreover, in the liver it is not as much the death of hepatocytes as the dysfunction of viable hepatocytes which is responsible for reduction of hepatic function calling for compensation, something which had been called anabolic liver injury. Thus the proliferative mechanism is active predominantly after hepatocellular injury.

Regeneration of the liver, for instance after hepatectomy, is delayed, but eventually catches up, not necessarily by recruitment of additional dividing hepatocytes, but rather by more mitotic cycles. In general, the growth restraints in regeneration are not disturbed in the aging liver. A practical question is whether older age implies a great susceptibility to cancer initiation. In view of the long promotion and progression time of most cancers, those which had been induced decades before appear in older age in greater numbers.

The most significant alteration of the aging liver is disturbed adaptation; that means the response to mediators, including modification of immunologic reactivity. It is not clear to what degree this depends on hepatic or extrahepatic factors, particularly since most hepatocellular mediators are formed by nonhepatic cells. Their hepatocellular receptor activity appears changed, their number and affinity decrease reflected in altered V_{max} and K_m. However, here again extensive variability is noted in that, for instance, insulin and glucagon receptors are not altered whereas their activity may be modified, seemingly from three-dimensional or conformational alteration rather than chemical modification. One can conclude reduced synthesis of immunologic mediators and of hormones outside the hepatocytes which to a great degree account for the main feature of aging of the human liver, namely altered adaptation.

The animal models of aging provide fascinating information, particularly as to genetic factors determining lifespan; this has been illuminated greatly in animals way down on the developmental scale. However, one must question to what degree these genetic observations apply to the human liver with the long lifespan of its hepatocytes and the relative low production of active oxygen species as compared to the small animals. Whether food restriction which endows rats with longevity is effective in man is another moot problem. The most sensible application derives from investigations of the heat shock protein of the *Drosophila* as a counterpart of the alarm reaction which may be modified in aging humans.

Turning now briefly to practical problems, the main one is the question of the altered drug metabolism which is applied in drug dosage. I want to give particular credit to the investigator who originally described the characteristic changes of the cytochrome P-450 system in aging male rats and who, himself, subsequently demonstrated that these alterations do not occur in primates and therefore probably not in humans. Thus the alterations of the drug metabolism in human aging are so far not adequately established and seem to vary with individual drugs. It appears that in the class I (mixed mono-oxygenase-dependent) reactions the different responses depend on the specific variant of the cytochrome P-450 involved and thus on variations in gene activation. In contrast to these variations in the class I or oxidative reactions, the class II conjugating or hydrating reactions are, in general, not altered in older age. Aging seems to modify several extra-hepatic factors in drug metabolism, in part, already referred to by Peter Holt. Besides gastrointestinal absorption and renal excretion, they include drug distribution, particularly of the lipid-soluble drugs distributed in the more extensive fat tissues of the aged, susceptibility of target organs such as the brain and, particularly applicable to the liver, reduced uptake of first-pass drugs because of reduced hepatic blood flow. The frequency of adverse drug reactions in the aged results seemingly from greater drug usage. The main rule therefore remains that each single drug should be tested in the individual aged person as to his or her susceptibility. But since interactions between drugs are far more important, and polypharmacy is really the rule in older age, the interactions may be far more important than the response to single drugs.

Secondly, liver function in the aged, as estimated by the routine hepatic tests, seems not to be significantly altered and it appears a safe rule, at this time, to ascribe altered results in routine hepatic tests to diseases rather than to aging, although the results of more sophisticated tests like galactose elimination and antipyrine breath tests tend to reflect reduced function.

Thirdly, only few experimental liver injuries are more severe in the aged animal.

Fourthly, greater susceptibility to non-primary hepatic diseases in advanced age is problematic, except possibly for bacterial infections and immunologic disorders. Hepatitis B vaccination required more booster doses, but autoimmunity diseases may be less rather than more common in the aged. There is no more an age limitation for hepatobiliary operations. Increased age-related susceptibility to endotoxin-related altered function of the sinusoidal cells may be important in the increase of alcohol-abuse related diseases in old people. Probably the increased alcohol consumption of the aged is more significant. The question of greater susceptibility to environmental factors is also not resolved. It is not questioned for lung and other diseases, but for liver diseases it is still not certain and we do not know whether cancer is initiated to higher or lesser degrees in aging.

Since the liver shows only limited disturbance of constitutive hepatic functions but reduced response to regulation, the question arises as to whether the human liver senesces or withers. Several reasons speak against a deterioration: one is the long lifespan of the hepatocytes; another, the reduced tendency to oxygen toxicity; a third is the absence of age-dependent liver diseases; and the most important may be the extensive supply of blood to the liver, far in excess for its own maintenance or integrity; it rather serves the action of the hepatocytes on the blood. We thus conclude that the human liver does not senesce but that reduced activities of the hepatocytes depend greatly on extrahepatic or, at least, extra-hepatocellular functions. This is important in the use of livers of older donors in organ transplantation; this recognition may be one of the most important practical contributions of hepatic geriatrics.

The future may see an interventional gerontology which would retard the senescence of the organism by therapeutic influences on the liver. Specific effects might include a control of toxic oxygen species by supplying anti-oxidants, particularly dismutases or vitamins E, C, and also A which may reduce, via the liver, toxic organ effects in other organs. Dietary provision of precursors of glutathione might be reasonable, since the liver distributes glutathione to other body sites which, particularly during injury, might require counteraction of local oxidative stress. A further possibility is the dietary modulation of phospholipid in membranes, and thus of microsomal enzymes and plasma membrane processes on both the sinusoidal and cana-licular membranes, the latter modulating bile secretion. Hepatic and general regulation of the production of toxic oxygen species and cytosolic calcium may enter the management of senescence of the body via the liver. Finally, food restriction in the prolongation of the lifespan may be related to a hepatic effect. Challenging hypotheses may, even if proven wrong, offer new vistas.

In closing, I, at least, have learned much. In the final conclusion of this summary, three main themes have emerged concerning the aging of the liver: (1) the variability of the alterations, possibly a reflection of faulty synchronization; (2) the junk macromolecules; and (3) their compensation, which still does not exclude increased susceptibility to stress. Aging may thus also serve as an experiment of nature in which one factor, time, has changed. The hope is expressed that the readers of this volume will enjoy it as much as the participants of the meeting who were most grateful to the sponsors and organizers.

Index